Clinical Toxicology

Editors

SILAS W. SMITH
DANIEL M. LUGASSY

EMERGENCY MEDICINE
CLINICS OF NORTH AMERICA

www.emed.theclinics.com

Consulting Editor
AMAL MATTU

February 2014 • Volume 32 • Number 1

ELSEVIER

1600 John F. Kennedy Boulevard ● Suite 1800 ● Philadelphia, Pennsylvania, 19103-2899

http://www.theclinics.com

EMERGENCY MEDICINE CLINICS OF NORTH AMERICA Volume 32, Number 1
February 2014 ISSN 0733-8627, ISBN-13: 978-0-323-26654-3

Editor: Patrick Manley
Developmental Editor: Donald Mumford

Emergency Medicine Clinics of North America (ISSN 0733-8627) is published quarterly by Elsevier Inc., 360 Park Avenue South, New York, NY, 10010-1710. Months of issue are February, May, August, and November. Business and Editorial Offices: 1600 John F. Kennedy Boulevard, Suite 1800, Philadelphia, PA 19103-2899. Customer Service Office: 6277 Sea Harbor Drive, Orlando, FL 32887-4800. Periodicals postage paid at New York, NY, and additional mailing offices. Subscription prices are $155.00 per year (US students), $315.00 per year (US individuals), $523.00 per year (US institutions), $220.00 per year (international students), $450.00 per year (international individuals), $642.00 per year (international institutions), $220.00 per year (Canadian students), $385.00 per year (Canadian individuals), and $642.00 per year (Canadian institutions). International air speed delivery is included in all *Clinics'* subscription prices. All prices are subject to change without notice. **POSTMASTER:** Send address changes to *Emergency Medicine Clinics of North America*, Elsevier Periodicals Customer Service, 11830 Westline Industrial Drive, St. Louis, MO 63146. Customer Service (orders, claims, online, change of address): Elsevier Periodicals Customer Service, 11830 Westline Industrial Drive, St. Louis, MO 63146. Tel: 1-800-654-2452 (U.S. and Canada); 314-453-7041 (outside U.S. and Canada). Fax: 314-453-5170. E-mail: journalscustomerservice-usa@elsevier.com (for print support); journalsonlinesupport-usa@elsevier.com (for online support).

Reprints. For copies of 100 or more of articles in this publication, please contact the Commercial Reprints Department, Elsevier Inc., 360 Park Avenue South, New York, NY 10010-1710. Tel.: 212-633-3874; Fax: 212-633-3820; E-mail: reprints@elsevier.com.

Emergency Medicine Clinics of North America is covered in *MEDLINE/PubMed (Index Medicus), Current Contents/Clinical Medicine, EMBASE/Excerpta Medica, BIOSIS, SciSearch, CINAHL, ISI/BIOMED,* and *Research Alert.*

Printed and bound by CPI Group (UK) Ltd, Croydon, CR0 4YY

Transferred to digital print 2013

Contributors

CONSULTING EDITOR

AMAL MATTU, MD
Professor and Vice Chair, Department of Emergency Medicine, University of Maryland
School of Medicine, Baltimore, Maryland

EDITORS

SILAS W. SMITH, MD, FACEP
Department of Emergency Medicine, Assistant Professor and Section Chief, Quality,
Safety, and Practice Innovation, New York University School of Medicine, Bellevue
Hospital Center; Associate Director, Fellowship in Medical Toxicology, New York City
Poison Control Center, New York, New York

DANIEL M. LUGASSY, MD
Department of Emergency Medicine, Assistant Professor and Director of Medical Student
Medical Toxicology Education, New York University School of Medicine, Bellevue Hospital
Center; Consultant, New York City Poison Control Center, New York, New York

AUTHORS

STEVEN E. AKS, DO
Department of Emergency Medicine, John H. Stroger Jr. Hospital of Cook County,
Toxikon Consortium, Illinois Poison Control Center, Chicago, Illinois

KAVITA BABU, MD
Department of Emergency Medicine, University of Massachusetts Medical School,
Worcester, Massachusetts

KAMNA S. BALHARA, MD
Department of Emergency Medicine, Johns Hopkins University, Baltimore, Maryland

SEAN M. BRYANT, MD
Department of Emergency Medicine, John H. Stroger Jr. Hospital of Cook County,
Toxikon Consortium, Illinois Poison Control Center, Chicago, Illinois

DIANE P. CALELLO, MD
Medical Toxicologist, New Jersey Poison Information and Education System, Rutgers,
the State University of New Jersey, New Brunswick; Attending Physician, Pediatric
Emergency Medicine, Department of Emergency Medicine, Morristown Medical Center,
Morristown; Emergency Medical Associates Research Foundation, Parsippany,
New Jersey

PETER CHAI, MD, MMS
Department of Emergency Medicine, Rhode Island Hospital, Providence, Rhode Island

DORAN M. CHRISTENSEN, DO
Associate Director/Staff Physician, Radiation Emergency Assistance Center/Training Site
(REAC/TS), Oak Ridge Institute for Science and Education (ORISE), U.S. Department of
Energy (DOE), Oak Ridge Associated Universities (ORAU), Oak Ridge, Tennessee

LINDSAY FOX, MD
Emergency Medicine Residency, Icahn School of Medicine at Mount Sinai, New York,
New York

ROBERT G. HENDRICKSON, MD
Medical Toxicologist, and Program Director of the Fellowship in Medical Toxicology;
Associate Professor, Department of Emergency Medicine, Oregon Health & Sciences
University; Associate Medical Director, Oregon Poison Center, Portland, Oregon

FRED M. HENRETIG, MD
Attending Physician and Director, Section of Clinical Toxicology, Division of Emergency
Medicine, Senior Toxicologist, The Poison Control Center, The Children's Hospital of
Philadelphia, Professor Emeritus of Pediatrics, Perelman School of Medicine, University
of Pennsylvania, Philadelphia, Pennsylvania

CAROL J. IDDINS, MD
Staff Physician, Radiation Emergency Assistance Center/Training Site (REAC/TS),
Oak Ridge Institute for Science and Education (ORISE), U.S. Department of Energy (DOE),
Oak Ridge Associated Universities (ORAU), Oak Ridge; Adjunct Clinical Faculty,
Lincoln Memorial University - DeBusk College of Osteopathic Medicine, Harrogate,
Tennessee

DAVID H. JANG, MD, MSc
Assistant Professor, Division of Medical Toxicology, Department of Emergency Medicine,
School of Medicine, New York University, New York, New York

MICHAEL LEVINE, MD
Section of Medical Toxicology, Department of Emergency Medicine, University of
Southern California, Los Angeles, California; Department of Medical Toxicology, Banner
Good Samaritan Medical Center, Phoenix, Arizona

ZHANNA LIVSHITS, MD
Assistant Professor of Medicine and Medical Toxicology, Weill Cornell Medical College,
New York Presbyterian Hospital, New York, New York

ANNETTE M. LOPEZ, MD
Fellow, Medical Toxicology; Adjunct Instructor, Department of Emergency Medicine,
Oregon Health and Sciences University, Portland, Oregon

ALEX F. MANINI, MD, MS, FACMT
Associate Professor, Division of Medical Toxicology, Department of Emergency
Medicine, Elmhurst Hospital Center, Icahn School of Medicine at Mount Sinai, New York,
New York

CHARLES A. MCKAY Jr, MD, FACMT, FACEP
Medical Director, Occupational Health Services; Section Chief, Division of Medical
Toxicology, Department of Emergency Medicine, Hartford Hospital, Hartford; Associate
Medical Director, Connecticut Poison Control Center, University of Connecticut Health
Center; Associate Professor of Emergency Medicine, University of Connecticut School of
Medicine, Farmington, Connecticut

MICHAEL E. NELSON, MD, MS
Department of Emergency Medicine, NorthShore University Health System, Evanston; Department of Emergency Medicine, John H. Stroger Jr. Hospital of Cook County, Toxikon Consortium, Illinois Poison Control Center, Chicago, Illinois

RAMA B. RAO, MD
Assistant Professor of Medicine and Director of Medical Toxicology, Weill Cornell Medical College, New York Presbyterian Hospital, New York, New York

ANNE-MICHELLE RUHA, MD
Director, Department of Medical Toxicology, Banner Good Samaritan Medical Center, Center for Toxicology and Pharmacology Education and Research, Clinical Associate Professor, University of Arizona College of Medicine, Phoenix, Arizona

SILAS W. SMITH, MD, FACEP
Department of Emergency Medicine, Assistant Professor and Section Chief, Quality, Safety, and Practice Innovation, New York University School of Medicine, Bellevue Hospital Center; Associate Director, Fellowship in Medical Toxicology, New York City Poison Control Center, New York, New York

MEGHAN B. SPYRES, MD
Emergency Medicine Residency, School of Medicine, New York University, New York, New York

ANDREW STOLBACH, MD
Assistant Professor, Department of Emergency Medicine, Johns Hopkins University, Baltimore, Maryland

STEPHEN L. SUGARMAN, MS, CHP, CHCM
Health Physics Project Manager and Coordinator, Cytogenetics Biodosimetry Laboratory, Radiation Emergency Assistance Center/Training Site (REAC/TS), Oak Ridge Institute for Science and Education (ORISE), U.S. Department of Energy (DOE), Oak Ridge Associated Universities (ORAU), Oak Ridge; Adjunct Clinical Faculty, Lincoln Memorial University - DeBusk College of Osteopathic Medicine, Harrogate, Tennessee

SAGE W. WIENER, MD
Assistant Professor, Director of Medical Toxicology, Department of Emergency Medicine, SUNY Downstate Medical Center; Assistant Professor, Director of Medical Toxicology, Department of Emergency Medicine, Kings County Hospital Center, Brooklyn, New York; Consultant and Faculty Staff, New York City Poison Control Center, New York City Department of Health and Mental Hygiene, New York, New York

Contents

Foreword: Clinical Toxicology   xv

Amal Mattu

Preface   xvii

Silas W. Smith and Daniel M. Lugassy

Emerging Drugs of Abuse   1

Michael E. Nelson, Sean M. Bryant, and Steven E. Aks

Many new emerging drugs of abuse are marketed as legal highs despite being labeled "not for human consumption" to avoid regulation. The availability of these substances over the Internet and in "head shops" has lead to a multitude of emergency department visits with severe complications including deaths worldwide. Despite recent media attention, many of the newer drugs of abuse are still largely unknown by health care providers. Slight alterations of the basic chemical structure of substances create an entirely new drug no longer regulated by current laws and an ever-changing landscape of clinical effects. The purity of each substance with exact pharmacokinetic and toxicity profiles is largely unknown. Many of these substances can be grouped by the class of drug and includes synthetic cannabinoids, synthetic cathinones, phenethylamines, as well as piperazine derivatives. Resultant effects generally include psychoactive and sympathomimetic-like symptoms. Additionally, prescription medications, performance enhancing medications, and herbal supplements are also becoming more commonly abused. Most new drugs of abuse have no specific antidote and management largely involves symptom based goal directed supportive care with benzodiazepines as a useful adjunct. This paper will focus on the history, epidemiology, clinical effects, laboratory analysis, and management strategy for many of these emerging drugs of abuse.

Pediatric Toxicology: Specialized Approach to the Poisoned Child   29

Diane P. Calello and Fred M. Henretig

The poisoned child presents unique considerations in circumstances of exposure, clinical effects, diagnostic approach, and therapeutic interventions. The emergency provider must be aware of the pathophysiologic vulnerabilities of infants and children and substances that are especially toxic. Awareness is essential for situations in which the risk of morbidity and mortality is increased, such as child abuse by poisoning. Considerations in treatment include the need for attentive supportive care, pediatric implications for antidotal therapy, and extracorporeal removal methods such as hemodialysis in children. In this article, each of these issues and emerging poison hazards are discussed.

Toxin-induced Coagulopathy   53

Peter Chai and Kavita Babu

Although warfarin and heparin have been mainstays of anticoagulation for almost 50 years, the recent introduction of multiple oral anticoagulants has led some practitioners to shift away from warfarin as the anticoagulant of choice for various diseases. Major advances have been made in targeting downstream clotting factors in the coagulation cascade, resulting in two major new classes of drugs: direct thrombin inhibitors and factor Xa inhibitors. Developed partially with the patient in mind, these drugs are taken orally and, because of their target specificity, have eliminated the need for routine blood monitoring, making them attractive to patients currently on warfarin.

Toxin-Induced Cardiovascular Failure   79

David H. Jang, Meghan B. Spyres, Lindsay Fox, and Alex F. Manini

Adverse cardiovascular events comprise a large portion of the morbidity and mortality in drug overdose emergencies. Adverse cardiovascular events encountered by emergency physicians treating poisoned patients include myocardial injury, hemodynamic compromise with shock, tachydysrhythmias, and cardiac arrest. Early signs of toxin-induced cardiovascular failure include bradycardia, tachycardia, and specific ECG findings. Treatment of toxicologic tachycardia relies on rapid supportive care along with proper use of benzodiazepines for sedation. Treatment of toxicologic bradycardia consists of the use of isotonic fluids, atropine, calcium salts, and glucagon. High-dose insulin euglycemia should be used early in the course of suspected severe poisoning and intravenous lipid emulsion given to patients who suffer cardiac arrest.

Toxin-Induced Hepatic Injury   103

Annette M. Lopez and Robert G. Hendrickson

Toxins such as pharmaceuticals, herbals, foods, and supplements may lead to hepatic damage. This damage may present as nonspecific symptoms in the setting of liver test abnormalities. Most cases involving toxin-induced damage are caused by acetaminophen. The most important step in the patient evaluation is to gather an extensive history that includes toxin exposure and excludes common causes of liver dysfunction. Patients whose hepatic dysfunction progresses to acute liver failure may benefit from transfer to a transplant service for further management. Currently, the mainstay in management for most exposures is stopping the offending agent. This manuscript will review the incidence, pathophysiology, diagnosis and management of the different forms of toxin-induced hepatic injury and exam in-depth the most common hepatic toxins.

Toxin-induced Respiratory Distress   127

Charles A. McKay Jr

This article describes the impact of various toxic substances on the airway and pulmonary system. Pulmonary anatomy and physiology provide the basis for understanding the response to toxin-induced injury. Simple asphyxiants displace oxygen from the inspired air. Respiratory irritants include water-soluble and water-insoluble compounds. Several inhaled agents produce direct airway injury, which may be mediated by caustic, thermal, and hydrocarbon exposures. Unique pulmonary toxins and toxicants are discussed, as well as inhaled toxin mixtures. Several inhaled toxins may also impair oxygen transport. The pulmonary system may also provide a mechanism for systemic toxin delivery on respiratory exposure.

Toxicologic Acid-Base Disorders   149

Sage W. Wiener

Acid-base disorders may complicate the presentation of patients with poisoning. This article summarizes an approach to acid-base disorders from a toxicologic perspective. It aims to assist the reader in identifying underlying acid-base processes, generating a differential diagnosis for each, and approaching that differential diagnosis in a systematic fashion. Understanding these processes will help to guide management and interventional strategies.

An Approach to Chemotherapy-Associated Toxicity   167

Zhanna Livshits, Rama B. Rao, and Silas W. Smith

The effects of chemotherapy in multiple organ systems may be challenging to discern from the sequelae of malignancy and systemic illnesses with concomitant immunocompromise. Chemotherapeutic agents typically affect multiple organ systems. Intrathecal medication errors may pose particularly devastating neurologic consequences and death, often requiring emergent intervention. This article provides an overview of commonly used chemotherapeutic drugs, indications for use, their adverse effects by organ system, and the management of commonly encountered toxicities. Intrathecal medication errors and specific antidotes are discussed in pertinent management sections. Emergency department management should focus on rapid patient assessment, immediate intervention following intrathecal medication errors, exclusion of infection, and excellent supportive care.

Central Nervous System Toxicity   205

Anne-Michelle Ruha and Michael Levine

Central nervous system toxicity caused by xenobiotic exposure is a common reason for presentation to the emergency department. Sources of exposure may be medicinal, recreational, environmental, or occupational; the means of exposure may be intentional or unintended. Toxicity may manifest as altered thought content resulting in psychosis or confusion; may affect arousal, resulting in lethargy, stupor, or coma; or may affect both elements of consciousness. Seizures may also occur.

Marine Envenomations   223

Kamna S. Balhara and Andrew Stolbach

This article describes the epidemiology and presentation of human envenomation from marine organisms. Venom pathophysiology, envenomation presentation, and treatment options are discussed for sea snake, stingray, spiny fish, jellyfish, octopus, cone snail, sea urchin, and sponge envenomation. The authors describe the management of common exposures that cause morbidity as well as the keys to recognition and treatment of life-threatening exposures.

Ionizing Radiation Injuries and Illnesses   245

Doran M. Christensen, Carol J. Iddins, and Stephen L. Sugarman

Although the spectrum of information related to diagnosis and management of radiation injuries and illnesses is vast and as radiation contamination

incidents are rare, most emergency practitioners have had little to no practical experience with such cases. Exposures to ionizing radiation and internal contamination with radioactive materials can cause significant tissue
damage and conditions. Emergency practitioners unaware of ionizing
radiation as the cause of a condition may miss the diagnosis of radiation-
induced injury or illness. This article reviews the pertinent terms, physics,
radiobiology, and medical management of radiation injuries and illnesses
that may confront the emergency practitioner.

Index   **267**

EMERGENCY MEDICINE
CLINICS OF NORTH AMERICA

FORTHCOMING ISSUES

May 2014
Endocrine and Metabolic Emergencies
George C. Willis, MD, and
M. Tyson Pillow, MD, *Editors*

August 2014
Hematology/Oncology Emergencies
John C. Perkins, MD, and
Jonathan E. Davis, MD, *Editors*

November 2014
Critical Care in the Emergency Department
Evie Marcolini, MD, and
Haney A. Mallemat, MD, *Editors*

RECENT ISSUES

November 2013
**Dangerous Fever in the Emergency
Department**
Emilie Calvello, MD, and
Christian Theodosis, MD, *Editors*

August 2013
Pediatric Emergency Medicine
Le N. Lu, MD, Dale Woolridge, MD, and
Ann M. Dietrich, MD, *Editors*

May 2013
**Head, Eyes, Ears, Nose, and Throat
Emergencies**
Alisa M. Gibson MD, and
Kip R. Benko MD, *Editors*

PROGRAM OBJECTIVE

The goal of *Emergency Medicine Clinics of North America* is to keep practicing emergency medicine physicians and emergency medicine residents up to date with current clinical practice in emergency medicine by providing timely articles reviewing the state of the art in patient care.

TARGET AUDIENCE

All practicing physicians and healthcare professionals who provide patient care utilizing findings from *Emergency Medicine Clinics of North America*.

LEARNING OBJECTIVES

Upon completion of this activity, participants will be able to:

1. Discuss toxin induced respiratory distress, hepatic injury, coagulopathy, and cardiovascular failure.
2. Recognize emerging drugs of abuse.
3. Review the specialized approach to pediatric toxicology.

ACCREDITATION

The Elsevier Office of Continuing Medical Education (EOCME) is accredited by the Accreditation Council for Continuing Medical Education (ACCME) to provide continuing medical education for physicians.

The EOCME designates this enduringmaterial for a maximum of 15 *AMA PRA Category 1 Credit*(s)™. Physicians should claim only the credit commensurate with the extent of their participation in the activity.

All other health care professionals requesting continuing education credit for this enduring material will be issued a certificate of participation.

DISCLOSURE OF CONFLICTS OF INTEREST

The EOCME assesses conflict of interest with its instructors, faculty, planners, and other individuals who are in a position to control the content of CME activities. All relevant conflicts of interest that are identified are thoroughly vetted by EOCME for fair balance, scientific objectivity, and patient care recommendations. EOCME is committed to providing its learners with CME activities that promote improvements or quality in healthcare and not a specific proprietary business or a commercial interest.

The planning committee, staff, authors and editors listed below have identified no financial relationships or relationships to products or devices they or their spouse/life partner have with commercial interest related to the content of this CME activity:

Steven Aks, DO, FACMT, FACOEP, FACEP; Kavita Babu, MD; Kamna Singh Balhara, MD, MA; Sean Bryant, MD, FACMT; Diane Calello, MD; Peter Chai, MD; Doran Michael Christensen, DO; Lindsay M. Fox, MD; Kristen Helm; Robert Hendrickson, MD; Fred Henretig, MD, FAAP, FACMT; Brynne Hunter; Carol J. Iddins, MD; David Jang, MD, MSc; Indu Kumari; Sandy Lavery; Michael Levine, MD; Zhanna Livshits, MD; Annette Meliza Lopez, MD; Daniel Lugassy, MD; Alex Manini, MD; Patrick Manley; Amal Mattu, MD; Charles A. McKay, Jr, MD; Jill McNair; Michael Nelson; Rama Rao, MD, FACMT; Anne-Michelle Ruha, MD, FACMT; Silas Smith, MD; Meghan Spyres, MD; Andrew Stolbach, MD; Stephen L. Sugarman, MS, CHP, CHCM; Sage W. Wiener, MD.

The planning committee, staff, authors and editors listed below have identified financial relationships or relationships to products or devices they or their spouse/life partner have with commercial interest related to the content of this CME activity:

UNAPPROVED/OFF-LABEL USE DISCLOSURE

The EOCME requires CME faculty to disclose to the participants:

1. When products or procedures being discussed are off-label, unlabelled, experimental, and/or investigational (not US Food and Drug Administration (FDA) approved); and
2. Any limitations on the information presented, such as data that are preliminary or that represent ongoing research, interim analyses, and/or unsupported opinions. Faculty may discuss information about pharmaceutical agents that is outside of FDA-approved labelling. This information is intended solely for CME and is not intended to promote off-label use of these medications. If you have any questions, contact the medical affairs department of the manufacturer for the most recent prescribing information.

TO ENROLL

To enroll in the *Emergency Medicine Clinics* Continuing Medical Education program, call customer service at 1-800-654-2452 or sign up online at http://www.theclinics.com/home/cme. The CME program is available to subscribers for an additional annual fee of $212 USD.

METHOD OF PARTICIPATION

In order to claim credit, participants must complete the following:
1. Complete enrolment as indicated above.
2. Read the activity.
3. Complete the CME Test and Evaluation. Participants must achieve a score of 70% on the test. All CME Tests and Evaluations must be completed online.

CME INQUIRIES/SPECIAL NEEDS

For all CME inquiries or special needs, please contact elsevierCME@elsevier.com.

Foreword

Clinical Toxicology

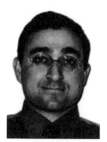

Amal Mattu, MD
Consulting Editor

Humans love drugs. Since the beginning of recorded history of medicine, laypersons and physicians alike have sought substances to cure maladies and to ease pain. Early natural substances eventually gave way to synthetic and chemical compounds as technology advanced, and with this advancement came increased potency of those substances. Increased potency of drugs resulted in increased side effects. In addition, with medical advances in our ability to ease pain came greater opportunity to abuse substances. Drugs originally intended to ease suffering were increasingly used to heighten pleasure and produce altered states of consciousness. In the modern day, our society's ability to create drugs has essentially produced a three-edged sword: on the one hand, drugs can cure disease and improve life; they can also produce dangerous side effects, and they can be intentionally abused and result in serious adverse social and medical consequences.

Compounding these issues are other changes in our society that have contributed to the number of cases of "adverse drug scenarios." The combination of a rapidly growing geriatric population along with medication over-prescribing has resulted in complications related to polypharmacy never before seen in human history. Advanced chemotherapy drugs, immunosuppressants, and anticoagulants have myriad side effects and deadly drug interactions. With regard to the substances of abuse, illicit drug use continues to be on the rise, fueled by an entertainment industry (music, movies and television, sports figures) that both implicitly and explicitly endorses "recreational" drug use. Clinical toxicologists and on-site clinical pharmacists have never before been in such high demand. For those emergency care providers that do not have immediate access to toxicology experts, it is imperative to know as much as possible about toxin-induced diseases.

In this issue of *Emergency Medicine Clinics of North America*, guest editors Drs Lugassy and Smith have assembled an outstanding group of authors to educate us on this increasing challenge in our specialty. An early, fairly comprehensive article is provided to update us on the newest, most "innovative" drugs of abuse. The authors

http://dx.doi.org/10.1016/j.emc.2013.10.005
0733-8627/14/$ – see front matter

then turn their attention to the tremendous problem of toxin-induced disease and drug side effects. They address the hot topic of drug-induced coagulopathy, clearly an almost daily problem we face in emergency departments today. They also address drug-induced maladies of various organ systems: the heart, the liver, the lungs, and the central nervous system. Separate articles are provided to address chemotherapeutic agents, acid-base abnormalities, radiation exposure, and marine envenomations. Finally, an article is provided to address some special concerns in pediatric patients.

This issue of *Emergency Medicine Clinics of North America* represents an important addition to the emergency medicine literature. The guest editors and authors are to be commended for providing a single resource that covers a broad spectrum of toxicologic emergencies in a succinct, clinically relevant, and cutting-edge manner.

Amal Mattu, MD
Department of Emergency Medicine
University of Maryland School of Medicine
Baltimore, MD, USA

E-mail address:
amattu@smail.umaryland.edu

Preface

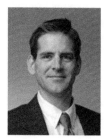 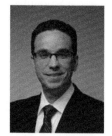

Silas W. Smith, MD, FACEP   Daniel M. Lugassy, MD
Editors

In the intervening years since the last issue of *Emergency Medicine Clinics of North America* dedicated to the topic of Medical Toxicology, poisoning has risen to become the leading cause of injury-related death in the United States. Poisoning surpassed deaths from motor vehicle crashes and further exceeds deaths from firearms, falls, and drowning. According to the Centers for Disease Control and Prevention, unintentional poisoning death rates in the United States have steadily increased each year since 1999. Despite the limitations of a spontaneous, voluntary self-reporting structure, National Poison Data System data reveal that over 2.3 million human exposure cases are managed by the nation's Poison Control Centers annually. These sad statistics highlight the clear and pervasive threat to the nation's public health posed by medications, household substances, environmental agents, occupational chemicals, drugs of abuse, and other toxic substances and should prompt rededicated efforts toward poisoning prevention, care, and research.

Tasked with selecting topics for inclusion, we were presented with the near-inexhaustible range of potentially toxic substances, as well as the possibility of mixed exposures, which confront the emergency practitioner and our own practice. We elected to focus less on particular toxins (although they are reviewed within the articles) and to shift the approach to toxic presentations in several specific organ systems, while recognizing that global dysfunction may be evident. We have also included a few selected topics that may initially seem outside of the scope of emergency medicine, but may either take on a more prominent role or require key initial critical actions by emergency practitioners. We hope that the dedicated work of our contributors will assist emergency practitioners challenged with the care of patients with potential poisoning.

Silas W. Smith, MD, FACEP
Department of Emergency Medicine
Assistant Professor and Section Chief
Quality, Safety, and Practice Innovation
New York University School of Medicine
Bellevue Hospital Center
462 First Avenue, Room A 345-A
New York, NY 10016, USA

Emerg Med Clin N Am 32 (2014) xvii–xviii
http://dx.doi.org/10.1016/j.emc.2013.10.004
0733-8627/14/$ – see front matter © 2014 Elsevier Inc. All rights reserved.
emed.theclinics.com

Daniel M. Lugassy, MD
Department of Emergency Medicine
Director of Medical Student Medical Toxicology Education
New York University School of Medicine
Bellevue Hospital Center
462 First Avenue, Room A 345-A
New York, NY 10016, USA

E-mail addresses:
Silas.Smith@nyumc.org (S.W. Smith)
Daniel.Lugassy@nyumc.org (D.M. Lugassy)

Emerging Drugs of Abuse

Michael E. Nelson, MD, MS[a,b,*], Sean M. Bryant, MD[b],
Steven E. Aks, DO[b]

KEYWORDS

- Synthetic cathinones • Synthetic cannabinoids • Phenethylamines • Piperazines
- Herbal drugs of abuse • Prescription drug abuse • Managing new drug exposures

KEY POINTS

- Emerging drugs of abuse are forever changing and involve manipulation of basic chemical structures to avoid legal ramifications.
- The individual names and chemical formulations of emerging drugs of abuse are not as important as a general understanding of the classes of drugs.
- Most of the synthetic new drugs of abuse result in psychoactive and sympathomimetic effects.
- Management generally involves symptom-based goal-directed supportive care with benzodiazepines as a useful adjunct.

INTRODUCTION

Remaining abreast of emerging drugs of abuse continues to challenge emergency practitioners (EPs). As law enforcement agencies classify certain drugs as illegal, street pharmacists rapidly adapt and develop new congeners of old drugs for distribution and use. It is essential that EPs have a solid foundation in the general classes of drugs of abuse. Many of the newer drugs have similar effects, and respond well to meticulous and aggressive supportive management. Sources of information and surveillance should be available so that EPs remain knowledgeable of current trends. Poison centers, along with local public health officials, should be important sources of current information. Internet sites, social media, and search engines may be additional tools for drugs of abuse trends.[1,2]

Legal highs present an ongoing issue. These products are sold in head shops, the Internet, and other sources.[3] Bath salts (cathinones, mephedrone, and others) and synthetic cannabinoids are two useful examples of the problem of legal highs and

[a] Department of Emergency Medicine, NorthShore University Health System, 2650 Ridge Avenue, Evanston, IL 60201, USA; [b] Department of Emergency Medicine, John H. Stroger Jr. Hospital of Cook County, Toxikon Consortium, Illinois Poison Control Center, 1900 West Polk Street, 10th Floor, Chicago, IL 60612, USA
* Corresponding author. Department of Emergency Medicine, John H. Stroger Jr. Hospital of Cook County, Toxikon Consortium, Illinois Poison Control Center, 1900 West Polk Street, 10th Floor, Chicago, IL 60612.
E-mail address: menelson4@gmail.com

Emerg Med Clin N Am 32 (2014) 1–28
http://dx.doi.org/10.1016/j.emc.2013.09.001
0733-8627/14/$ – see front matter © 2014 Elsevier Inc. All rights reserved.

are discussed later. These substances tend to be slightly altered chemicals derived from other known drugs of abuse. They were easily obtained on the Internet and in tobacco head shops, and were finally banned once public health and law enforcement officials identified these compounds and adapted laws. Recent legislation shows that authorities can act quickly to implement important public health laws. The Synthetic Drug Abuse Prevention Act of 2012 included synthetic cannabinoids in the schedule I category, which subsequently diminished their availability considerably.[4]

One article nicely summarizes the cycle of one drug of abuse.[5] Ecstasy (MDMA, 3,4-methylenedioxy-N-methylamphetamine) has been abused for several decades. Its street use was complicated by adulteration and substitution. However, there has been a resurgence of this drug as "Molly," which is touted to be a pure form of ecstasy. Much of this street information is unreliable, but the fact that Molly appeared in the fashion section of a notable newspaper is remarkable.

PRESCRIPTION DRUG ABUSE EPIDEMIC

Another major perspective for EPs to maintain is the current prescription drug epidemic. Beginning in 2004, prescription opioids have outstripped street heroin and cocaine as causes of death.[6] Physician prescriptions can and are being used as emerging drugs of abuse. Opioids and benzodiazepines are frequent diversion targets.[6,7] Patients prescribed these medications and other controlled substances such as medications for attention deficit hyperactivity disorder (ADHD) should be screened for at-risk substance abuse.[8]

Most physicians are aware of prescription-monitoring programs and can use this as a tool to detect diversion and to identify multiple prescriptions of controlled substances.[9,10] Although it is controversial whether prescription-monitoring programs are effective in reducing rates of drug overdose mortality, they are an important tool to prevent the inappropriate use and diversion of these medications.[9]

Unfortunately, the problem expands far beyond the prescription drug arena. There is widespread over-the-counter drug abuse and misuse.[11] Weight-control drugs and laxatives are just two such examples. Further attention on how a product is sold, such as behind-the-counter (BTC) status, is appropriate to assure age-appropriate use.[11]

Performance-enhancing drugs are and will continue to be emerging drugs of abuse. The incentives to perform at high levels are profound and with increasingly sophisticated techniques of drug detection, it is logical that this will be an evolving arena. These substances are widely available on the Internet.[12] The World Anti-Doping Agency (WADA) modifies its prohibited list on an annual basis in response to this ongoing issue.[13] This discussion, however, is immense in itself and beyond the scope of this article.

Not only are performance-enhancing drugs abused, but so too are drugs that are used to improve appearance. Examples include weight loss and melanotan products. Melanotan products are Internet-purchased substances used to improve tanning, and have been reported to cause significant sympathomimetic signs and symptoms, along with rhabdomyolysis and renal dysfunction.[14]

In addition to the substances covered in this article, there are numerous other examples of drugs of abuse that continue to emerge and evolve. Methoxetamine, a ketamine analogue, has become a drug of abuse. It carries the purported advantage over ketamine of being less toxic to the urologic system, although animal studies call this into question.[15] Krokodil, or desomorphine, is a drug of abuse that is typically used when heroin or poppy straw is in short supply. Significant abuse has been described in Ukraine.[16] Even common substances found in convenience stores can be misused. A recent example includes the abuse of energy drinks. These beverages can contain caffeine, taurine, niacin, and other substances. Some individuals coingest these drinks with ethanol, and this pattern of misuse has resulted in mixed toxic effects.[17]

As the number of potential substances for abuse is immense and beyond the scope of a single article, the following sections cover the most significant recent and emerging drugs of abuse. These substances include the synthetic cannabinoids, bath salts, amphetamines and phenethylamine substances, piperazines, and emerging herbs of abuse. General toxicity as well as overall supportive measures are also reviewed.

SYNTHETIC CANNABINOIDS
Introduction

Cannabis is one of the most widely used illicit substances worldwide and in the United States, possession and distribution carry legal ramifications.[18] In the last decade, synthetic cannabinoids (SCs, also referred to as synthetic cannabinoid receptor agonists) gained popularity as a legal alternative to achieve euphoric effects similar to cannabis. These products were sold at head shops, convenience stores, and on the Internet as herbal incense or air fresheners, and were marketed as not for human consumption.[19,20] The most common street names for SCs are K2 and Spice.[21] They did not originally come under initial legal regulations from the US Federal Controlled Substances Act because of their structural dissimilarity to Δ^9-tetrahydrocannabinol (Δ^9-THC). In addition, many other biological herbs besides SC are contained in these products.[21–23] Packaging notoriously contains minimal information regarding the chemical composition of the plant products and no standard exists for the ingredients or concentrations.[24] SCs are typically sold in metal foil sachets as a mixture of dried vegetable matter with the SC substance sprayed onto the herbal mixture.[25] SCs are comprised of many substances (**Box 1**), with dozens of different assigned street names (**Box 2**).

History and Epidemiology

The first synthetic Δ^9-THC was produced in 1967, and in 1985, dronabinol (Marinol) was approved as an antiemetic in the United States.[21] Subsequently, other SCs including nabilone (Cesamet) and nabiximols (Sativex) were used for refractory emesis in chemotherapy, as adjuncts for neuropathic pain, and for anorexia in patients with

Box 1	
Various synthetic cannabinoids	
JWH-015	(C8)-CP-47,497
JWH-018	HU-210
JWH-073	CP-55,490
JWH-200	AM-2201
JWH-081	WIN-48,098
JWH-122	WIN-54,461
JWH-210	WIN-55,212-2
JWH-250	XLR-11
JWH-398	UR-144
CP-47,497	—

Box 2
Common street/brand names for substances containing synthetic cannabinoids

Spice	Bombay blue
K2	Blaze
Happy tiger incense	Bliss
Spice gold	Chill zone cherry
Spice silver	Chaos mint
Spice diamond	Clover spring
Spice Egypt	Fake weed
Spice arctic synergy	Genie
SpicyXXX	Eclipse
Smoke	Krypton
Banana cream nuke	Moon rocks
Aroma	Mr Smiley
Aztec fire	Sensation vanilla
Black mamba	Yucatan fire
Blueberry posh	Zohai

AIDS.[21,26,27] Another classic cannabinoid is HU-210, which is structurally similar to Δ^9-THC, but much more potent.[20,21] Other nonclassic cannabinoids, called cyclohexophenols (CP) and aminoalkylindoles (AAIs), were developed in the 1960s to 1980s and have similar clinical effects as Δ^9-THC.[20,21,24,28,29] The SCs fall into seven major structural groups: naphthoylindoles (eg, JWH-015, JWH-018, JWH-073), naphthylmethylindoles, naphthoylpyrroles, naphthylmethylindenes, phenylacetylindoles (eg, JWH-250), cyclohexophenols (eg, CP-47,497), and classic cannabinoids.[24,25,30]

John William Huffman, a chemist at Clemson University and namesake of many SCs (JWH compounds), synthesized multiple AAIs with varying degrees of affinity for cannabinoid receptors (CBRs).[19,31–33] Of the various JWH compounds created, the pharmacology is similar to Δ^9-THC, JWH-018 is reported to have the greatest potency at CBRs.[21,29,33–35] JWH-018 was the first and most widely reported substance uncovered in SCs.[24,34–36] These SC-containing products emerged in European markets in 2004 and in the United States in 2008, with the first cases reported to US poison centers in 2009.[22,36,37] In November 2010, the US Drug Enforcement Administration designated five popular SCs (JWH-018, JWH-073, JWH-200, CP-47,497, and a C8 homologue of CP-47,497) temporarily schedule I status effective March 2011 "to avoid an imminent hazard to the public safety."[38]

A unique property of SC products is the frequently changing chemical composition and development of new derivatives, perhaps as a means to avoid legal ramifications. Regardless, these products are lipid-soluble, nonpolar, and volatilized chemicals that mimic the action of Δ^9-THC.[20] This variable composition of SC products makes development of standardized tests and confirmatory analysis in patients difficult.[20,39] Furthermore, because of this variability, obtaining pharmacologic and pharmacokinetic profiles of SCs with adverse effects is more difficult.[20] Hundreds of different SCs may be incorporated into the various constituents being used.[30]

The exact prevalence of societal SC use is unknown. According to 2012 data, SC use in US 12th graders remained constant from 2011 to 2012 at an annual prevalence rate of 11.3%, but had a low level of perceived risk in 23% to 25% of respondents.[40] Even among athletes tested in 2010, JWH-018 and JWH-073 metabolites were detected in 4.5% of samples.[41] Nearly 11,000 exposures to SC have been reported to US poison centers between 2009 and mid-2012, with overall reported exposures increasing until July 2011. Since then, reported exposures to SCs have remained increased at roughly 500 to 700 per month, higher than exposures to synthetic cathinone.[37] The most common reason for use is intentional abuse, and inhalational exposure predominates.[37,42,43] Most SC users tend to be male and in their teens to early 20s.[24,37,42–44] More severe clinical effects have been observed in SC users than in marijuana users; up to 7.3% of exposures were life-threatening.[42,43] In a recent large global sample of nearly 15,000 participants, 17% reported SC use, with 99% of these individuals having used natural cannabis.[44] During the increase in popularity of SCs, EPs had little knowledge of common names for SC products, with most of their knowledge originating from nonmedical sources. Eighty percent of clinicians felt unprepared to care for patients with SC poisoning in the emergency department (ED).[45]

Pharmacology

Cannabinoid receptors are diverse with a large number of biological targets. CB_1 G-protein coupled receptors are abundant in the brain and modulate γ-aminobutyric acid and glutamate neurotransmission. A high density of CB_1 receptors exists in the basal ganglia. CB_2 receptors are typically found in the peripheral tissues (spleen and immune cells) and possibly mediate immunosuppression, but may also be present in the central nervous system (CNS).[20,30,46] CBRs are also complexed with other receptors, including opioid and dopamine receptors. Cannabinoids themselves can modulate various receptors including acetylcholine, opioid, serotonin, glycine, glutamatergic, and nuclear peroxisome proliferation-activated receptor α receptors.[20,47] Cannabinoids' main metabolic pathway occurs through oxidation via the hepatic cytochrome P450 pathway and conjugation with glucuronic acid to achieve renal excretion.[48]

Synthetic cannabinoids have varying degrees of affinity for CBRs.[49] The potency of HU-210 is reported to be 100 to 800 times greater than Δ^9-THC at CBRs and CP-47,497 and its C8 homologue is 30 times more potent.[21,49] In addition, different SCs have greater affinity for CB_2 receptors, such as JWH-015 and JWH-133.[21] Because of this wide variability, the pharmacodynamics and kinetic profiles of many SCs are unknown.[20,30] One of the more common SCs, JWH-018, reaches peak serum concentrations rapidly via inhalation, has a short half-life, and is five times more potent than Δ^9-THC. This pharmacologic profile, however, cannot be extrapolated to all SCs.[50,51] SC users report a quicker peak and shortened duration of effects compared with natural cannabis.[44] Furthermore, unlike Δ^9-THC, SC metabolites have varying degrees of activity (agonistic, antagonistic, or neutral) at CBRs, potentially explaining the mixed effects observed clinically.[20,51,52] Activity at receptors other than CBRs for SCs is unknown and implications are undetermined, but the potential exists given the many receptors where natural cannabinoids exert their effects.[20,47]

Clinical Effects

A wide variety of clinical effects have been reported, from mild symptoms to severe sympathomimeticlike effects and seizures (**Table 1**). Because of the variability of SC concentration and substances, recreational use can result in unintentional overdose.[22] The most common findings reported to poison centers include tachycardia, agitation, vomiting, drowsiness, confusion, hallucinations, hypertension, dizziness, and chest pain.[42,43]

A multitude of psychoactive SC effects are described and range from a desired euphoria to severe anxiety and psychosis.[20,22,24,53] A case series of 10 otherwise healthy men developed auditory hallucinations, visual hallucinations, paranoid delusions, odd affect, disorganized speech and behavior, with suicidal ideation lasting days to months after smoking SC products.[54] Spice use has also triggered an acute

Table 1
Clinical effects of synthetic cannabinoids

System	Effects
CNS	Seizures, agitation, anxiety, irritability, sedation, confusion, paranoia, psychosis
Cardiovascular	Tachycardia, dysrhythmia, chest pain, myocardial infarction, elevated blood pressure
Gastrointestinal	Nausea, vomiting
Renal	Acute kidney injury
Metabolic	Hypokalemia, hyperglycemia
Ophthalmologic	Mydriasis, conjunctivitis
Other	Hyperthermia, tolerance, withdrawal, dependence

exacerbation of cannabis-induced recurrent psychosis, paranoid delusions, and an enhanced risk of psychosis in susceptible individuals.[53,55,56] Anxiety-like reactions can occur, necessitating treatment in the ED.[56,57]

Synthetic cannabinoid use is also associated with additional CNS effects including confusion, tremors, sedation, memory changes, and seizures.[20,36,53,57–60] Although rare for natural cannabis, the mechanism of action for seizure induction with SC is still unknown, but may occur through release of excitatory neurotransmitters or a decrease in inhibitory neurotransmitters.[36,58] This effect may be dose related.[36]

Cardiovascular effects commonly include hypertension and tachycardia.[36,42,43] Cases have involved refractory supraventricular tachycardia requiring electrical cardioversion.[36] Chest pain with electrocardiogram (ECG) changes typical for ST elevation myocardial infarction and increased troponin levels have been observed in teenagers despite normal coronary arteries.[61]

Additional effects reported include gastrointestinal upset with nausea and emesis.[42,58,62,63] Ophthalmologic examination generally reveals normal to mydriatic pupils and injected conjunctiva.[22,57,62] Xerostomia and flushing can occur with development of hyperthermia.[21,22,50] Appetite changes have been reported including both increased and decreased appetite.[53] A case of diffuse pulmonary infiltrates with acute respiratory distress syndrome (ARDS) has been attributed to chronic SC use.[64] Metabolic changes may not be observed in many cases, but have included hypokalemia, hyperglycemia, and leukocytosis.[21,36,57,58,62–65] Recent reports from several states include cases of acute kidney injury requiring hemodialysis from SC use (in particular the SCs XLR-11, UR-144, AM-2201).[63] According to voluntary, spontaneous reporting to the National Poison Data System (NPDS) from 2011, a total of 4 deaths were related to THC homologues. One ingestion was coded as "probably responsible" for the death and described a 19-year-old man with postmortem urinalysis positive solely for metabolites of JWH-018.[66]

Chronic effects of SC use are unknown.[20] Chronic cannabis use has been associated with neuropsychological decline with impaired concentration and greater IQ decline.[67] Cannabis influences emotional and sensory processing and SCs may have similar cognitive effects.[20] The chronic psychiatric symptoms or effects are unknown, but SCs have triggered psychotic symptoms with suicidal ideations.[54,55] Natural cannabis withdrawal symptoms have been described and include insomnia, anxiety, irritability, malaise, myalgias, shakiness, nausea, vomiting, and drug craving for 1 to 2 weeks.[68,69] Chronic use of SCs can result in a similar withdrawal syndrome on cessation.[70,71]

Among users, natural cannabis is preferred to SCs by an overwhelming majority because of the more negative effects produced by SCs, including paranoia and hangover effects.[44] Consumers of SCs also self-reported concomitant use of other substances including alcohol, cocaine, benzodiazepines, amphetamines, MDMA, ketamine, and mephedrone.[44] Mixed ingestions may create complex clinical situations and complicate care.

Testing and Imaging

No specific testing is recommended or indicated for synthetic cannabinoid ingestion. Laboratory testing and imaging should be directed toward clinical observations and symptoms as needed. Routine qualitative drug testing of urine for Δ^9-THC is generally negative.[22,36,57–60] SCs can, however, be detected by gas chromatography-mass spectrophotometry (GC-MS) or by liquid chromatography-tandem mass spectrometry (LC-MS/MS).[20,22,24,30,39,50,60] Independent laboratories have commercial tests for both the SC product and for SCs in human blood and urine samples.[72] These tests generally are time-consuming, must be sent to referral laboratories, and the results are not readily available for the treating EPs.

Treatment

No specific antidote exists for SCs.[30] Treatment consists of symptom-based goal-directed supportive care with patient education and abstinence from further use. Specific treatment options are discussed in greater detail in the section on management principles.

Summary

SCs are a diverse group of heterogeneous compounds with a wide variety of clinical effects. Their use has increased over the past decade, as they have been viewed as a legal and safe alternative to natural cannabis.[65] Although true prevalence rates are unknown, young men tend to be the highest risk group of individuals to use SCs. In addition, diverse SCs exist with different potency at CBRs and potentially other receptors. The clinical presentation of SC intoxication varies greatly but generally involves tachycardia, hypertension, alteration in cognition and mood, and potentially seizures. No specific antidote exists and patients should be treated based on symptoms. Despite public awareness and legal action, SC use has remained popular.[30]

SYNTHETIC CATHINONES (BATH SALTS)
Introduction

Synthetic cathinones, commonly sold as bath salts, have recently emerged as a popular drug of abuse. They were marketed as legal highs similar to SCs and "not for human consumption" to avoid legal and regulatory oversight.[30] They are sold at head shops and on the Internet similar to SCs. Cathinone occurs naturally in the leaves of the khat plant (*Catha edulis*). Khat leaves contain phenylalkylamine compounds (cathinone, cathine, and norephedrine) structurally related to amphetamine and noradrenaline and produce stimulant effects.[73,74] Cathinone, however, seems to be the main constituent responsible for the amphetaminelike euphoria.[75] Synthetic cathinones are derivatives of cathinone with various chemical alterations affecting pharmacokinetics and pharmacodynamics.[30] They comprise many various substances (**Box 3**) and are referred to by a wide variety of street names (**Box 4**).

Box 3
Common synthetic cathinones

Methcathinone	Ethylone
Mephedrone	Methedrone
Methylenedioxypyrovalerone (MDPV)	Naphyrone
Methylone	3-Fluoromethcathinone
Butylone	4-Fluoromethcathinone (flephedrone)
Brephedrone	α-Pyrrolidinovalerophenone
Pyrovalerone	3,4-Methylenedioxy-α-
Dimethylecathinone	pyrrolindinopropiophenone (MDPPP)
Ethcathinone	—

History and Epidemiology

Individuals have chewed khat leaves to obtain the stimulant effects of natural-occurring cathinone (S-(−)-2-amino-1-phenyl-1-propanone) for centuries.[30] Chewing natural khat remains local to areas where it is grown, particularly in Middle Eastern nations such as Yemen and in East African nations such as Somalia and Ethiopia, as only the fresh leaves contain the active cathinone.[75,76] Khat chewing itself has reportedly been associated with higher risk of stroke and death.[76] The first synthetic cathinone, methcathinone, was created in 1928, with mephedrone soon following in 1929.[74,77] Shortly after, the Advisory Committee on the Traffic in Opium and Other Dangerous Drugs of the League of Nations discussed the potential of khat and cathinone as a health hazard.[73] In the 1930s and 1940s, methcathinone was used as an antidepressant in the Soviet Union and subsequently has been used recreationally.[78] In the 1970s, pyrovalerone was studied for treating fatigue and obesity, but the study had to be discontinued because users developed dependency and abuse.[74] The cathinone derivative chloro-α-t-butylaminopropiophenone was patented in 1974 and currently is marketed as bupropion (Wellbutrin, Zyban) for prescription use to treat depression and nicotine craving.[74,79] Cathinone abuse outbreaks occurred in the United States and Europe in the 1990s, and in 1993 methcathinone was designated as a schedule I substance.[30,78,80]

Around the same time as the SC epidemic, synthetic cathinones also gained popularity. First reports in Internet drug chat forums of mephedrone use occurred in 2007 and were detected by a web-mapping research group in 2008.[81] The increased popularity of mephedrone and other synthetic cathinones was driven by lack of availability or poor purity of other recreational stimulants such as cocaine and MDMA combined with availability over the Internet and no legal regulation.[82] US poison centers began receiving calls related to bath salts in 2010 with a peak in volume in mid-2011.[37]

Box 4
Common street names for synthetic cathinones

Khat	Meow meow
Bath salts	MCAT
Ivory wave	Bubbles
Vanilla sky	Cloud 9
White rush	Explosion
White lightning	Impact
White dove	Energy-1

The exact prevalence of use of synthetic cathinones in society is unknown. Synthetic cathinone use in US 12th graders in 2012 had an annual prevalence rate of 1.3% (compared with 11.3% for SC).[40] A survey of 1006 secondary and university school students in the United Kingdom reported 20.3% of respondents used mephedrone with 4.4% reporting daily use. Sixty-six percent of individuals surveyed found mephedrone easily obtainable.[82] A survey of 2700 UK dance club frequenters reported 41.3% used mephedrone, 10.8% used methylone, and 1.9% used methylenedioxypyrovalerone (MDPV).[83] A 1-year review of data from 9 US Midwest poison centers relating to bath salts involved 1633 patients. Males (68%) dominated and most (54%) were younger than 30 years.[84] Synthetic cathinone users tend to be younger males, the same demographic as SC users.

In the United States, calls to poison centers related to bath salts totaled 303 in 2010, 6062 in 2011, 2656 in 2012, and 450 in the first 5 months of 2013. The number of calls thus far in 2013 is nearly one-third of the number during the same time period in 2012 (450 calls compared with 1304 calls).[85] An increase in call numbers occurred in June 2011 and again in June 2012 for unclear reasons. From September 2012 to May 2013, calls to poison centers regarding bath salts have averaged roughly 93 per month.[85] By comparison, calls to poison centers regarding synthetic marijuana during the same time period have averaged 240 calls per month.[86]

Legislative measures have been taken against synthetic cathinones to address these once legal highs. In April 2010, the Misuse of Drugs Act classified mephedrone and other similar substances as Class B substances.[87,88] This legal action caused the price of mephedrone to double in the United Kingdom and increased purchasing from street dealers as presumably Internet purchasing was limited.[87] In September 2011, the US Drug Enforcement Agency (DEA) temporarily scheduled 3 synthetic cathinones (mephedrone, methylone, and MDPV) as schedule I.[89] The Synthetic Drug Abuse Prevention Act of 2012 extended the schedule I status of various SCs and phenethylamines including MDPV and mephedrone.[90] Calls to US poison centers for bath salts decreased from nearly 500 in September 2011 to just over 200 in November 2011.[85]

Pharmacology

Synthetic cathinones are β-ketophenethylamines structurally similar to amphetamines and catecholamines but with subtle variations that alter chemical properties and potency.[30,88] The ketone on the β-carbon of the phenethylamine constituent leads to increased polarity with reduction in CNS penetration.[88] This property may lead to higher dosing with more profound adverse peripheral effects.[88,91] The serum concentration of synthetic cathinone alone cannot determine the toxicity observed.[92]

Many routes of administration occur for bath salts. Most commonly, synthetic cathinones are insufflated (snorting) or ingested orally.[84,93,94] Intravenous, intramuscular, and rectal routes of administration also occur.[94,95] Duration of action, dosing, and time of onset of symptoms can vary with routes of administration.[94]

Limited pharmacokinetic data on synthetic cathinones are available.[30,74,91,96] Each synthetic cathinone has variable effects on neurotransmitters (serotonin, dopamine, and norepinephrine), with differing degrees of potency. The ability to modulate these monoamines creates psychoactive and sympathomimetic effects.[74,91,96,97] Synthetic cathinones inhibit monoamine uptake transporters and cause release of intracellular stores of monoamine neurotransmitters, leading to increased amounts of these neurotransmitters in the synapse.[96,98,99]

Understanding of metabolism is also limited, but animal models provide some principles. Metabolism of mephedrone generally occurs through phase I pathways with generation of multiple metabolites through N-demethylation to the primary amine, reduction of the ketone, and oxidation of the totyl group into its corresponding alcohol and carboxylic acid.[74,91,100,101] In addition, various hepatic cytochromes (CYPs) are involved in the demethylation process of MDPV, including CYP1A2, 2D6, and 2C19.[102] Many phase II metabolites of MDPV are also possible thus providing a complex process for metabolism.[102]

Clinical Effects

Cathinones create amphetaminelike sympathomimetic effects with tachycardia, hypertension, and euphoria.[75,103] The degree of hyperadrenergic effects varies based on the substance and amount ingested. Many clinical effects are possible (**Table 2**). The most common adverse effects reported involve the cardiac, neurologic, and psychiatric systems.[74] The most common clinical findings reported to poison centers include agitation, tachycardia, hallucination, hypertension, confusion, mydriasis, tremor, and fever. Additional serious effects reported include rhabdomyolysis, renal failure, seizures, and death.[84,93,104]

Cardiovascular effects are related to the stimulant effect of cathinones. Common signs and symptoms include chest pain, palpitations, hypertension, and tachycardia.[84,93–95] Mephedrone reportedly caused ECG changes, with ST segment elevation and myocardial inflammation.[105] Synthetic cathinones can potentially result in fatal cardiac dysrhythmias.[106]

Psychoactive and CNS effects most commonly involve agitation and aggression.[84,93] Many reports exist that detail psychosis and excited delirium with various synthetic cathinones.[107–111] Visual, auditory, and tactile hallucinations can occur.[108,109] Patients may become severely agitated and display violent behavior that requires physical or chemical restraint.[107] Additional findings include confusion, dysphoria, delusions, insomnia, nightmares, changes in concentration, and altered mental status.[83,94] Seizures are one of the most severe CNS effects that occur.[84,112]

Additional effects observed mimic stimulant-like symptoms with euphoria, talkativeness, desire to move, bruxism, insomnia, and reduced appetite.[113] Gastrointestinal effects include nausea, vomiting, abdominal discomfort, and xerostomia.[94] Ingestion of methylone and butylone resulted in a case of serotonin syndrome, disseminated intravascular coagulation (DIC), ARDS, and death.[114] Metabolic abnormalities have been observed, including acidosis and hyponatremia.[95,111,112] Compartment syndrome

Table 2
Clinical effects of synthetic cathinones

System	Effects
Psychiatric	Agitation, aggression, confusion, anxiety, insomnia, dysphoria, hallucinations, paranoia, delusions
CNS	Altered mental status, hyperreflexia, nystagmus, tremors, seizures
Cardiovascular	Tachycardia, hypertension, myocarditis, chest pain
Gastrointestinal	Abdominal pain, nausea, vomiting, xerostomia
Renal	Acute renal failure
Metabolic	Hyponatremia, acidosis
Ophthalmologic	Mydriasis, blurred vision
Other	Hyperthermia, diaphoresis, body odor, bruxism, epistaxis, rhabdomyolysis

has been reported.[115] Further serious effects include renal dysfunction, rhabdomyolysis, hyperthermia, and multiorgan system failure.[110,115,116] Drug-induced hyperthermia has historically been associated with poor neurologic outcomes and increased mortality.[117] Unfortunately, multiple deaths related to various synthetic cathinones are evident.[92,104,106,110,111,114,118–120]

The long-term effects of synthetic cathinone use are unknown. MDPV users reported tolerance, with consumption of higher doses.[96] Nearly 25% of mephedrone users reported a persistent desire to use and would continue to use despite physical and psychological problems, indicating a compulsion.[113] Fifty-six percent of mephedrone users reported at least one undesired effect with use.[82] Discontinuation of mephedrone has led to withdrawallike symptoms with nasal congestion, tiredness, insomnia, and impaired concentration.[113] Additional withdrawal syndromes have been self-reported with MDPV and methcathinone.[96] Nearly 30% of mephedrone users involved in the dance music scene had indicative findings of stimulant dependence.[113] Serotonergic and dopaminergic neuron toxicity in has been demonstrated in rodent models with methcathinone.[121] In humans, abstinent methcathinone users had decreased dopamine transporters on positron emission tomography scans similar to methamphetamine users and patients with Parkinson disease, suggesting the potential risk for long-term neuropsychiatric problems.[122]

Testing and Imaging

No specific testing is recommended or indicated for synthetic cathinone ingestion. Laboratory testing and imaging should be directed toward clinical observations and symptoms as needed. Despite the structural similarity to amphetamine, routine urinary qualitative drug testing and enzyme immunoassays for amphetamines are generally negative.[30,95,96,107,110,116,123] False-positive assays for methamphetamine may occur with mephedrone.[118] Synthetic cathinones and metabolites can be detected by GC-MS, LC-MS, or LC-MS/MS.[30,100–102,124] Independent laboratories have commercial tests for both the synthetic cathinone product and human blood and urine samples.[125] These tests generally are time consuming, must be sent to the referral laboratories, and results are not readily available for treating EPs.[114] Correlation of drug concentrations with observed clinical effects is not well defined or understood.[74]

Treatment

No specific antidote exists for synthetic cathinones.[30,74,111] Treatment consists of symptom-based goal-directed supportive care with patient education and abstinence from further use. The most common treatment provided for synthetic cathinones reported to poison centers is benzodiazepines.[84,104] Specific treatment options are discussed in greater detail in the section on management principles.

Summary

Synthetic cathinones are a broad group of compounds with amphetaminelike effects. Their use has increased over the past decade because they were marketed as legal highs. Many synthetic cathinones exist with variable potency but mainly affect monoamine neurotransmitters, resulting in sympathomimetic signs and symptoms. No specific antidotes exist, and treatment should be focused mainly on supportive care. Despite numerous reports of adverse events and legislative efforts, synthetic cathinone use remains popular.

OTHER PHENETHYLAMINES (2C DRUGS)
Introduction

The basic chemical structure of phenethylamine is shared among catecholamines, amphetamines, synthetic cathinones, and many other drugs.[91,126] Another class of synthetic phenethylamines abused for recreational highs are the 2C class of drugs; the name relates to the two carbons between the benzene ring and the terminal amine group.[126] Alexander T. Shulgin has often been credited with the discovery of various 2C drugs and the father of MDMA after the publication of his book *PiHKAL, A Chemical Love Story*.[127,128] The PiHKAL acronym stands for "Phenethylamines I Have Known and Loved."[128] In this text, Shulgin describes the synthesis, production, and dosages of various phenethylamines.[127] Various substitutions of the base phenethylamine structure can alter its pharmacologic and clinical effects, creating a vast array of chemical derivatives (**Table 3**).

The true prevalence of 2C and other phenethylamine use is unknown.[129] A survey of UK dance club frequenters reported 17.6% used 2C-B and 11.2% used 2C-I.[83] 2C-B was present in roughly 3% of drug materials analyzed in Spain between 2006 and 2009, and generally comes in a tablet or powder form.[129] Individuals that seek ecstasy at dance raves and other music festivals may inadvertently be exposed to 2C drugs as contaminants or MDMA substitutes.[130–132] These substances can be purchased on the Internet and can be listed as research chemicals.[132] As with SC and synthetic cathinones, 2C users tend to be younger males and may have a history of polydrug use.[129,132,133]

Many 2C substances are listed as schedule I substances.[90] Newer phenethylamine compounds, however, are continuously being designed and introduced to evade existing legislation and regulatory oversight.[130] This challenges treating providers in terms of being aware of new street names for these drugs.

Pharmacology

Complete pharmacologic and pharmacokinetic profiles of all the 2C drugs are unknown. Little modification, however, is needed to the basic phenethylamine structure

Table 3 Selected 2C phenethylamine drugs	
2C-B	4-Bromo-2,5-dimethoxyphenethylamine
2C-B-Fly	8-Bromo-2,3,6,7-benzo-dihydro-difuran-ethylamine
2C-C	4-Chloro-2,5-dimethoxyphenethylamine
2C-D	4-Methyl-2,5-dimethoxyphenethylamine
2C-E	4-Ethyl-2,5-dimethoxyphenethylamine
2C-F	4-Fluoro-2,5-dimethoxyphenethylamine
2C-G	3,4-Dimethyl-2,5-dimethoxyphenethylamine
2C-I	4-Iodo-2,5-dimethoxyphenethylamine
2C-I-Fly	8-Iodo-2,3,6,7-benzo-dihydro-difuran-ethylamine
2C-N	4-Nitro-2,5-dimethoxyphenethylamine
2C-P	4-Propyl-2,5-dimethoxyphenethylamine
2C-SE	4-Methylseleno-2,5-dimethoxyphenethylamine
2C-T	4-Methylthio-2,5-dimethoxyphenethylamine
2C-T-2	4-Ethylthio-2,5-dimethoxy-β-phenethylamine

to create significant alterations in neurochemical actions.[91] Frequently, the fourth carbon position on the benzene ring is substituted to create a different compound (see **Table 3**). Furthermore, by making alterations to the substituents at the second, third, fifth, and sixth positions of the aromatic ring, even more compounds can be created (eg, Fly compounds). Most of the 2C drugs show affinity for serotonin receptors, in particular 5-hydroxytryptamine 2 receptors with variable action at receptor subtypes.[134] In addition, 2C-B has α_1-adrenergic receptor agonistic properties.[134,135] Some 2C drugs inhibit reuptake of dopamine, serotonin, and norepinephrine.[99]

Metabolism of 2C drugs occurs via O-demethylation with oxidative deamination to a corresponding acid or reduction to a corresponding alcohol.[134,136–138] Deamination mainly occurs via monoamine oxidase (MAO). As an important consequence of this metabolism, 2C drugs may create drug interactions with MAO inhibitors.[138] 2C drugs tend to have a higher affinity for MAO-A than for MAO-B.[138] Hepatic cytochrome P450 enzymes, in particular 2D6, also play a role in metabolism.[136]

Clinical Effects

Phenethylamines create a clinical picture of both stimulatory and hallucinogenic effects.[91,126] Signs and symptoms observed may include hallucinations, nausea, vomiting, dizziness, diarrhea, headaches, body aches, depression, and confusion.[132] 2C-B use resulted in a case of diffuse cerebral vasculopathy likely from vasospasm.[139] 2C-I ingestion led to reported recurrent seizures and serotonin syndrome with hyperthermia.[140] A case series of 10 patients using 2C-E displayed sympathomimetic and neurologic symptoms with tachycardia, hypertension, euphoria, agitation, psychosis, and hallucinations. Other effects seen with serotonergic and sympathomimetic toxicity can also be observed. One patient experienced fatal cardiac arrest one hour after snorting 2C-E.[133] 2C-E was reported as "undoubtedly responsible" for the death of a 19-year-old man in 2011.[66] Other various 2C compounds have resulted in deaths.[91,126] There is little to no literature on the long-term effects of 2C use.[126]

Testing and Imaging

No specific testing or imaging is recommended or indicated for phenethylamine ingestion. Laboratory testing and imaging should be directed toward clinical observations and symptoms as needed. 2C phenethylamines are not detected with standard commercial immunoassays.[141] GC/MS or LC-MS/MS can be used to confirm the substance or exposure.[137,141]

Treatment

No specific antidote exists for 2C phenethylamine drugs.[126] Treatment consists of symptom-based goal-directed supportive care with patient education and abstinence from further use. Specific treatment options are discussed in greater detail in the section on management principles.

Summary

2C phenethylamines share the structure of catecholamines, amphetamines, synthetic cathinones, The may be purposefully used or unintentionally encountered as MDMA substitutes. Some 2C drugs show affinity for serotonin receptors, which may impart additional properties in addition to sympathomimetic effects. Specific antidotes are lacking and treatment is primarily supportive.

PIPERAZINES

Piperazine recreational drugs are fully synthetic substances; they do not have natural counterparts. They were initially developed as antihelminthic drugs but later studied as antidepressants.[141] Two main groups of piperazines are used recreationally: benzylpiperazines and phenylpiperazines.[91] Commonly used substances in this class of recreational drugs include 1-benzylpiperazine (BZP), 1-methyl-4-benzylpiperazine, 1-(3-trifluoromethylphenyl)piperazine (TFMPP), 1-(3-chlorophenyl)piperazine, and 1-(2-methoxy-phenyl)piperazine.[30] Piperazines may be found as constituents or substitutes in pills sold as ecstasy or amphetamine.[91,142] Piperazines can be sold in pill or powder form. They may also be obtained as mixtures of piperazine (such as BZP/TFMPP) or in combination with other drugs of abuse.[142] A UK survey demonstrated that piperazines are some of the most common active substances found in drugs purchased on the Internet.[143] Typical users are young males.[144,145]

BZPs enhance neurotransmitter release and reuptake inhibition of dopamine, serotonin, and norepinephrine. In contrast, phenylpiperazines (eg, TFMPP) act directly at serotonin receptors, at serotonin reuptake transporters, and at the serotonin transporter to enhance release of serotonin, but have variable to little effects on dopamine or norepinephrine.[99,146,147] BZP doses typically range from 50 to 250 mg, with effects lasting 6 to 8 hours.[30,141] Dosing, time to onset of symptoms, and duration of effect are variable among piperazines. BZP is not extensively metabolized and is typically excreted unchanged, but may undergo hydroxylation via CYP450 enzymes with methylation by catechol-O-methyltransferase and glucuronidation or sulfation.[148] By comparison, TFMPP undergoes extensive hepatic metabolism and is mainly excreted as metabolites. It primarily undergoes hydroxylation, particularly by CYP 2D6 but also 1A2 and 3A4, followed by glucuronidation or sulfation, and partial N-acetylation.[148]

BZP produces psychomotor stimulant effects in humans similar to dexamphetamine.[149] The combination of BZP/TFMPP mimics the actions of MDMA.[150] Overall, most symptoms with piperazine use resemble a sympathomimetic toxidrome.[141,151] Toxicity is difficult to predict on an individual basis despite taking recommended doses.[141] Commonly experienced symptoms include insomnia, anxiety, headaches, nausea, tremors, shakiness, diaphoresis, dizziness, palpitations, shortness of breath, confusion, hallucinations, and paranoia.[145,148,152] Other potential serious effects include seizures, QT interval prolongation, and hyponatremia.[145,153] Because of the serotonergic effects of piperazines, serotonin syndrome is a risk, especially if combined with other serotonergic agents.[141,151] Additional life-threatening complications of BZP use include status epilepticus, hyperthermia, disseminated intravascular coagulation, rhabdomyolysis, and renal failure.[141,148,151] BZP fatalities have been reported and piperazines have been detected in postmortem samples.[154,155] The long-term effects of piperazine are unknown.[141]

No commercial immunoassays are presently available for piperazine detection, but piperazine use may result in a false-positive test for amphetamines.[148,151] Routine qualitative urinary drug screens may be negative. Confirmation of exposure to piperazines can be done via GC-MS, LC-MS, or thin-layer chromatography (TLC).[141,148,151] These testing methods are time consuming and rarely available to aide in the acute management of patients.

No specific antidote exists for piperazine drugs and treatment consists of symptom-based goal-directed supportive care. There is no information on methods for enhancing elimination of piperazines.[141] Specific treatment options are discussed in greater detail in the section on management principles.

KRATOM

Originating from a tree in southeast Asian (*Mitragyna speciosa* Korth), kratom was traditionally used as early as the late 1800s by manual laborers from Thailand and Malaysia for the purposes of euphoria, stimulation, analgesia, and opium withdrawal.[156] Other beneficial effects of kratom include antipyretic, antihypertensive, antiinflammatory, antidiarrheal, hypoglycemic, procirculatory, and sexual prowess properties.[30] Currently, kratom is readily available for purchase on the Internet and has notoriously gained popularity in its use and abuse.[157]

Kratom is most commonly used for the hallucinogenic effects, but may also be used less commonly for management of opioid withdrawal. Mitragynine is merely 1 of more than 2 dozen alkaloids within the plant, and is believed to be the 1 responsible for the opioidlike effects encountered when higher doses are taken.[158] Lower dosing regimens primarily result in a stimulant effect, but these cocainelike effects are not well described. The drug is frequently smoked or ingested after being brewed into a tea. Like its pharmacologic profile, the time of onset and duration of effect (5 minutes and 1 hour, respectively) are dose dependent. These dual properties would lead to inclusion of kratom within a differential diagnosis for several presentations (eg, sympathomimetic, opioid, opioid withdrawal); however, most writings focus on its use for opioid withdrawal. Thus, the most likely patient in the ED will present with either opioid effects or withdrawal. Because this agent is used for opioid withdrawal, and mitragynine has been described to have a potency greater than 10 times that of morphine, kratom withdrawal is also a possibility. Not only can this be a finding in patients who use kratom for opioid withdrawal relief but also has been reported in patients who use kratom for chronic pain syndromes.[159] Kratom withdrawal is indistinguishable from opioid withdrawal and may exhibit identical symptomatology (yawning, rhinorrhea, diarrhea, and irritability).

Generalized tonic-clonic seizurelike activity has also been reported from kratom use.[160] A report describes a 64-year-old man with chronic abdominal pain using kratom in the form of a tea. He seized 30 minutes after ingestion and required mechanical ventilation. Mitragynine was subsequently detected in his urine. Overall, seizures seem exceedingly rare, and other causes such as cerebral hypoxia might have accounted for his condition.[160] One particular form of kratom, named Krypton, may be associated with more severe toxicity and resulting morbidity or mortality. A Swedish case series detailed 9 fatalities in a 1-year period.[161] It was speculated that O-desmethyltramadol (an active tramadol metabolite) was intentionally added for greater opioid potency. The combination effect of adding a pharmaceutical to a herb blend for superior potency is of great concern. Herbal regulations differ significantly from pharmaceuticals, and a dose of an active ingredient is rarely standardized.

Care for patients presenting after kratom use is primarily supportive. Attention to airway control is vital in any patient with mental status or respiratory depression. Reports of naloxone reversing kratomlike opioid effects are absent from the literature. However, standard therapy should be implemented for withdrawal symptoms. In the rare event of seizures, benzodiazepines are the first-line therapy.

SALVIA

Although there are hundreds of species of salvia, *Salvia divinorum* is the most relevant to EPs and is the specific species reviewed. A member of the mint family, salvia is native to Mexico and has historically been used during religious ceremonies.[162] The hallucinogenic properties after smoking, ingesting a tea, or chewing the plant leaves are attributed to salvinorin A. Slang terms used for salvia include magic mint, mystic sage, and Sally D. Head shops or the Internet are a source of prepackaged crushed leaves.

The hallucinogenic properties of salvia differs from many other hallucinogens. Classically, serotonin receptor agonism is the common pharmacologic mechanism producing hallucinations. This includes lysergic acid diethylamide (LSD) and magic mushrooms (psilocybin). Salvia, however, stimulates kappa opioid receptors and is noted to result in perceptual distortions, pseudohallucinations, and an altered sense of self and environment.[163] Chewing and allowing buccal absorption will result in these effects. Oral ingestion, however, will not permit them due of first-pass metabolism or enzymatic degradation of salvia by multiple cytochrome oxidases (eg, CYP 2D6, 2E1).[164]

Classically, salvia is smoked with deep inhalation with valsalva, similar to smoking marijuana.[163] The effects are rapid in onset (30 seconds to 10 minutes depending on exposure route) and quickly dissipate within 30 minutes.[162,163] This brief and intense experience seems to be exaggerated in younger adults and adolescents, and many report visual distortions of body image, out of body experiences, and hearing colors.[162] Most people who use salvia do not seek treatment at a health care facility. One retrospective poison center study documented 37 intentional exposures to salvia over a 10-year period in California.[165] Among these cases, vital sign abnormalities were present in only 2 patients (hypertension and tachycardia in one and isolated tachycardia in the other). Approximately 50% of cases managed included isolated salvia exposure. The most common symptoms recognized among this group included confusion, disorientation, hallucinations, giddiness or dizziness, and a flushed sensation. Benzodiazepine administration was the most common therapeutic intervention.[165] Another case reported from southern California described a 21-year-old man who had no previous medical history or use of psychoactive medications who presented for acute psychosis and paranoia shortly after smoking salvia.[166] He experienced echolalia, paranoia, flight of ideas, and psychomotor agitation for two full days, and then experienced relapsing negative effects after being weaned from risperidone. This may demonstrate salvia's ability to unmask, precipitate, and exacerbate psychiatric disease in vulnerable users. EPs can be expected to offer supportive measures for those who do present after intoxication and provide appropriate follow-up (ie, addiction and psychiatric services) that may ultimately benefit the patient.

MUSHROOMS

Magic shrooms refer to the class of mushrooms that contain the hallucinogenic chemical psilocybin, which is subsequently metabolized to psilocin. Because these compounds resemble serotonin, the subsequent clinical effects are similar to LSD. In most cases, these mushrooms are ingested and result in hallucinations, illusions, and ataxia within one hour.[167] One case reports a rare alleged intravenous injection of fresh psilocybe juice in a 30-year-old man who was at a party. He subsequently experienced vomiting, myalgias, tachycardia, and hyperpyrexia.[168] EPs manage only a small number of cases of hallucinogenic mushroom use. Those who do present are likely manifesting severe nausea, vomiting, diaphoresis, tachycardia, hyperthermia, and rarely seizures.[169]

Classically, patients presenting to the ED might be from a concert setting where ingested mushrooms leads to a bad trip. Another source could be from a college setting, where recreational use is common. According to one survey of nearly 900 undergraduates from a liberal arts college in upstate New York, college students frequently experimented with hallucinogenic mushrooms.[170] Although less than half responded to the survey, the main factor influencing the decision to try hallucinogenic mushrooms for the first time was curiosity, and users were more likely to have used other drugs (marijuana, cocaine, ecstasy, opiates, nonprescribed prescription drugs, and other hallucinogens).[170]

The goals of management in the clinical setting are like other hallucinogens. Rigorous supportive care, benzodiazepines, and a safe, quiet environment to protect the patient from behavioral toxicity (eg, inappropriately acting on hallucinations) are likely all that is required. Patients with seizures, vital sign abnormalities, or evidence of ongoing psychosis warrant further workup and observation.

HAWAIIAN BABY WOODROSE (*ARGYREIA NERVOSA*)

Lysergamide (LSA) originating in plants may be abused as a hallucinogen, as it is chemically similar to synthetic lysergamide or LSD. Woodrose (*Argyreia nervosa*) chemically differs from morning glory (*Ipomoea violacea*) in that it is contains a higher percentage of ergoline constituents.[171] The seeds from the woodrose are eaten or consumed from an extract after being soaked in water. A commonly ingested dose is five to 10 seeds, which may yield a dose of 2 to 5 mg of LSA, sufficient to result in hallucinations for a duration of four to six hours.[171] Head shops and Internet distribution account for the largest available market of seeds throughout Europe and the United States.[172]

Characteristic symptoms after use are typical of other hallucinogens, however, the effects may be differentiated from the anticipated LSDlike experience. Although increased insight and positive emotional states (eg, euphoria, happiness, delight, altered perceptions of colors and textures, mood elevations) may occur after exposure; tachycardia, hypertension, nausea, vertigo, mydriasis, anxiety, sedation, and a sense of derealization can be considered negative effects.[171,173,174] In recreational users, feelings of loneliness, depression, and suicidal thoughts have also been reported.[174] One case describes a 29-year-old man who ingested an unknown number of seeds after soaking them in water for 2.5 to three hours and then proceeded to become severely agitated and defenestrate a fourth floor window.[171] This patient reportedly had smoked cannabis with another man who witnessed the traumatic death. It is unclear from the report to what extent the ingestion of woodrose seeds contributed to the suicide.

Treatment of intoxication in the emergency setting consists of addressing abnormal vital signs, sedation for anxiety or deliriousness with benzodiazepines, protection, and potentially merely sensory isolation for mild poisoning. Obtaining a psychiatric history and assessing suicidal risk may also be important in the chronic recreational abuser, and may alter ultimate disposition.

MANAGEMENT PRINCIPLES

Many patients presenting under the influence of a drug or substance abused for recreational purposes have an altered sensorium and are unable to provide a robust history surrounding the ingestion. Ideally, knowing the time, route, and intent of use assists in ultimate disposition. For instance, a delayed presentation with ongoing delirium may warrant a computed tomography scan of the brain to rule out another cause of continuing symptomatology. Understanding the route of ingestion is potentially helpful in determining likely symptom duration. In addition, recognizing the patient's intent (ie, recreational vs suicidal) is vital for the purposes of specialty consultation with psychiatry and/or admission or transfer for mental health care.

Much like treating many emergency patients, the management of the poisoned patient consists of sound common sense and aggressive supportive care. The standard

A, B, C approach is a common framework to use when managing a poisoned patient (**Table 4**). Airway and breathing management are paramount, and any patient with impaired oxygenation and/or ventilatory drive warrants intubation. Likewise, a common indication for intubation and mechanical ventilation is the absence of protective airway reflexes. Emesis and aspiration can further complicate any obtunded patient's course and can be prevented with anticipatory airway management. Circulatory status can be assessed through evaluation of the patient's vital signs and perfusion status. Intravenous crystalloids are a standard first-line attempt to treat hypotension. Infrequently, this patient population may require pressors to increase perfusion. In addition to pulse and blood pressure, a vital sign of fundamental concern is core temperature. Poisoned patients with a high core temperature are prone to have poor outcomes, including major morbidity (eg, multisystem organ failure) and mortality.[117,175] When managing a toxin-induced hyperthermic patient, excess heat generation coupled with impaired heat dissipation is primarily the cause of the hyperthermia rather than a classic pyrogen-induced fever. Treatment with antipyretics is therefore futile. The goal should be to actively and aggressively cool the patient. Ice immersion, mist and fanning, and pharmacologic interventions such as liberal benzodiazepines are principal approaches. This will likely result in normalization of tachycardia as well.

Benzodiazepines serve many useful functions in the agitated patient. Even with absent complex and poor side effect profile (eg, hypotension, anticholinergic effects, increasing serotonergic tone), benzodiazepines are considered a first-line agent in any delirious, altered, seizing, and/or hyperthermic poisoned patient. The dose can be titrated to produce an effect much like ethanol withdrawal.

Decontamination (D) of this patient population is unlikely to provide much benefit. If presenting in the ED, symptomatology is likely already present. Gastric lavage should not be used routinely in this patient population, and activated charcoal only benefits a patient with a protected airway who presents early after ingestion and before the onset of symptomatology. Enhancing elimination (E), through hemodialysis, sodium bicarbonate infusions, and multiple doses of activated charcoal, of xenobiotics is not routinely used in these patients. Hemodialysis, however, should still be considered for severe acid-base or electrolyte disturbances.

The F in the poisoned patient algorithm, refers to focused therapy. Beyond the use of benzodiazepines, as discussed previously, no specific antidotal treatment is likely to benefit most patients within this particular patient group.

Specific diagnostic tests that are likely beneficial include an ECG, specifically taking note of rhythm and interval abnormalities. Sodium bicarbonate boluses for QRS widening (like a tricyclic antidepressant overdose), electrolyte evaluation (potassium,

Table 4 Poisoned patient algorithm	
A	Airway
B	Breathing
C	Circulation
D	Decontamination
E	Enhanced elimination
F	Focused therapy (antidotal therapy)
G, H	Get help (consult regional poison center)

calcium, and magnesium concentrations), and correction for patients with a prolonged QTc is reasonable. Acid-base status, urine pregnancy testing, and renal function testing linked to creatinine phosphokinase are important as well. Aggressive hydration is warranted for any patient demonstrating rhabdomyolysis to prevent kidney injury. In addition to intubated patients, those with abnormal vital signs, renal insufficiency, altered mental status, concerning ECG changes, and hemodynamic instability warrant intensive care disposition. Obtaining a concentration of the specific drug ingested is not helpful. Most assays must be sent out and will not guide treatment in real time. Although obtaining the forensic data may help to explain why a patient presented and the corresponding reasons for their pathophysiology, even timely results are unlikely to change the EPs evaluation, management, and/or disposition of such patients. Likewise, a qualitative urine toxicology screen will not be an adequate diagnostic test to rule in or out the agents discussed within this review.

Getting help (G, H) is useful when dealing with patients with exposure to emerging drugs of abuse. Seeking regional poison center assistance (1-800-222–1222 in the United States), discussion with affiliated staff toxicologists, and/or speaking to experts regarding the patient's presentation and treatment schemata are important steps to promote positive patient outcomes. Speaking to an expert in poisoning and overdose helps to direct care and focus on essentials. In addition to providing treatment advice, poison centers provide an essential public health function through surveillance. Some centers are active at legislative levels to help assist law enforcement with emerging trends.[84] Interfacing with other public health agencies and disseminating health alerts and educational materials to facilities when these newer agents are identified is a core public health function of poison centers.

SUMMARY

Drugs of abuse are ever changing and EPs are at the forefront of recognition of these substances. In the Internet age, substances from around the world are available for individuals to use recreationally. Some of these drugs include SCs, synthetic cathinones, phenethylamines, piperazines, herbal products, prescription drugs, and many other substances. These substances also go by a multitude of common street names. Many of the current emerging drugs of abuse result in psychoactive and sympathomimetic effects with excited delirium. Benzodiazepines remain an effective tool to assist in controlling delirium and combating sympathomimetic excess. Regardless of the drug ingested, the mainstay of management includes symptom-based goal-directed supportive care.

REFERENCES

1. Chary M, Genes N, McKenzie A, et al. Leveraging social networks for toxicovigilance. J Med Toxicol 2013;9:184–91.
2. Deluca P, Davey Z, Corazza O, et al. Identifying emerging trends in recreational drug use; outcomes from the Psychonaut Web Mapping Project. Prog Neuropsychopharmacol Biol Psychiatry 2012;39:221–6.
3. Gibbons S. "Legal highs" – novel and emerging psychoactive drugs: a chemical overview for the toxicologist. Clin Toxicol 2012;50:15–24.
4. Sutter ME, Chenoweth J, Albertson TE. Alternative drugs of abuse. Clin Rev Allergy Immunol 2013. http://dx.doi.org/10.1007/s12016-013-8370-2.
5. Aleksander I. Molly: pure but not so simple. 2013. Available at: http://www.nytimes.com/2013/06/23/fashion/molly-pure-but-not-so-simple.html?pagewanted=1&_r=1&hpw&. Accessed June 24, 2013.

6. Okie S. The flood of opioids: a rising tide of deaths. N Engl J Med 2010;363: 1981–5.
7. Ibanez GE, Levi-Minzi MA, Rigg KK, et al. Diversion of benzodiazepines through healthcare sources. J Psychoactive Drugs 2013;45:48–56.
8. Nelson A, Galon P. Exploring the relationship among ADHD, stimulants, and substance abuse. J Child Adolesc Psychiatr Nurs 2012;25:113–8.
9. Paulozzi LJ, Kilbourn EM, Desai HA. Prescription drug monitoring programs and death rates from drug overdose. Pain Med 2011;12:747–54.
10. Manchikanti L. National drug control policy and prescription drug abuse: facts and fallacies. Pain Physician 2007;10:399–424.
11. Pomeranz JL, Taylor LM, Austin SB. Over-the-counter and out-of-control: legal strategies to protect youths from abusing products for weight control. Am J Public Health 2013;103:220–5.
12. Brennan BP, Kanayama G, Pope HG. Performance-enhancing drugs on the web: a growing public-health issue. Am J Addict 2013;22:158–61.
13. Thevis M, Kuuranne T, Geyer H, et al. Annual banned-substance review: analytical approaches in human sports drug testing. Drug Test Anal 2013; 5:1–19.
14. Nelson ME, Bryant SM, Aks SE. Melanotan II injection resulting in systemic toxicity and rhabdomyolysis. Clin Toxicol 2012;50:1165–8.
15. Ward J, Rhyee S, Plansky J, et al. Methoxetamine: a novel ketamine analog and growing health-care concern. Clin Toxicol 2011;49:874–5.
16. Booth RE. Krokodil and other home-produced drugs for injection: a perspective from Ukraine. Int J Drug Policy 2013;24:277–8.
17. Wolk BJ, Ganetsky M, Babu KM. Toxicity of energy drinks. Curr Opin Pediatr 2012;24:243–51.
18. Adams IB, Martin BR. Cannabis: pharmacology and toxicology in animals and humans. Addiction 1996;91:1586–614.
19. Gunderson EW, Haughey HM, Ait-Daoud N, et al. "Spice" and "K2" herbal highs: a case series and systematic review of the clinical effects and biopsychosocial implications of synthetic cannabinoid use in humans. Am J Addict 2012;21: 320–6.
20. Seely KA, Lapoint J, Moran JH, et al. Spice drugs are more than harmless herbal blends: a review of the pharmacology and toxicology of synthetic cannabinoids. Prog Neuropsychopharmacol Biol Psychiatry 2012;39:234–43.
21. Seely KA, Prather PL, James LP, et al. Marijuana-based drugs: innovative therapeutics or designer drugs of abuse. Mol Interv 2011;11:36–51.
22. Auwärter V, Dresen S, Weinmann W, et al. Spice and other herbal blends: harmless incense or cannabinoid designer drugs? J Mass Spectrom 2009;44:832–7.
23. European Monitoring Centre for Drugs and Drug Addiction (EMCDDA). EMCDDA 2009 thematic paper – understanding the 'Spice' phenomenon. Luxembourg: Office for Official Publications of the European Communities; 2009.
24. Vardakou I, Pistos C, Spiliopoulou CH. Spice drugs as a new trend: mode of action, identification and legislation. Toxicol Lett 2010;197:157–62.
25. European Monitoring Centre for Drugs and Drug Addiction (EMCDDA). Synthetic cannabinoids and 'Spice.' Available at: http://www.emcdda.europa.eu/publications/drug-profiles/synthetic-cannabinoids. Accessed September 2, 2013.
26. Einhorn L, Nagy C, Furnas B, et al. Nabilone: an effective antiemetic in patients receiving cancer chemotherapy. J Clin Pharmacol 1981;21:64S–9S.

27. United States Adopted Names Council: Statement on a nonprioprietary name. Available at: http://www.ama-assn.org/ama1/pub/upload/mm/365/nabiximols. pdf. Accessed June 4, 2013.
28. Weissman A, Milne GM, Melvin LS Jr. Cannabimimetic activity from CP-47,497, a derivative of 3-phenylcyclohexanol. J Pharmacol Exp Ther 1982;223:516–23.
29. Bell MR, D'Ambra TE, Kumar V, et al. Antinociceptive (aminoalkyl)indoles. J Med Chem 1991;34:1099–110.
30. Rosenbaum CD, Carreiro SP, Babu KM. Here today, gone tomorrow... and back again? A review of herbal marijuana alternatives (K2, Spice), synthetic cathinones (bath salts), Kratom, Salvia divinorum, methoxetamine, and piperazines. J Med Toxicol 2012;8:15–32.
31. Huffman JW, Dai D. Design, synthesis and pharmacology of cannabimimetic indoles. Bioorg Med Chem Lett 1994;4:563–6.
32. Huffman JW, Yu S, Showalter V, et al. Synthesis and pharmacology of a very potent cannabinoid lacking a phenolic hydroxyl with high affinity for the CB2 receptor. J Med Chem 1996;39:3875–7.
33. Wiley JL, Comptom DR, Dai D, et al. Structure-activity relationships of indole- and pyrrole-derived cannabinoids. J Pharmacol Exp Ther 1998;285: 995–1004.
34. Huffman JW. Cannabimimetic indoles, pyrroles, and indenes: structure-activity relationships and receptor interactions. In: Reggio PH, editor. The cannabinoid receptors, 1. New York: Humana Press; 2009. p. 49–94.
35. Atwood BK, Huffman J, Straiker A, et al. JWH018, a common constituent of 'Spice' herbal blends, is a potent and efficacious cannabinoid CB_1 receptor agonist. Br J Pharmacol 2010;160:585–93.
36. Lapoint J, James LP, Moran CL, et al. Severe toxicity following synthetic cannabinoid ingestion. Clin Toxicol 2011;49:760–4.
37. Wood KE. Exposure to bath salts and synthetic tetrahydrocannabinol from 2009 to 2012 in the United States. J Pediatr 2013;163:213–6.
38. Schedules of controlled substances: temporary placement of five synthetic cannabinoids into schedule I [FR Doc No: 11075–11078]. Drug Enforcement Administration (DEA). Available at: http://www.deadiversion.usdoj.gov/fed_regs/rules/ 2011/fr0301.htm. Accessed June 5, 2013.
39. Moran CL, Le VH, Chimalakonda KC, et al. Quantitative measurement of JWH-018 and JWH-073 metabolites excreted in human urine. Anal Chem 2011;83: 4228–36.
40. Johnston LD, O'Malley PM, Bachman JG, et al. Monitoring the future national results on drug use: 2012 overview, key findings on adolescent drug use. Ann Arbor (MI): Institute for Social Research, The University of Michigan; 2013. Available at: http://www.monitoringthefuture.org/pubs/monographs/mtf-overview2012.pdf. Accessed June 6, 2013.
41. Heltsley R, Shelby MK, Crouch DJ, et al. Prevalence of synthetic cannabinoids in U.S. athletes: initial findings. J Anal Toxicol 2012;36:588–93.
42. Hoyte CO, Jacob J, Monte AA, et al. A characterization of synthetic cannabinoid exposures reported to the national poison data system in 2010. Ann Emerg Med 2012;60:435–8.
43. Forrester MB, Kleinschmidt K, Schwarz E, et al. Synthetic cannabinoid and marijuana exposures reported to poison centers. Hum Exp Toxicol 2012;31:1006–11.
44. Winstock AR, Barratt MJ. Synthetic cannabis: a comparison of patterns of use and effect profile with natural cannabis in a large global sample. Drug Alcohol Depend 2013;131:106–11.

45. Lank PM, Pines E, Mycyk MB. Emergency physicians' knowledge of cannabinoid designer drugs. West J Emerg Med 2013;14(5):1–4. Available at: http://www.escholarship.org/uc/item/9mk2951f. Accessed September 2, 2013.

46. Ameri A. The effects of cannabinoids on the brain. Prog Neurobiol 1999;58: 315–48.

47. Pertwee RG. Receptors and channels targeted by synthetic cannabinoid receptor agonists and antagonists. Curr Med Chem 2010;17:1360–81.

48. Gronewold A, Skopp G. A preliminary investigation on the distribution of cannabinoids in man. Forensic Sci Int 2011;210:e7–11.

49. Shim JY, Welsh WJ, Howlett AC. Homology model of the CB1 cannabinoid receptor: sites critical for nonclassical cannabinoid agonist interaction. Biopolymers 2003;71:169–89.

50. Teske J, Weller JP, Fieguth A, et al. Sensitive and rapid quantification of the cannabinoid receptor agonist naphthalen-1-yl-(1-pentylindol-3-yl) methanone (JWH-018) in human serum by liquid chromatography-tandem mass spectrometry. J Chromatogr B Analyt Technol Biomed Life Sci 2010; 878:2659–63.

51. Brents LK, Reichard EE, Zimmerman SM, et al. Phase I hydroxylated metabolites of the K2 synthetic cannabinoid JWH-018 retain in vitro and in vivo cannabinoid 1 receptor affinity and activity. PLoS One 2011;6:e21917.

52. Rajasekaran M, Brents LK, Franks LN, et al. Human metabolites of synthetic cannabinoids JWH-018 and JWH-073 bind with high affinity and act as potent agonists at cannabinoid type-2 receptors. Toxicol Appl Pharmacol 2013;269: 100–8.

53. Castellanos D, Singh S, Thornton G, et al. Synthetic cannabinoid use: a case series of adolescents. J Adolesc Health 2011;49:347–9.

54. Hurst D, Loeffler G, McLay R. Psychosis associated with synthetic cannabinoid agonists: a case series. Am J Psychiatry 2011;168:1119.

55. Müller H, Sperling W, Köhrmann M, et al. The synthetic cannabinoid Spice as a trigger for an acute exacerbation of cannabis induced recurrent psychotic episodes. Schizophr Res 2010;118:309–10.

56. Every-Palmer S. Synthetic cannabinoid JWH-018 and psychosis: an explorative study. Drug Alcohol Depend 2011;117:152–7.

57. Schneir AB, Cullen J, Ly BT. "Spice" girls: synthetic cannabinoid intoxication. J Emerg Med 2011;40:296–9.

58. Schneir AB, Baumbacher T. Convulsions associated with the use of a synthetic cannabinoid product. J Med Toxicol 2012;8:62–4.

59. Tofighi B, Lee JD. Internet highs – seizures after consumption of synthetic cannabinoids purchased online. J Addict Med 2012;6:240–1.

60. Pant S, Deshmukh A, Dholaria B, et al. Spicy seizure. Am J Med Sci 2012;344: 67–8.

61. Mir A, Obafemi A, Young A, et al. Myocardial infarction associated with use of the synthetic cannabinoid K2. Pediatrics 2011;128(6):e1622–7.

62. Simmons JR, Skinner CG, Williams J, et al. Intoxication from smoking "Spice". Ann Emerg Med 2011;57(2):187–8.

63. Centers for Disease Control and Prevention (CDC). Acute kidney injury associated with synthetic cannabinoid use – multiple states 2012. MMWR Morb Mortal Wkly Rep 2012;62:93–8.

64. Alhadi S, Tiwari A, Vohra R, et al. High times, low sats: diffuse pulmonary infiltrates associated with chronic synthetic cannabinoid use. J Med Toxicol 2013; 9:199–206.

65. Fattore L, Fratta W. Beyond THC: the new generation of cannabinoid designer drugs. Front Behav Neurosci 2011;5:1–12.
66. Bronstein AC, Spyker DA, Cantilena LR, et al. 2011 annual report of the American Association of Poison Control Centers' National Poison Data System (NPDS): 29th annual report. Clin Toxicol 2012;50:911–1164.
67. Meier MH, Caspi A, Ambler A, et al. Persistent cannabis users show neuropsychological decline from childhood to midlife. Proc Natl Acad Sci U S A 2012; 109:E2657–64.
68. Duffy A, Milin R. Case study: withdrawal syndrome in adolescent chronic cannabis users. J Am Acad Child Adolesc Psychiatry 1996;35:1618–21.
69. Haney M. The marijuana withdrawal syndrome: diagnosis and treatment. Curr Psychiatry Rep 2005;7:360–6.
70. Nacca N, Vatti D, Sullivan R, et al. The synthetic cannabinoid withdrawal syndrome. J Addict Med 2013;7:296–8.
71. Zimmermann US, Winkelmann PR, Philhatsch M, et al. Withdrawal phenomena and dependence syndrome after the consumption of "Spice Gold". Dtsch Arztebl Int 2009;106:464–7.
72. National Medical Services (NMS) labs. NMS Labs Online Test Catalog. 2013. Available at: http://www.nmslabs.com/test-catalog/synthetic%20cannabinoids@0. Accessed June 10, 2013.
73. World Health Organization Expert Committee on Drug Dependence. Assessment of khat (*Catha edulis* Forsk). 34th ECDD. Geneva (Switzerland): WHO Expert Committee on Drug Dependence; 2006. Available at: http://www.who.int/medicines/areas/quality_safety/4.4KhatCritReview.pdf. Accessed June 11, 2013.
74. Prosser JM, Nelson LS. The toxicology of bath salts: a review of synthetic cathinones. J Med Toxicol 2012;8:33–42.
75. Brenneisen R, Fisch HU, Koelbing U, et al. Amphetamine-like effects in humans of the khat alkaloid cathinone. Br J Clin Pharmacol 1990;30:825–8.
76. Ali WM, Zubaid M, Al-Motarreb A, et al. Association of khat chewing with increased risk of stroke and death in patients presents with acute coronary syndrome. Mayo Clin Proc 2010;85:974–80.
77. Hyde JF, Browning E, Adams R. Synthetic homologs of D,L-ephedrine. J Am Chem Soc 1928;50:2287–92.
78. Emerson TS, Cisek JE. Methcathinone: a Russian designer amphetamine infiltrates the rural Midwest. Ann Emerg Med 1993;22:1897–903.
79. Mehta MB. United States patent 3,819,706: Meta-chloro substituted α-butylaminopropiophenones. United States Patent and Trademark Office (USPTO). 1974. Available at: http://patimg1.uspto.gov/.piw?Docid=03819706&homeurl=http%3A%2F%2Fpatft.uspto.gov%2Fnetacgi%2Fnph-Parser%3FSect1%3DPTO1%2526Sect2%3DHITOFF%2526d%3DPALL%2526p%3D1%2526u%3D%25252Fnetahtml%25252FPTO%25252Fsrchnum.htm%2526r%3D1%2526f%3DG%2526l%3D50%2526s1%3D3819706.PN.%2526OS%3DPN%2F3819706%2526RS%3DPN%2F3819706&PageNum=&Rtype=&SectionNum=&idkey=NONE&Input=View+first+page. Accessed June 13, 2013.
80. United States Drug Enforcement Administration. Methcathinone. 2013. Available at: http://www.justice.gov/dea_old/concern/methcathinone.html. Accessed June 13, 2013.
81. Psychonaut Web Mapping Research Group. Mephedrone. London: Institute of Psychiatry, King's College London; 2009. Available at: http://www.psychonautproject.eu/newsletters/n2.php. Accessed June 13, 2013.

82. Dargan PI, Albert S, Wood DM. Mephedrone use and associated adverse effects in school and college/university students before the UK legislation change. QJM 2010;103:875–9.

83. Winstock AR, Mitcheson LR, Deluca P, et al. Mephedrone, new kid for the chop? Addiction 2010;106:154–61.

84. Warrick BJ, Hill M, Hekman K, et al. A 9-state analysis of designer stimulant, "bath salt, " hospital visits reported to poison control centers. Ann Emerg Med 2013;62:244–51.

85. American Association of Poison Control Centers. Bath salts data. 2013. Available at: https://aapcc.s3.amazonaws.com/files/library/Bath_Salts_Data_for_Website_5.31.2013.pdf. Accessed June 14, 2013.

86. American Association of Poison Control Centers. Synthetic marijuana data. 2013. Available at: https://aapcc.s3.amazonaws.com/files/library/Synthetic_Marijuana_Data_for_Website_5.31.2013.pdf. Accessed June 14, 2013.

87. Winstock A, Mitcheson L, Marsden J. Mephedrone: still available and twice the price. Lancet 2010;376:1537.

88. Gibbons S, Zloh M. An analysis of the 'legal high' mephedrone. Bioorg Med Chem Lett 2010;20:4135–9.

89. US Department of Justice DEA. Notice of intent – scheduled of controlled substances: temporary placement of three synthetic cathinones into schedule I. Microgram Bulletin 2011;44:57–65.

90. 112th Congress. S. 3190: Synthetic Drug Abuse Prevention Act of 2012. Sec 2. Addition of Synthetic Drugs to Schedule I of the Controlled Substances Act. Washington, DC: Library of Congress [May 16, 2012]. Available at: http://www.govtrack.us/congress/bills/112/s3190/text. Accessed July 2, 2013.

91. Hill SL, Thomas SH. Clinical toxicology of newer recreational drugs. Clin Toxicol 2011;49:705–19.

92. Marinetti LJ, Antonides HM. Analysis of synthetic cathinones commonly found in bath salts in human performance and postmortem toxicology: method development, drug distribution and interpretation of results. J Anal Toxicol 2013;37:135–46.

93. James D, Adams RD, Spears R, et al. Clinical characteristics of mephedrone toxicity reported to the UK National Poisons Information Service. Emerg Med J 2011;28:686–9.

94. Schifano F, Albanese A, Fergus S, et al. Mephedrone (4-methylmethcathinone; 'meow-meow'): chemical, pharmacological and clinical issues. Psychopharmacology 2011;214:593–602.

95. Wood DM, Davies S, Greene SL, et al. Case series of individuals with analytically confirmed acute mephedrone toxicity. Clin Toxicol 2010;48:924–7.

96. Coppola M, Mondola R. Synthetic cathinones: chemistry, pharmacology, and toxicology of a new class of designer drugs of abuse marketed as "bath salts" or "plant food". Toxicol Lett 2012;211:144–9.

97. Cameron K, Kolanos R, Vekariya R, et al. Mephedrone and methylenedioxypyrovalerone (MDPV), major constituents of "bath salts, " produce opposite effects at the human dopamine transporter. Psychopharmacology 2013;227:493–9.

98. Cozzi NV, Sievert MK, Shulgin AT, et al. Inhibition of plasma membrane monoamine transporters by β-ketoamphetamines. Eur J Pharmacol 1999;381:63–9.

99. Nagai F, Nonaka R, Satoh Hasashi Kamimura K. The effects of non-medically used psychoactive drugs on monoamine neurotransmission in rat brain. Eur J Pharmacol 2007;559:132–7.

100. Meyer MR, Wilhelm J, Peters FT, et al. Beta-ketoamphetamines: studies on the metabolism of the designer drug mephedrone and toxicological detection of mephedrone, butylone, and methylone in urine using gas chromatography-mass spectrometry. Anal Bioanal Chem 2010;397:1225–33.
101. Zaitsu K, Katagi M, Tatsuno M, et al. Recently abused β-keto derivatives of 3,4-methylenedioxyphenylalkylamines: a review of the metabolisms and toxicological analysis. Forensic Toxicol 2011;29:73–84.
102. Meyer MR, Du P, Schuster F, et al. Studies on the metabolism of the α-pyrrolidinophenone designer drug methylenedioxy-pyrovalerone (MDPV) in rat and human urine and human liver microsomes using GC-MS and LC-high resolution MS and its detectability in urine by GC-MS. J Mass Spectrom 2010;45:1426–42.
103. Wood DM, Davies S, Puchnarewicz M, et al. Recreational use of mephedrone (4-methylmethcathinone, 4-MMC) with associated sympathomimetic toxicity. J Med Toxicol 2010;6:327–30.
104. Murphy CM, Dulaney AR, Beuhler MC, et al. "Bath Salts" and "Plant Food" products: the experience of one regional US Poison Center. J Med Toxicol 2013;9:42–8.
105. Nicholson PJ, Quinn MJ, Dodd JD. Headshop heartache: acute mephedone 'meow' myocarditis. Heart 2010;96:2051–2.
106. Wyman JF, Lavins ES, Engelhart D, et al. Postmortem tissue distribution of MDPV following lethal intoxication by "Bath Salts". J Anal Toxicol 2013;37:182–5.
107. Penders TM, Gestring RE, Vilensky DA. Excited delirium following the use of synthetic cathinones (bath salts). Gen Hosp Psychiatry 2012;34:647–50.
108. Thornton SL, Gerona RR, Tomaszewksi CA. Psychosis from a bath salt product containing flephedrone and MDPV with serum, urine, and product quantification. J Med Toxicol 2012;8:310–3.
109. Stoica MV, Felthous AR. Acute psychosis induced by bath salts: a case report with clinical and forensic implications. J Forensic Sci 2013;58:530–3.
110. Murray BL, Murphy CM, Beuhler MC. Death following recreational use of designer drug "Bath Salts" containing 3,4-methylenedioxypyrovalerone (MDPV). J Med Toxicol 2012;8:69–75.
111. Olives TD, Orozco BS, Stellpflug SJ. Bath salts: the ivory wave of trouble. West J Emerg Med 2012;13:58–62.
112. Boulanger-Gobeil C, St-Onge M, Laliberté M, et al. Seizures and hyponatremia related to ethcathinone and methylone poisoning. J Med Toxicol 2012;8:59–61.
113. Winstock A, Mitcheson L, Ramsey J, et al. Mephedrone: use, subjective effects and health risk. Addiction 2011;106:1991–6.
114. Warrick BJ, Wilson J, Hedge M, et al. Lethal serotonin syndrome after methylone and butylone ingestion. J Med Toxicol 2012;8:65–8.
115. Levine M, Levitan R, Skolnik A. Compartment syndrome after "Bath Salts" use: a case series. Ann Emerg Med 2012;61:480–3.
116. Borek HA, Holstege CP. Hyperthermia and multiorgan failure after abuse of "Bath Salts" containing 3,4-methylenedioxypyrovalerone. Ann Emerg Med 2012;60:103–5.
117. Rosenberg J, Pentel P, Pond S, et al. Hyperthermia associated with drug intoxication. Crit Care Med 1986;14:964–9.
118. Torrance H, Cooper G. The detection of mephedrone (4-methylmethcathinone) in 4 fatalities in Scotland. Forensic Sci Int 2010;202:e62–3.
119. Carbone PN, Carbone DL, Carstairs SD, et al. Sudden cardiac death associated with methylone use. Am J Forensic Med Pathol 2013;34:26–8.

120. Maskell PD, De Paoli G, Seneviratne C, et al. Mephedrone (4-methylmethcathinone)-related deaths. J Anal Toxicol 2011;35:188–91.

121. Sparago M, Wlos J, Yaun J, et al. Neurotoxic and pharmacologic studies on enantiomers of the N-methylated analog of cathinone (methcathinone): a new drug of abuse. J Pharmacol Exp Ther 1996;279:1043–52.

122. McCann UD, Wong DF, Yokoi F, et al. Reduced striatal dopamine transporter density in the abstinent methamphetamine and methcathinone users: evidence from positron emission tomography studies with [11C]WIN-35,428. J Neurosci 1998;18:8417–22.

123. Petrie M, Lynch KL, Ekins S, et al. Cross-reactivity studies and predictive modeling of "Bath Salts" and other amphetamine-type stimulants with amphetamine screening immunoassays. Clin Toxicol 2013;51:83–91.

124. Swortwood MJ, Boland DM, DeCaprio AP. Determination of 32 cathinone derivatives and other designer drugs in serum by comprehensive LC-QQQ-MS/MS analysis. Anal Bioanal Chem 2013;405:1383–97.

125. National Medical Services (NMS) labs. NMS Labs Online Test Catalog. 2013. Available at: http://www.nmslabs.com/test-catalog/bath%20salts@0. Accessed June 18, 2013.

126. Dean BV, Stellpflug SL, Burnett AM, et al. 2C or Not 2C: phenethylamine designer drug review. J Med Toxicol 2013;9:172–8.

127. Shulgin AT, Shulgin A. PiHKAL - a chemical love story. Berkley (CA): Transform Press; 1991.

128. Benzenhöfer U, Passie T. Rediscovering MDMA (ecstasy): the role of the American chemist Alexander T. Shulgin. Addiction 2010;105:1355–61.

129. Caudevilla-Gálligo F, Riba J, Ventura M, et al. 4-Bromo-2,5-dimethoxyphenethylamine (2C-B): presence in the recreational drug market in Spain, pattern of use and subjective effects. J Psychopharmacol 2012;26:1026–35.

130. de Boer D, Bosman I. A new trend in drugs-of-abuse; the 2C series of phenethylamine designer drugs. Pharm World Sci 2004;26:110–3.

131. Giroud C, Augsburger M, Rivier L, et al. 2C-B: a new psychoactive phenethylamine recently discovered in Ecstasy tablets sold on the Swiss black market. J Anal Toxicol 1998;22:345–54.

132. Sanders B, Lankenau SE, Bloom JJ, et al. "Research Chemicals": tryptamine and phenethylamine use among high-risk youth. Subst Use Misuse 2008;43:389–402.

133. Topeff JM, Ellsworth H, Willhite LA, et al. A case series of symptomatic patients, including one fatality, following 2C-E exposure. Clin Toxicol 2011;49:526.

134. Maurer HH. Chemistry, pharmacology, and metabolism of emerging drugs of abuse. Ther Drug Monit 2010;32:544–9.

135. Saez P, Borges Y, Gonzalez E, et al. Alpha-adrenergic and 5-HT2-serotonergic effects of some beta-phenylethylamines on isolated rat thoracic aorta. Gen Pharmacol 1994;25:211–6.

136. Carmo H, Hengstler JG, de Boer D, et al. Metabolic pathways of 4-bromo-2,5-dimethoxyphenethylamine (2C-B): analysis of phase I metabolism with hepatocytes of six species including human. Toxicology 2005;206:75–89.

137. Theobald DS, Maurer HH. Studies on the metabolism and toxicological detection of the designer drug 2,5-dimethoxy-4-methyl-β-phenethylamine (2C-D) in rat urine using gas chromatographic/mass spectrometric techniques. J Mass Spectrom 2006;41:1509–19.

138. Theobald DS, Maurer HH. Identification of monoamine oxidase and cytochrome P450 isoenzymes involved in the deamination of phenethylamine-derived designer drugs (2C-series). Biochem Pharmacol 2007;73:287–97.
139. Ambrose JB, Bennett HD, Lee HS, et al. Cerebral vasculopathy after 4-bromo-2,5-dimethoxyphenethylamine ingestion. Neurologist 2010;16:199–202.
140. Bosak A, LoVecchio F, Levine M. Recurrent seizures and serotonin syndrome following "2C-I" ingestion. J Med Toxicol 2013;9:196–8.
141. Schep LJ, Slaughter RJ, Vale JA, et al. The clinical toxicology of the designer "party pills" benzylpiperazine and trifluoromethylphenylpiperazine. Clin Toxicol 2011;49:131–41.
142. Staack RF. Piperazine designer drugs of abuse. Lancet 2007;369:1411–3.
143. Davies S, Wood DM, Smith G, et al. Purchasing 'legal highs' on the Internet – is there consistency in what you get? QJM 2010;103:489–93.
144. Wilkins C, Sweetsur P, Girling M. Patterns of benzylpiperazine/trifluoromethyl-phenylpiperazine party pill use and adverse effects in a population sample in New Zealand. Drug Alcohol Rev 2008;27:633–9.
145. Gee P, Gilbert M, Richardson S. Toxicity from the recreational use of 1-benzylpiperazine. Clin Toxicol 2008;46:802–7.
146. Baumann MH, Clark RD, Budzynski AG, et al. Effects of "Legal X" piperazine analogs on dopamine and serotonin release in rat brain. Ann N Y Acad Sci 2004;1025:189–97.
147. Baumann MH, Clark RD, Budzynski AG, et al. N-substituted piperazines abused by humans mimic the molecular mechanism of 3,4-methylenedioxymethamphetamine (MDMA, or 'Ecstasy'). Neuropsychopharmacology 2005;30:550–60.
148. Arbo MD, Bastos ML, Carmo HF. Piperazine compounds as drugs of abuse. Drug Alcohol Depend 2012;122:174–85.
149. Bye C, Munro-Faure AD, Peck AW, et al. A comparison of the effects of 1-benzylpiperazine and dexamphetamine on human performance tests. Eur J Clin Pharmacol 1973;6:163–9.
150. de Boer D, Bosman IJ, Hidvégi E, et al. Piperazine-like compounds: a new group of designer drugs-of-abuse on the European market. Forensic Sci Int 2001;121:47–56.
151. Gee P, Jerram T, Bowie D. Multiorgan failure from 1-benyzlpiperazine ingestion – legal high or lethal high? Clin Toxicol 2010;48:230–3.
152. Wilkins C, Sweetsur P. Differences in harm from legal BZP/TFMPP party pills between North Island and South Island users in New Zealand: a case of effective industry self-regulation? Int J Drug Policy 2010;21:86–90.
153. Wood DM, Dargan PI, Button J, et al. Collapse, reported seizure – and an unexpected pill. Lancet 2007;369:1490.
154. Balmelli C, Kupferschmidt H, Rentsch K, et al. Fatal brain edema after ingestion of ecstasy and benzylpiperazine. Dtsch Med Wochenschr 2001;126:809–11.
155. Elliott S, Smith C. Investigation of the first deaths in the United Kingdom involving the detection and quantification of the piperazines BZP and 3-TFMPP. J Anal Toxicol 2008;32:172–7.
156. Shellard EJ. Ethnopharmacology of Kratom and the mitragyna alkaloids. J Ethnopharmacol 1989;25:123–4.
157. Boyer EW, Babu KM, Macalino GE, et al. Self-treatment of opioid withdrawal with a dietary supplement, Kratom. Am J Addict 2007;16:352–6.
158. Thongpradichote S, Matsumoto K, Tohda M, et al. Identification of opioid receptor subtypes in antinociceptive actions of supraspinally-administered mitragynine in mice. Life Sci 1998;62:1371–8.

159. Suwanlert S. A study of Kratom eaters in Thailand. Bull Narc 1975;27:21–7.
160. Nelson JL, Lapoint J, Hodgman MJ, et al. Seizures and coma following Kratom (*Mitragynina speciosa* Korth) exposure. J Med Toxicol 2010;6:424–6.
161. Kronstrand R, Roman M, Thelander G, et al. Unintentional fatal intoxications with mitragynine and O-desmethyltramadol from the herbal blend Krypton. J Anal Toxicol 2011;35:242–7.
162. Kelly BC. Legally tripping: a qualitative profile of *Salvia divinorum* use among young adults. J Psychoactive Drugs 2011;43:46–54.
163. Baggott MJ, Erowid E, Erowid F, et al. Use patterns and self-reported effects of *Salvia divinorum*: an internet-based survey. Drug Alcohol Depend 2010;111: 250–6.
164. Tsujikawa K, Kuwayama K, Miyaguchi H, et al. In vitro stability and metabolism of Salvinorin A in rat plasma. Xenobiotica 2009;39:391–8.
165. Rais V, Seefeld A, Cantrell L, et al. *Salvia divinorum*: exposures reported to a statewide poison control system over 10 years. J Emerg Med 2011;40:643–50.
166. Przekop P, Lee T. Persistent psychosis associated with *Salvia divinorum* use. Am J Psychiatry 2009;166:832.
167. Hatfield GM, Brady LR. Toxins of higher fungi. Lloydia 1975;38:36–55.
168. Curry SC, Rose MC. Intravenous mushroom poisoning. Ann Emerg Med 1985; 14:900–2.
169. McClintock RL, Watts DJ, Melanson S. Unrecognized magic mushroom abuse in a 28-year-old man. Am J Emerg Med 2008;26:972.e3–4.
170. Hallock RM, Dean A, Knecht ZA, et al. A survey of hallucinogenic mushroom use, factors related to usage, and perceptions of use among college students. Drug Alcohol Depend 2013;130:245–8.
171. Klinke HB, Muller IB, Steffenrud S, et al. Two cases of lysergamide intoxication by ingestion of seeds from Hawaiian baby woodrose. Forensic Sci Int 2010;197: e1–5.
172. Schmidt MM, Sharma A, Schifano F, et al. "Legal highs" on the net: evaluation of UK-based websites, products and product information. Forensic Sci Int 2011; 206:92–7.
173. Kremer C, Paulke A, Wunder C, et al. Variable adverse effects in subjects after ingestion of equal doses of *Argyreia nervosa* seeds. Forensic Sci Int 2012;214: e6–8.
174. Juszczak GR, Swiergiel AH. Recreational use of D-lysergamide from the seeds of *Argyreia nervosa*, *Ipomoea tricolor*, *Ipomoea violacea*, and *Ipomoea purpurea* in Poland. J Psychoactive Drugs 2013;45:79–93.
175. Rusyniak DE, Sprague JE. Toxin-induced hyperthermic syndromes. Med Clin North Am 2005;89:1277–96.

Pediatric Toxicology
Specialized Approach to the Poisoned Child

Diane P. Calello, MD[a,b,c],*, Fred M. Henretig, MD[d]

KEYWORDS

- Detergent pods • ECG • Hemodialysis • Pediatric • Poisoning • Salicylate
- Supportive care

KEY POINTS

- Pediatric poison exposures most commonly occur in children 1 to 5 years of age and are exploratory in nature. In recent years, incidence and morbidity of these exposures have been increasing.
- Child abuse by poisoning should be considered when the patient is outside this age range, when multiple substances are involved, with recurrent episodes, and when the history is inconsistent with clinical picture.
- Because of inherent differences in physiology and pharmacokinetics, certain substances are more dangerous to young children than would be expected based on adult experience.
- Supportive care and adherence to resuscitation principles are the cornerstone of treatment in the poisoned child.
- The administration of antidotes and use of enhanced elimination techniques have specific implications in the young pediatric patient.
- Pediatric poison fatalities, although rare compared with adult statistics, are in many cases inherently preventable and involve the same substances year after year.
- Newer poison hazards include magnetic foreign bodies, laundry detergent pods, and button batteries. Continued toxicosurveillance is essential for awareness of emerging dangers.

Funding Sources: None.
Conflict of Interest: None.
[a] New Jersey Poison Information and Education System, Rutgers, the State University of New Jersey, New Brunswick, NJ, USA; [b] Department of Emergency Medicine, Morristown Medical Center, 100 Madison Avenue, Morristown, NJ 07960, USA; [c] Emergency Medical Associates Research Foundation, Parsippany, NJ, USA; [d] Section of Clinical Toxicology, Division of Emergency Medicine, The Poison Control Center, The Children's Hospital of Philadelphia, Perelman School of Medicine, University of Pennsylvania, 34th Street and Civic Center Boulevard, Philadelphia, PA, USA
* Corresponding author. Department of Emergency Medicine, Morristown Medical Center, 100 Madison Avenue, Morristown, NJ 07960.
E-mail address: dianepcalello@yahoo.com

Emerg Med Clin N Am 32 (2014) 29–52
http://dx.doi.org/10.1016/j.emc.2013.09.008   **emed.theclinics.com**

INTRODUCTION

A child is rushed into the emergency department (ED) by anxious parents after the witnessed ingestion of a household product or medication. Such a scenario unfolds nearly 90,000 times per year in the United States,[1] yet it remains a uniquely compelling event for all the actors involved: patient, family, and medical staff. In the most dramatic of cases, the child's life depends on the ED staff's ability to rapidly recognize the poisoning, institute life support, and provide definitive initial treatment. For most such visits, the family returns home within a few hours, after a period of benign observation, with perhaps a few laboratory tests obtained, or a dose of charcoal administered. Parents might even be advised that next time a quick call to the regional poison control center (PCC) would have obviated the ED visit in the first place. However, in every case, it is likely that the patient and family bear some lasting impression of their ED experience.[2] Young children fear strangers (especially physicians) and are made uncomfortable by even the prospect of the most minor medical interventions. Parents are the natural protectors and sources of comfort for their children when sick, and yet, in the ED setting they often feel obligated to serve in a quasi-professional helping role. In the context of childhood poisoning, they may also feel considerable anxiety about their child's outcome and guilt for allowing the incident to have occurred. In essence, they too are patients. Emergency providers (EPs) may appropriately dread having to draw blood, insert an intravenous (IV) line, or place a nasogastric (NG) tube into a screaming toddler, and would gladly omit such interventions if they were medically unnecessary. In the rare context of the critically ill poisoned child, EPs also welcome the knowledge and confidence to initiate potentially lifesaving treatment appropriately. This article therefore attempts to guide EPs confronted with the wide spectrum of pediatric exposures to potentially toxic substances, with a focus on exploratory ingestions in young children and selected toxins that have proved to be particularly dangerous in this age group. In addition, some attention is given to special pediatric topics, including particularly poisons that are deadly in small dose; child abuse by poisoning; pediatric medication errors; approach to the well-appearing child who may have ingested a toxic substance; and new (or resurgent) toxic household products and medication formulations.

CAUSE, EPIDEMIOLOGY, AND PREVENTION

Children may be poisoned by numerous mechanisms, including ingestion, inhalation, dermal contact, envenomation, and transplacental exposure. The focus of this is article is on the most common of these mechanisms: ingestion. The ingestion of a nonfood, potentially poisonous substance by a young child typically represents a complex interplay of child-related, substance-related, and environmental factors.[3] The term accidental ingestion was formerly used to describe these common events[4–6] but has fallen out of favor and is now replaced by inadvertent, unintentional, or perhaps most properly, exploratory ingestion.[7] This usage emphasizes the modern injury model that views injuries as predictable events based on several critical factors, not unlike the infectious disease model, with a victim (or host), agent (or microbe), and a conducive environment, as elucidated by Haddon in 1980.[8] Typical poisoning victims are between 1 and 5 years of age, at a developmental stage that allows mobility and expression of normal exploratory behavior, yet too young to learn what is dangerous.[9] They tend to be more hyperactive and impulsive, and more pica prone.[5,10,11] Some agents are more likely to be ingested, either because of ease of access or attractiveness to the youngster.[12] A classic example was adult-intended iron tablets that simulated candy, were small, smooth-coated and easy for toddlers to swallow intact, were available over the counter, and were typically prescribed to pregnant or postpartum women, who often have an older toddler-aged child in the home. As a result, acute iron poisoning had been one of the leading causes of childhood poisoning mortality until 1997, when the US Food and Drug Administration (FDA) required most iron preparations to be blister packaged (the regulation was subsequently suspended, but many manufacturers have voluntarily continued this practice, and pediatric iron-related morbidity has since remained low).[13] A recent example of a new product that has proved enticing, and dangerous, to children is laundry detergent pods.[14,15] Certain environmental changes or stresses are also highly poisoning-prone, including the arrival of a new baby, moving to a new home or apartment, parental illness or disability, and grandparent caretaking or visiting.[16–19] The concordance of two or three such factors likely further increases the probability of exploratory ingestion.

Given the propensity to exploratory ingesting, many physicians (and parents) swear that "kids will eat anything." The number of childhood ingestions are compelling, and the scope of drugs and nonpharmaceutical agents involved in childhood poisoning is broad. The American Association of Poison Control Centers (AAPCC) National Poison Data System (NPDS) data reveal an average of more than 1.2 million exposures per year in children younger than 6 years between 2009 and 2011, the 3 most recent years for which tabulated data were available.[20–22] These data typically represent more than 50% of all poison-related calls to the nation's PCCs. **Table 1** summarizes the most commonly ingested agents reported in 2011. Among these agents are cosmetics and personal care products, noncorrosive cleaners, and plants, all with a low likelihood of causing serious effects. An excellent effort to stratify the litany of pediatric exposures into those with real toxicologic hazard potential, based on frequency of occurrence and inherent toxicity of particular agents (hazard factor), was published in 1992.[23] For pharmaceuticals, the most hazardous agents at that time were iron supplements, antidepressants, cardiovascular agents, and salicylates (of these, iron in particular has diminished as a threat through decreased accessibility, as noted earlier). Additional hazardous drugs included opioids, anticonvulsants, chloroquine,

Table 1	
Major substances most often involved in exposures to young children	
Substance Category	**Percent of Total Substances**[a]
Cosmetics and personal care products	14
Analgesics	10
Cleaning products	9
Foreign bodies, toys, and so forth	7
Topical preparations	7
Vitamins	4
Antihistamines	4
Pesticides	3
Cold and cough medications	3
Antimicrobials	3
Gastrointestinal medications	3
Plants	3

[a] Rounded to nearest integer.

Data from Bronstein AC, Spyker DA, Cantilena LR Jr, et al. 2011 annual report of the American Association of Poison Control Centers' National Poison Data System (NPDS): 29th annual report. Clin Toxicol 2012;50:911–1164.

isoniazid, theophylline, oral hypoglycemics, and diphenoxylate/atropine. The most hazardous nonpharmaceutical household products were hydrocarbons, pesticides, alcohols/glycols, drain and oven cleaners, and gun bluing agents that contain selenious acid; several of these remain highly hazardous today. Button batteries would now also rank near the top of the list of nonpharmaceutical hazards.[24] These and several new threats are discussed in more detail later.

Of those 3.6 million childhood exposures reported in the United States from 2009 to 2011, more than 2500 developed a life-threatening illness, and 109 died of exposure-related effects.[20–22] Yet, these summary data represent a vast improvement in morbidity and mortality from a half-century ago, when 300 to 500 childhood poisoning deaths per year were routine. Pediatricians, public health authorities, and consumer advocates rightfully take great pride in this evolution, believed largely caused by the widespread use of child-resistant packaging for many medications and hazardous household products after passage of the Poison Prevention Packaging Act in 1970.[25] Conceptualizing the accidental poisoning of the 1950s in the modern injury model has allowed for substantial inroads in poison prevention efforts, primarily by attacking the toxic agent via decreased accessibility through regulation with child-resistant packaging and household product reformulation to less toxic forms. Additional decreases in childhood morbidity are undoubtedly caused by the poison center movement and advances in emergency and hospital-based care for the poisoned patient.

Despite these enormous gains, recent data suggest a disturbing trend since 2000 that pediatric ingestions, and in particular, related ED visits and hospital admissions are increasing again.[26–28] Analysis of AAPCC data from 2001 to 2008 determined that pharmaceutical exposures and related ED visits increased significantly, with parallel increases in injuries and hospital admissions.[26] The agents most often involved in serious exposures were prescription medications, particularly oral hypoglycemics, opioid analgesics, sedative/hypnotics, and cardiovascular drugs. It was postulated that the best explanation for this disturbing trend was the general increase in such potent medications in current use, and thus in the environment of young children. This hypothesis was tested by researchers who compared AAPCC data for pediatric exposures with data from the National Ambulatory Medical Care Surveys for adult-intended prescriptions written for 2000 to 2009.[28] A striking association of these variables was found, particularly for children 0 to 5 years old, and again, for opioid analgesics, oral hypoglycemics and cardiovascular medications. Thus, challenges remain to further decrease pediatric toxic exposures, and new efforts are being addressed, including so-called next-generation safety packaging, which limits flow rate of liquid medications, or use of a blister packet within a traditional child-resistant container for pill-form medications.[29]

Two etiologic considerations deserve special comment: malicious poisoning in young children and pediatric medication errors. Child abuse by poisoning is uncommon, occurring in only 0.007% to 0.02% of pediatric poisonings reported to the AAPCC.[30,31] However, the frequency may be higher when hospital-based cases are analyzed. One investigation determined that 13% of ED and in-patient pediatric poisonings resulted in consultation to their hospital's child abuse team, and 4% were referred to the regional child protective services agency (although many of these were for concern of poor supervision, neglect or exposure to illicit substances, rather than truly malicious intent).[32] Such cases might be especially suspected in poisoned children younger than 1 year, or between 5 and 11 or so years old (eg, preadolescent), and when the history is inconsistent or otherwise arouses clinician discomfort. Additional risk factors include previous history of poisoning or siblings who were poisoned; massive overdose; ingestion of multiple agents (unless perhaps the child was found with an open pill minder or equivalent); exposure to illicit drugs; unusual poisonings from common household substances such as salt, pepper, and even water; and evidence of other forms of child abuse or neglect.[33-35] The morbidity of such cases tends to be higher,[30,31] and if child abuse is suspected, these patients require prompt reporting to child protective services, meticulous documentation of clinical and laboratory findings, and careful attention to chain-of-custody procedures for handling of toxicology specimens.

Drug toxicity in young children may also be the result of iatrogenic or parental medication error.[35] Children may be more prone to these errors because of several factors, including the inevitable necessity of calculating weight-based or age-based dosing, and the fact that they cannot speak for themselves regarding allergy history or early symptoms of an adverse event. Moreover, medically complex children in hospital settings may be at increased risk.[36,37] A not uncommon scenario is a 10-fold overdose caused by calculation error of a mg/kg dose. Alternatively, compounding of medications lacking a standardized pediatric formulation presents the opportunity for errors in the compounded concentration or on administration of alternative concentrations. Furthermore, potentially toxic medications with multiple pediatric oral suspension concentrations exist, such as verapamil, atenolol, carvedilol, labetalol, propranolol, and tacrolimus.[38] The frequency and morbidity from pediatric medication errors are considerable.[39] They account for as many as 6% of all exposures in young children, and for 12% of poisoning deaths in this age group.[35] Prevention strategies include computerized order entry systems, unit-based clinical pharmacists, and enhanced efforts at communication among health care team providers.[40,41]

PEDIATRIC PATHOPHYSIOLOGIC CONSIDERATIONS

Pediatric patients respond differently to poisoning than adults, the reasons for which extend beyond their comparatively smaller size. Myriad differences in the child's anatomy and physiology affect vulnerability to toxic exposures. In addition, developmental changes in drug disposition and effect render some agents unusually toxic in the very young child.

Dermal absorption is clearly increased in children, who have a higher body surface area/weight ratio, increased skin perfusion, and increased skin hydration.[42] There is greater potential for toxicity from dermal exposures and greater susceptibility to dehydration and insensible losses. Absorption by inhalation is also a particular pediatric vulnerability; the increased respiratory rate and minute ventilation of young children deliver a higher dose in a shorter time for many airborne toxins. The most common of these toxins is carbon monoxide, in which a group of exposed persons have varying degrees of symptom severity, the most severe of which are often found in the smallest child.

Because of a higher metabolic rate and decreased reserve, children are more sensitive to hypoxia and respiratory failure. Increased reliance on the diaphragm and limited capacity of other accessory muscles lead to the abdominal breathing so often seen in young children with respiratory distress, and an increased tendency to fatigue and respiratory failure. This situation can affect a child's resilience to a direct respiratory toxin (such as an aspirated hydrocarbon), as well as the ability to compensate for acid-base disturbances. As a result, children may be more acidemic at initial presentation with salicylism and may have more severe acidemia with other clinical scenarios, such as toxic alcohol poisoning. An additional metabolic vulnerability is a relative lack of glycogen stores, which significantly increases the likelihood of fasting hypoglycemia from ethanol, β-receptor antagonists, and other agents altering glucose homeostasis.

Children have more limited cardiovascular reserve in response to stress. Cardiac output is heavily reliant on heart rate, with limited capacity to augment stroke volume. However, increased adrenergic tone allows for maintenance of normal blood pressure until the advanced stages of shock. Thus, a child in impending circulatory failure may appear deceptively stable, with a normal blood pressure, and tachycardia as a lone vital sign abnormality. When a drug is ingested that alters this fragile balance, a precipitous decline may ensue. For example, drugs inducing bradycardia such as calcium channel antagonists or organophosphorus pesticides may precipitate circulatory arrest in very small doses.

Although a detailed discussion of pediatric pharmacokinetics and pharmacodynamics is beyond the scope of this review, it is becoming increasingly clear that the manner in which a given drug is absorbed, distributed, metabolized, and excreted changes considerably throughout childhood.[43] Various neurotransmitter receptors and ion channels also undergo maturation in this period. These developmental alterations in drug distribution and response may explain the long-observed phenomenon of agents that cause specific toxicity only in young children. Several opioid receptor agonists or their structural isomers cause enhanced central nervous system (CNS) and respiratory depression in children, including dextromethorphan cough syrups, clonidine, diphenoxylate antidiarrheals, codeine, and buprenorphine.[44–47] Young infants are more prone to paradoxical reactions to benzodiazepines[48] and increased tendency to QT_c prolongation with sotalol and other prodysrhythmic drugs.[49]

EMERGENCY MANAGEMENT OVERVIEW

Despite the relative infrequency of serious clinical toxicity resulting from most common pediatric exploratory ingestions, as noted earlier, some become seriously ill. Thus, it remains incumbent for EPs to recognize and treat poisoned children.

Readily available recent literature offers excellent summaries of the general approach to the poisoned patient.[50–53] Little modification is necessary in expanding these overviews to focus on the pediatric situation.[54–56] Several comments are offered that represent our experience and method of conceptualizing this approach, particularly as it applies to the child who is critically ill or at risk for precipitous decline. This suggested approach offers an updated improvement of the senior author's previous effort in this regard 20 years ago.[3]

Severe poisoning in a young child may be considered analogous to the modern multiple trauma model and approached in a similar manner.[57] A previously well child is potentially injured in multiple organ systems, with a great variance in the degree of (chemical) injury at each site. There is often a brief window of opportunity for emergency medical services personnel and EPs to make dramatic interventions that prove lifesaving. Prompt and thorough evaluation of life-threatening conditions accompanied by sequential immediate intervention (or primary survey) allows for a more detailed secondary evaluation and detoxification phase (secondary survey). This approach is summarized in **Table 2**. EPs are well versed in this paradigm, and only a few comments are here annotated.

Life Support

The initial phase of management includes attention to the traditional ABCs (airway, breathing, circulation) well known to the EP, with some toxicologic expansion to $ABCD_3EF$. Additional Ds in this mnemonic stand for disability assessment (eg, brief neurologic examination, such as a level of consciousness, pupillary size, and reactivity), empirical drug therapy (especially oxygen, dextrose, and naloxone), and initial

Table 2
Emergency management of the poisoned child

Phase	Actions and Considerations
Initial Life Support Phase (ABCD$_3$EF)	
Airway	Emphasis on protection in obtunded child Possible compromise in caustic exposures
Breathing	Adequate oxygenation and ventilation
Circulation	Close monitoring of vital signs, capillary perfusion Early IV access
Disability	Level of consciousness Pupillary size, reactivity
Drugs	Dextrose ($\pm$ rapid bedside testing) Oxygen Naloxone Other ACLS medications as needed
Decontamination	Ocular: copious saline lavage Skin: remove contaminated clothes, copious water, then soap and water GI: consider options (often none)
Electrocardiogram	Rate and rhythm QRS width, QTc length Terminal R wave in lead AVR
Fever	Core temperature check for hyperthermia Emergent cooling as needed
Evaluation, Decontamination, and Supportive Care Phase	

History	Brief, focused
	Known toxin
	   Estimate amount, elapsed time, early symptoms, home treatment, PMH?
	Suspected but unknown toxin, consider if
	   Acute onset of illness; age 1–5 y
	   PMH of pica, ingestions
	   Current household stressors
	   Multiorgan system dysfunction
	   Puzzling clinical picture
	   New medication access
	Suspicious HPI, PMH, or FH for child abuse
	   Institute hospital protocols
	   Consider expanded laboratory testing with chain-of-custody procedures

Physical Examination	Vital signs, pulse oximetry (with core temperature) Level of consciousness, neuromuscular status Eyes: pupillary size and reactivity, extraocular movements, nystagmus Mouth: corrosive lesions, odors on breath, hydration of mucous membranes Cardiovascular: rate, rhythm, capillary perfusion Respiratory: rate, chest excursion, air entry, auscultatory signs GI: tenderness, bowel sounds Skin: color, bullae, burns, autonomic signs (eg, diaphoretic, flushed, dry) Odors: breath, clothing, vomitus

(*continued on next page*)

Table 2
(continued)

Phase	Actions and Considerations
Laboratory (individualize)	CBC, co-oximetry ABG or VBG, ± serum osmolarity Chest radiograph, abdominal radiograph Electrolytes, BUN, creatinine, glucose, calcium, magnesium, liver function tests Rapid overdose toxicology screen Quantitative toxicology tests (especially acetaminophen, salicylate, ethanol) Comprehensive toxicology testing at reference laboratory
Assessment of severity and diagnosis	Clinical findings (see **Table 3** toxidromes) Laboratory and ECG abnormalities
Specific detoxification and continued supportive care	Reassess ABCD$_3$EF (always) Consider GI decontamination options Antidotal therapy, as indicated Enhance elimination, as indicated Supportive care (in every case!)

Abbreviations: ABG, arterial blood gas; ACLS, advanced cardiac life support; BUN, blood urea nitrogen; CBC, complete blood count; ECG, electrocardiogram; FH, family history; GI, gastrointestinal; HPI, history of present illness; PMH, past medical history; VBG, venous blood gas.

decontamination, with urgent emphasis on ocular and dermal decontamination and consideration of gastrointestinal decontamination options. E is added to address a more detailed electrocardiogram evaluation, and an F reminds the practitioner to check core temperature, which may be critically increased (hyperthermia) in many intoxications.

As noted earlier, the poisoned child shows the same precariousness of airway and respiratory function that complicates infectious (eg, croup, epiglottitis) and other CNS-depressed (eg, cranial injury) states. Seriously poisoned children often pass rapidly from obtundation with minimally impaired respiration to deep coma and apnea, and even those with seemingly normal respiratory drive may suffer airway obstruction because of narrow airway caliber, copious secretions, and depressed airway protective reflexes. Patients may vomit or be selected to undergo NG tube administration of activated charcoal (AC), which poses aspiration risks. Blood gas analysis may help in assessing ventilatory status, but in our view, EPs should usually rely on clinical judgment and maintain a low threshold for endotracheal intubation for definitive airway protection and to ensure adequate ventilation in the significantly obtunded, poisoned child. This approach allows for an orderly, if urgent, elective intubation, and obviates the chaos of a precipitous pediatric arrest.

Similarly, any symptomatic poisoned child deserves early assessment of cardiac rate and rhythm (including a 12-lead electrocardiogram [ECG]), blood pressure and capillary perfusion, and rapid attainment of IV access. The poisoned child in cardiac arrest or with severe hemodynamic compromise requires an approach that generally follows established American Heart Association guidelines for pediatric advanced life support.[58] Occasional exceptions to this rule include the early use of sodium bicarbonate in advanced cyclic antidepressant (or other sodium channel blocking agent) toxicity or additional specific antidotal therapy for other cardiotoxic drugs, such as digitalis antibodies for severe digoxin overdose, glucagon for β-adrenergic blocker (BB) toxicity, and calcium and insulin/glucose therapy for severe calcium channel blocker (CCB) toxicity.[59,60] For the child who has not arrested, but is in shock, the initial management usually begins with IV crystalloid fluids (eg, 20 mL/kg bolus, repeated and titrated to clinical effect), again followed by specific antidotes if such are appropriate. Cautious use of inotropes is warranted for persistent shock after circulatory filling has been achieved. Such severe cases should prompt seeking emergent toxicology advice from an in-house consultant or a call to the PCC.

The use of empirical drug therapy in obtunded young children who are poisoned, or potentially so, is similar to that in adults, with the exception of the routine use of thiamine. Although pediatricians and emergency physicians are usually timely in their consideration and use of dextrose, they may occasionally omit a trial of naloxone in toddlers. However, many opioids are available to toddlers in the form of prescription analgesics (which increased in the past decade, as noted earlier), antidiarrheal preparations, cough medicines, or illicit drugs, as well as the partially naloxone-responsive antihypertensive agent clonidine.[61] All potentially poisoned obtunded children deserve a trial of naloxone. Toddlers who are deeply obtunded or apneic may be treated immediately with relatively high doses, by adult standards, with little fear of precipitating withdrawal; we routinely initiate therapy with 0.1 mg/kg (or 1–2 mg) IV.[62] This therapy may be repeated when necessary if opioid toxicity is highly suspected, especially for agents such as methadone, fentanyl, buprenorphine, and clonidine.

As mentioned earlier, dextrose administration is a potentially critical intervention, and should be considered early in the approach to the comatose or seizing child. A rapid bedside test for blood glucose may be useful if it is clearly in the normal range, but one should be wary of relying on a borderline reading. In addition to coma or seizures, patients with hypoglycemia may show an atypical neuropsychiatric picture, with aphasia, slurred speech, and focal neurologic signs. Hypoglycemia is frequently seen after ethanol ingestions in toddlers (as opposed to adults),[63] as well as in ingestions of oral hypoglycemics, and occasionally with β-blocker and salicylate intoxication. The initial dose is 0.5 g/kg dextrose, which is provided as a 25% solution (2 mL/kg) in toddlers or as a 10% solution (5 mL/kg) in infants in order to minimize osmotic shifts from the typical 50% adult solution.

Additional advanced life support medications and anticonvulsants are used as needed. Dysrhythmias caused by poisonings are often the result of sodium channel or potassium channel blockade and may be worsened by traditional antiarrhythmic drugs. The former are often effectively treated with sodium bicarbonate and the latter by magnesium infusion or override pacing. Toxin-induced seizures tend to respond best to benzodiazepine therapy, titrated to effect. A barbiturate is often a preferred second-line agent. Phenytoin is relatively ineffective for almost all toxin-induced seizures. Blood glucose should be checked in all seizing patients. Pyridoxine is a specific antidote for isoniazid-induced seizures. The occurrence of toxin-induced dysrhythmias or seizures, especially if refractory to initial therapy, should again suggest the potential value of an emergent toxicology consult or call to the regional PCC.

Rarely, a young poisoned child might manifest extreme hyperthermia. This complication may occur after overdose of several classes of drugs, including sympathomimetics, anticholinergics, salicylates, and other uncouplers of oxidative phosphorylation, as well as in the context of the specific drug-induced hyperthermic syndromes, including malignant hyperthermia, serotonin syndrome, and neuroleptic malignant syndrome.[64] One additional hyperthermic scenario, that of alcohol or sedative/hypnotic withdrawal, is highly unlikely in a toddler presenting to the ED. Treatment consists of high-dose benzodiazepine administration (with ventilatory support as necessary) in most such cases, and rapid external cooling with consideration for neuromuscular paralysis. Specific antidotes (eg, bromocriptine for neuroleptic malignant syndrome; cyproheptadine for serotonin syndrome) might be of value and should be considered after toxicology consultation.

Within a few minutes of presentation, the poisoned child should be carefully assessed by the ABCD$_3$EF approach, and life-support interventions should be initiated as appropriate. Patients with significantly altered mental status should be considered for airway intubation, have IV access, and undergo empirical trials (or relevant rapid bedside testing) of oxygen, naloxone, and glucose. Additional advanced life-support medications such as anticonvulsants or antiarrhythmic agents, and cooling interventions for hyperthermic patients, should be instituted as necessary. Decontamination options should be considered.

Evaluation, decontamination, and supportive care

History A brief, focused history should be obtained as soon as the life-support phase has been completed. In the child with a known or suspected exposure, the usual questions regarding what, when, and how much was ingested are asked. However, young poisoned children often do not present to the ED with a clear history of toxin exposure, but rather with an acute illness of questionable origin. Features highly suggestive of occult poisoning in such cases include patient-related factors, such as age 1 to 5 years; history of pica-prone behavior; acute onset; multiple organ system dysfunction; altered sensorium; and any puzzling clinical picture.[57] Family and social history factors may also be helpful. Have any environmental stressors occurred, as noted earlier? Was the child visiting a grandparent's home, or vice versa, allowing the introduction of new medications into the household in a context that might be less child-proofed? Are siblings or parents ill or taking newly prescribed medications, such as the pregnant or postpartum mother with the nearly universal prescription of iron supplementation? Holiday gatherings, with numerous relatives of all ages visiting and a general lessening of parental availability to supervise toddlers, are also high-risk occasions, as are recent moves in residence with boxes full of medications and household products often temporarily on the floor. As mentioned earlier, a history that is inconsistent, or a concerning past medical or family history, might suggest malicious poisoning.

Physical examination The usual features on physical examination of any poisoned patient should be sought in the young child. A careful reassessment of vital signs and capillary perfusion should be performed, including measurement of core temperature. The examination should focus on central and autonomic nervous system findings, pupillary size and reactivity, and any obvious abnormalities of the skin, mucous membranes, and cardiorespiratory or gastrointestinal tracts. Characteristic odors of the breath or clothing ought to be sought. The classic constellations of clinical findings (toxidromes) seen in many categories of poisoning (eg, opioids, sympathomimetics, cholinergics, and anticholinergics)[65] are just as characteristic in young children as in adults when appropriate adjustment is made for age-corrected vital signs and baseline developmental status.[61,66] Several of the more common toxidromes are outlined in **Table 3**. As noted earlier, examination findings suggestive of child abuse or neglect might raise the possibility of malicious poisoning.

Laboratory and ECG evaluation The same issues regarding both rapid overdose toxicology panels and quantitative drug levels apply to toddlers as well as to adolescents or adults and are not commented on in detail. Toxicology screens have limited value in the emergency management of most poisoned patients.[61,65,67] This observation is particularly true for the toddler with a witnessed ingestion of a single agent. In the

Table 3
Major pediatric toxidromes

Toxidrome	Examples	Significant Clinical Findings
Anticholinergic	Atropine Antihistamines Cyclic antidepressants	VS: ↑T, ↑HR, ↑BP (↓BP, dysrhythmias with CAs) CNS: delirium, coma, seizures Eyes: mydriasis (sluggishly reactive), blurred vision Skin: flushed, hot, dry Misc.: ileus, urinary retention
Cholinergic	Organophosphorus and carbamate pesticides Military nerve agents	VS: ↑ or ↓HR, ↑RR (with pulmonary effects) CNS: confusion/drowsiness to coma, seizures Eyes: miosis, blurry vision, lacrimation Skin: diaphoresis Misc.: SLUDGE; bronchorrhea, bronchospasm, pulmonary edema; muscle fasciculations, weakness to paralysis
Sympathomimetic	ADHD medications Amphetamines Cathinones Cocaine	VS: ↑T, ↑HR, ↑BP CNS: agitation, delirium, psychosis Eyes: mydriasis (normally reactive) Skin: diaphoresis Misc.: tremor, myoclonus
Opioid	Prescription analgesics Antitussives Antidiarrheals Antihypertensives (clonidine) ADHD medication	VS: ↓T, ↓HR, ↓BP, ↓RR CNS: euphoria to coma Eyes: miosis (pinpoint pupils) Skin: normal Misc.: hyporeflexia

Abbreviations: ↑, increased; ↓, decreased; ADHD, attention-deficit/hyperactivity disorder; BP, blood pressure; CA, cyclic antidepressants; HR, heart rate; Misc., miscellaneous; RR, respiratory rate; SLUDGE, salivation, lacrimation, urination, defecation, gastric cramping, emesis; T, temperature; VS, vital signs.

patient with an unknown ingestion, the toxicology screen may be of some value (especially for forensic purposes if child abuse is suspected), but routine chemistries, blood gas analysis (± co-oximetry), and serum osmolarity (to evaluate pH disturbances, anion, and osmolal gaps) are more helpful in case management. A quantitative acetaminophen level is often indicated for the adolescent with an intentional overdose, because this may be an unreported or unrecognized coingestant. Routine screening for unreported acetaminophen ingestion is not usually indicated in small children.

Several clinically important drugs that are commonly ingested by toddlers, which can produce coma or disturbed cardiovascular function, and for which the usual toxicology screen is negative, are clonidine, digoxin, CCBs, and BBs, and iron.[68] However, each of these has characteristic clinical, ECG, or routine laboratory abnormality patterns. Clonidine resembles an opioid overdose, with variable response to naloxone, and a seemingly disproportionate degree of hypotension and bradycardia. Iron toxicity may produce marked vomiting, diarrhea, and hypotension, with an anion gap metabolic acidosis, hyperglycemia, and leukocytosis; CCBs and BBs often present with a history of drug availability from family members, especially grandparents, with combined bradycardia and hypotension, whereas digoxin more typically manifests sinus bradycardia with typical ECG findings, and hyperkalemia and ventricular dysrhythmias in severe cases.

A closer ECG examination is indicated during this evaluation and supportive care phase. Numerous drugs and toxins are capable of causing subtle ECG abnormalities, which provide clues to diagnosis and represent pathophysiologic changes that contribute to hemodynamic instability and dysrhythmia potential.[65] In particular, many drug classes result in sodium channel blockade (resulting in hypotension and propensity to ventricular tachycardia or fibrillation) or potassium efflux channel blockade, resulting in potential torsades de pointes. These conditions are manifested by lengthened QRS and QTc durations, respectively. Sodium channel blocking agents may also cause a significant rightward axis deviation in the terminal 40 milliseconds of the QRS complex, noted particularly with a significant terminal upright R wave in lead AVR, which is not typically present in normal children beyond the neonatal period. Common examples of sodium channel blockers include cyclic antidepressants, carbamazepine, chloroquine and hydroxychloroquine, class Ia and Ic antiarrhythmics, and diphenhydramine. A similar list of potassium channel blocking agents includes several nonsedating antihistamines, phenothiazines and butyrophenones, other antipsychotics, some serotonin selective antidepressants, such as citalopram and escitalopram, some macrolide and quinolone antibiotics, and again, class Ic antiarrythmics.

Assessment For the child with a known exposure, a careful clinical evaluation, and at times, additional laboratory input and ECG interpretation, allow the emergency physician to formulate an assessment of the potential severity of the intoxication. In the context of an occult poisoning, the same approach should allow an educated guess as to the likely agent or class of agents responsible for the child's condition. In either case, the practitioner may at this point consider further input from the PCC or a local toxicology consultant, for assistance in the management of those children exposed to the more exotic substances or who are more critically ill.

Specific detoxification issues Children with significant ocular or dermal contamination need rapid topical decontamination, as appropriate for any aged patient based on substance and clinical criteria. Gastrointestinal decontamination recommendations have evolved considerably over the past decade and are similar for children and adults.[57,69] Overall, most poisoned patients are managed safely and effectively in the ED without any gastrointestinal decontamination. Gastric emptying with syrup of ipecac is no longer recommended for in-home or hospital use. Gastric lavage is rarely indicated except for high-lethality ingestions in patients presenting within 30 to 60 minutes and is technically more difficult and complication prone in small children.

Similarly, single-dose AC administration is no longer a routine ED intervention but may be considered for patients who present soon after ingestion of agents that bind to AC, for whom supportive care or antidotal therapy may not be sufficient to prevent serious toxicity. AC is contraindicated for ingestions of caustics and hydrocarbons, because systemic toxicity is less consequential than direct mucosal injury or pulmonary aspiration risk, respectively. When elected, the pediatric dose is typically 1 g/kg, or an average of 10 to 15 g for toddlers. Many children swallow this amount, or close to it, when it is mixed in a fruit-flavored beverage and offered by mouth, especially if a cup with a plastic top and straw can be used to mitigate the unpleasant appearance. AC administration, especially by NG tube, results in vomiting in about 20% of children, so is relatively contraindicated in obtunded patients without previous airway protection.[70] In addition, NG tube use adds the potential for the life-threatening complication of inadvertent tracheal placement in a struggling child. We rarely use an

NG tube for administration of AC in toddlers, except in the most highly lethal overdoses, and in such cases, confirmation of gastric placement is crucial before its use, as well as serious consideration of previous endotracheal intubation for relative airway protection.

Of the several substances not well adsorbed to AC but ingestion of which is potentially mitigated by gastrointestinal decontamination, only iron is commonly of clinical importance in young children. Most children vomit profusely after a significant iron exposure but may still benefit from abdominal radiography to evaluate for remaining iron pills, fragments, or concretions. If present, whole bowel irrigation (WBI) with a polyethylene glycol balanced electrolyte solution, warrants consideration. WBI in toddlers does typically require NG tube placement, and is administered at a rate of 250 to 500 mL/h until the rectal effluent is clear, usually within 3 to 4 hours. WBI may also be used for the uncommon ingestion of various medications in patch formulations, the child who ingests illicit drug packets or vials, the young patient found to have large amounts of lead paint chips in the gastrointestinal tract, or large overdoses of significantly toxic medications, especially if in extended-release formulation (such a scenario is uncommon in toddlers; exceptions include several CCBs and β-blockers).

Antidotal therapy Although most poisonings are managed optimally with supportive care alone, specific antidotal therapy is warranted in select cases. The indications for and choice of antidotes in children are similar to those in adults, with some additional considerations.[51,71] Like many newer or limited-use therapies, pediatric experience is often limited, and the pediatric indication is off label. The potential for medication errors is high, because these are uncommonly administered medications that require weight-based dosing and diluent volume. Some medications, such as calcium salts and ethanol infusions, require large-bore IV access for continued administration, which is technically difficult to obtain in a small child. Nevertheless, many essential antidotes have shown a wide safety margin and in situations in which specific antidotal therapy may be lifesaving should not be withheld. **Table 4** highlights those antidotes with an occasional but critical role in pediatric toxicology management, a few of which deserve special mention.

The rapid administration of atropine can be vital to survival from organophosphorus pesticide or nerve agent poisoning, and pralidoxime likely plays a consequential adjunctive role in severe cases. For this reason, adult-dose autoinjectors are widely stocked by emergency medical services squads, which deliver higher doses than recommended for a small child.[72] Reduced-dose pediatric atropine autoinjectors may be available, and adult-dose kits can be easily modified to provide a reduced pralidoxime dose.[73] However, safety data from asymptomatic children inadvertently given adult atropine autoinjectors showed anticholinergic symptoms but no serious effects,[74] and in the event of severe nerve agent or organophosphorus pesticide poisoning, the doses needed may be higher than anticipated.[72] In this scenario, the therapeutic benefit of treating a child with a higher but immediately available dose exceeds the risk of toxicity.

N-acetylcysteine (NAC) for acetaminophen toxicity was FDA approved in an IV formulation in 2004. The development of a specific IV formulation has simplified the management of many acetaminophen-poisoned patients, eliminating issues of odor, unpalatability, and noncompliance associated with the enteral formulation. However, several pediatric therapeutic errors have been reported, with inappropriate dosing and diluent volume, which highlight the perils of pediatric antidote administration. Children receiving the adult diluent volume in error have developed hyponatremia and seizures.[75] Overdosage of NAC itself in the IV formulation may be fatal in young

Table 4
Major antidotes in pediatric poisonings

Drug or Toxin	Antidote
Acetaminophen	*N*-acetylcysteine
Benzodiazepines	Flumazenil
β-Adrenergic antagonists (β-blockers)	Glucagon[a]
CCBs	Calcium[a] High-dose insulin euglycemia (insulin and glucose)[a] IV lipid emulsion[a]
Coumadin (and similar rodenticides)	Vitamin K_1
Cyanide	Hydroxocobalamin (preferred) Sodium nitrite and sodium thiosulfate
Digoxin	Digoxin immune Fab
Ethylene glycol	Fomepizole (preferred) Ethanol[a]
Iron	Deferoxamine
Isoniazid	Pyridoxine
Lead	British anti-Lewisite CaNa$_2$EDTA (versenate) Succimer (dimercaptosuccinic acid)
Methanol	Fomepizole (preferred) Ethanol[a]
Methemoglobinemia	Methylene blue
Opioids	Naloxone
Organophosphorus insecticides and nerve agents	Atropine Pralidoxime
Sulfonylureas	Dextrose Octreotide[a]
Rattlesnake (and other crotalid) envenomations	Crotalidae polyvalent immune Fab
Tricyclic antidepressants	Sodium bicarbonate IV lipid emulsion[a]

[a] Without specific FDA approval for this indication.

children.[76,77] Meticulous adherence to prescribing information and consultation with a toxicologist are advised to ensure appropriate administration.

In patients with toxic alcohol poisoning, alcohol dehydrogenase inhibition is the mainstay of therapy to prevent toxic metabolite formation, with attendant organ injury and metabolic acidosis. This treatment is most commonly accomplished by the administration of fomepizole, which has shown efficacy and safety in the pediatric population.[78] Before the development of fomepizole, IV or oral ethanol administration achieved the same enzyme inhibitory effects and is still used in areas where fomepizole is not available. IV ethanol administration can be technically complicated, requiring central venous access and careful attention to dose titration, mental status depression, and the potential for fasting hypoglycemia. Although young children are more prone to hypoglycemia and CNS depression in the context of ethanol poisoning, therapeutic ethanol administration may have fewer adverse effects. One study of 60 methanol-poisoned children treated with IV or oral ethanol[79] reported no symptomatic hypoglycemia or significant CNS depression, which likely reflects the impact of close monitoring.

The cyanide antidotes are essential to survival in the event of poisoning from inhalation of fire smoke or other sources. Historically, cyanide antidotes available in the United States have included amyl nitrite, sodium nitrite, and sodium thiosulfate. However, nitrites, which generate methemoglobin to form nontoxic excretable cyanomethemoglobin, pose substantial risk for pediatric use. An increased proportion of fetal hemoglobin and decreased activity of methemoglobin reductase both engender high concentrations of methemoglobin with nitrite therapy.[80,81] In inhalation of fire smoke, the additive effects of methemoglobinemia, carboxyhemoglobinemia, and hypoxemia can overwhelm a child's already reduced respiratory and metabolic reserve. As a result, only sodium thiosulfate has traditionally been recommended for pediatric cyanide poisoning caused by smoke inhalation. In 2006, the vitamin B_{12} precursor hydroxocobalamin gained FDA approval in IV formulation for this indication and has long been used elsewhere with efficacy that seems comparable with if not superior to sodium nitrite combined with thiosulfate.[82] It is therefore the preferred agent if available for treatment of cyanide toxicity. Pediatric safety data are limited but reassuring with both hydroxocobalamin and sodium thiosulfate.[83] Both agents should be considered appropriate in the context of pediatric cyanide poisoning, for which expeditious antidote administration is vital.

Resuscitative IV lipid emulsion has been the focus of much investigation since its successful use first with local anesthetic toxicity and then with other poisonings causing cardiovascular collapse.[84] Clear indications are still evolving, but it seems to be an effective therapy for severe poisoning caused by certain lipophilic drugs, including bupropion, calcium channel antagonists, and tricyclic antidepressants.[85] Reported adverse effects include pancreatitis, fat embolus, acute respiratory distress syndrome (ARDS), and digit amputation.[86,87] Although the rate of these events is unknown, and pediatric data are even more scant, it seems a reasonable option for refractory cardiovascular collapse.

Enhanced elimination The ability to enhance toxin elimination in specific cases may be a critical adjunct to therapy after several important poisonings. Urinary alkalinization is a mainstay of therapy for moderate to severe salicylate intoxication.[88] Multiple-dose AC (MDAC) has been shown to increase clearance of several agents, including barbiturates, salicylate, carbamazepine, and theophylline via intestinal dialysis.[89] However its use was associated with complications of repeated AC administration, such as vomiting, aspiration, and intestinal obstruction, and it is not clear that the apparent pharmacokinetic benefit confers improved clinical outcomes. In our experience, MDAC was most useful when mild to moderate theophylline intoxications were common in children, and occasionally staved off the need for hemodialysis (HD); because this is no longer the case, there are few absolute indications for MDAC in young children, although it might be considered in moderately severe salicylate or carbamazepine intoxications.

For patients in whom a highly toxic substance has been absorbed and achieves a significant serum concentration, extracorporeal toxin removal methods can prevent worsened organ injury, metabolic compromise, or organ system collapse. High-flux HD clears solutes and toxins from the blood by diffusion and convection across a semipermeable membrane, and is the primary modality for expeditious toxin removal. Other methods such as charcoal hemoperfusion, exchange transfusion, plasmapheresis, and peritoneal dialysis have little role and are significantly less effective in both the amount and rate of toxin removal. Continuous renal replacement therapies, such as continuous venovenohemofiltration, also have slower clearance rates and are indicated only for the hemodynamically unstable patient who cannot tolerate acute HD.

Acute HD should be considered for poison removal if: (1) there is clinical benefit to faster removal than would be expected from endogenous clearance, (2) there is a clear relationship between serum concentrations and toxicity, and (3) the toxin itself can be removed in significant amounts. Highly dialyzable toxins generally have low molecular weight, are not significantly protein bound, and have low volumes of distribution. The classic examples of these toxins are the toxins for which HD is most often used: salicylates, toxic alcohols, lithium, and theophylline. Other toxins in which HD achieves some removal and may confer some benefit include valproic acid, barbiturates, and methotrexate. HD may also be lifesaving to reverse metabolic derangements and electrolyte disturbances without appreciable toxin clearance, as in the case of metformin-associated lactic acidosis.[90]

The use of acute HD in pediatrics is common for chronic and acute renal insufficiency, and it can be safely performed in conjunction with an experienced nephrologist. Adverse events include those associated with central venous access (insertion trauma, infection, anticoagulation), as well as electrolyte disturbances and hemodynamic instability. In very young infants, volume considerations may require specific small-volume tubing, specialized priming solutions, and close monitoring of the amount of fluid removed to prevent hypotension.[91] Despite these technical challenges, most pediatric tertiary-care centers are capable of performing HD, even in the neonate. It should be used without hesitation in the critically ill child in urgent need of toxin removal, even if transport to such a center is necessitated.

Supportive care In 1994, it was opined that the "most important aspect of managing poisoned children remains meticulous attention to detail in both routine and intensive supportive care."[3] We hold the same opinion today.[57] This treatment includes close observation of vital signs, cardiac monitoring, and pulse oximetry. Respect for the precipitous nature of respiratory failure in children has already been mentioned. Careful monitoring of fluid and electrolyte balance and responsive adjustment of fluid therapy is especially important in young children, whose large body surface area/mass ratio and immature renal function put them at increased risk of fluid overload or dehydration. Some intoxications warrant frequent serial drug levels (eg, salicylate, lithium, digoxin), and others necessitate close monitoring of organ system function (eg, liver function tests after toxic acetaminophen exposure). Much of this ongoing supportive care takes place after the child is admitted, but can be initiated in the ED, and with long boarding times, may need to be maintained for several hours by EPs. Severely poisoned children are most likely to receive optimal definitive care in specialized centers with experienced pediatric critical care staff and access to toxicology consultation.

THE WELL-APPEARING CHILD WITH POISON EXPOSURE

In contrast to the patient with overt signs of poisoning, the asymptomatic child with a feared or presumed exposure poses a different set of challenges. The nature of exploratory ingestions often entails an unsupervised period when a drug or chemical was accessible and unwitnessed ingestion may have occurred. Many of the substances involved in exposures to children younger than 6 years are nontoxic,[20–22,57] and many of these cases if called to the regional poison center are not referred to a health care facility.[20–22] However, once the patient presents to the ED, the emergency physician is tasked with evaluating the significance of the exposure.

A detailed history is most important, including the timing, nature, and estimated amount of the feared exposure. An exploratory ingestion generally can be expected to involve a few pills, or a small volume of an unpalatable liquid. More appealing liquids, chewable or dissolving tablets, and longer unsupervised periods may allow for ingestion of larger amounts. Important circumstantial evidence may include number and type of missing pills, residue in the child's mouth or on clothing, presence of coughing, gagging, or emesis after ingestion, and what the child states occurred, if the child is sufficiently verbal. Questions regarding medications in the home should include all potential exposures, not just those medications that the caretaker believes to be the likely exposure.

The child without clinical symptoms or signs of poisoning after a reasonable period of observation can be safely discharged in most cases, with a few caveats. First, the ingestion should be either of inconsequential amount, or a substance of inconsequential toxicity. Second, an observation period must sufficiently account for the pharmacokinetics of the presumed exposure (eg, formulation, absorption time, onset time to clinical effects, coingestants). The circumstances of ingestion need raise no red flags for suspicious circumstances, as detailed earlier.[34] Adequate follow-up must be in place. Consultation with a regional poison center may be helpful in determining the need for observation and appropriateness of discharge, and may provide follow-up by telephone as needed.

DEADLY IN SMALL DOSES: PERSISTENT PERILS AND EMERGING EXPOSURES

Although many substances ingested by young children may be nontoxic, certain exposures warrant extreme caution for potentially fatal effects in small doses.[23,92,93] It is advisable in these cases to presume the worst-case scenario in terms of amount and type of toxin ingested, and admit children for observation. This advice is especially true in the case of sustained-release preparations of highly dangerous pharmaceuticals. **Box 1** lists some of these most hazardous exposures.

New hazards are ever emerging of which the emergency physician needs to be aware. The first of these hazards involves foreign body ingestions with propensity for severe tissue damage. Button batteries, long known to require urgent endoscopic removal if lodged in the esophagus, have been associated with an increased number of exsanguination deaths from aortoesophageal fistula formation. This condition seems to be largely caused by increased availability of the 20-mm lithium disk battery. Often, the child is evaluated several times before the final ED visit, in which the child presents with massive hematemesis, shock, or asystole. In several cases, there is no known history of battery ingestion, which is then discovered post mortem.[24]

Other dangerous foreign bodies include small magnet toys, which can attract one another in the intestine, causing bowel obstruction and necrosis. The same risk is posed by expanding foam toys and flower fertilizer pellets, which increase in size on water exposure. Laundry detergent pods, which have entered the US consumer market over the past few years, are an enticing, colorful, compact package of highly concentrated detergent enclosed in a thin membrane, which dissolves in the presence of moisture. Shortly after they became available, cases of pediatric exposures began to appear, in which even a mouthful of the pod caused oral and aerodigestive tract burns, aspiration, respiratory distress, and CNS depression.[14,15] Although similar in appearance to dishwashing detergent packets, they seem to cause more severe clinical effect, and caution is advised in treating these children, who may develop toxicity in the hours after exposure. **Box 2** indicates several other pediatric exposures that have been reported in recent years.

In 2010, as a cooperative effort to the annual report published from NPDS, a specific review of pediatric poisoning fatalities was instituted to advance the detection of trends, prevention targets, and sentinel events in these most tragic cases.[36,37]

Box 1
Drugs and chemicals that may be fatal in small doses

Alcohols

Antidysrhythmics

Antimalarials

Benzocaine

Beta-receptor antagonists

Button batteries[a]

Calcium channel antagonists

Clonidine and other imidazolines

Cyclic antidepressants

Hydrocarbons, petroleum distillates

Laundry detergent pods[a]

Lomotil (diphenoxylate/atropine)

Magnetic or expanding foreign bodies[a]

Organophosphorus pesticides

Opioids and opiates

Salicylates (methylsalicylate)

Sulfonylurea oral hypoglycemics

  [a] Indicates new or worsening potentially fatal hazards.

Box 2
Illustrative cases of poisonings in young children[a]

Substance

  Alcohol (infant)[94]

  Alcohol (toddler)[63]

  Benzocaine (methemoglobinemia)[95]

  Carbamazepine (child abuse)[33]

  Clonidine[61]

  Lamp oil (hydrocarbon)[96]

  Laundry detergent pods[15]

  Mercury[97]

  Opioids[62]

  Sertraline[64]

  [a] These and additional cases are accessible in the "Pick your poison" section in *Pediatric Emergency Care*.

Although pediatric poisoning fatalities comprise only a few poison-related deaths each year, a closer evaluation of exposure circumstances shows that many are distinctly preventable. First, opioids continue to be among the most common responsible substances, with a disproportionate number of methadone and buprenorphine cases, highlighting the still unrelenting risk to these youngest victims of the opioid abuse epidemic. Therapeutic errors persistently appear, most of which involve medically complex children in health care facilities. Torch fuel and other hydrocarbon ingestions continue to rank among the most prevalent fatalities, often in the face of immediate and optimal airway management, ventilatory support, and exhaustive ICU care. There have been several exploratory ingestions of refrigerated medications, including liquid methadone, and several cases in which toddlers ingested their own antidysrhythmics, with rapidly ensuing cardiac arrest. Because of frequent use throughout the day by multiple members of the household, a refrigerator is more difficult to secure than a single medicine cabinet. This observation should promote caution to prescribers, who may elect an alternative medication not requiring refrigeration, a closer look at the true necessity of refrigerated storage for these compounds, and improved anticipatory guidance for families with these medications in the home.

SUMMARY

Pediatric poisoning cases require knowledge on the part of EPs of all the critical management principles for poisoned patients but also of where important differences lie in the epidemiology, toxicology, and optimal therapy for poisoned children compared with their adult counterparts. The circumstances of the exposure, the impact on the child and family, the physiologic response to poisoning, and the implications for evaluation and management all present unique considerations, which merit a specialized approach. This article provides a framework for this practice and shows the need for ongoing vigilance to remain current with evolving pediatric hazards and advances in diagnosis, treatment, and prevention.

REFERENCES

1. Schille SF, Shehab N, Thomas KE, et al. Medication overdoses leading to emergency department visits among children. Am J Prev Med 2009;37:181–7.
2. Henretig FM. Patient and family issues. In: Henretig FM, King C, editors. Textbook of pediatric emergency procedures. Baltimore (MD): Williams & Wilkins; 1997. p. 3–7.
3. Henretig FM. Special considerations in the poisoned pediatric patient. Emerg Med Clin North Am 1994;12:549–67.
4. Sobel R. Traditional safety measures and accidental poisoning in childhood. Pediatrics 1969;44:811–6.
5. Turbeville DT, Fearnow RG. Is it possible to identify the child who is a "high risk" candidate for the accidental ingestion of a poison? Clin Pediatr (Phila) 1976;15: 918–9.
6. Sibert JR, Newcombe RG. Accidental ingestion of poisons and child personality. Postgrad Med J 1977;53:254–6.
7. Osterhoudt KC. The lexiconography of toxicology. J Med Toxicol 2006;2:1–2.
8. Haddon W Jr. Advances in the epidemiology of injuries as a basis for public policy. Public Health Rep 1980;95:411–21.
9. Deeths TM, Breeden JT. Poisoning in children—a statistical study of 1057 cases. J Pediatr 1971;78:299–305.

10. Baltimore C, Meyer RJ. A study of storage, child behavioral traits, and mother's knowledge of toxicology in 52 poisoned families and 52 comparison families. Pediatrics 1969;44:816–20.
11. Margolis JA. Psychosocial study of childhood poisoning: a 5-year follow up. Pediatrics 1971;47:439–44.
12. Schum TR, Lachman BS. Effects of packaging and appearance on childhood poisoning. Vacor rat poison. Clin Pediatr (Phila) 1982;21:282–5.
13. Tenenbein M. Unit dose packaging of iron supplements and reduction of iron poisoning in young children. Arch Pediatr Adolesc Med 2005;159:593–5.
14. Beuhler MC, Gala PK, Wolfe HA, et al. Laundry detergent "pod" ingestions: a case series and discussion of recent literature. Pediatr Emerg Care 2013;29: 743–7.
15. Hepner J, Vohra R. Household "HazMat": a pair of sudsy siblings. Pediatr Emerg Care 2013;29:773–7.
16. Maragos GD, Greene CA, Mitchell JR. Accidental poisoning of children in transit. J Pediatr 1971;79:125–6.
17. Sibert JR. Stress of families of children who have ingested poisons. Br Med J 1975;3:87–9.
18. McFee RB, Caraccio TR. "Hang up your pocketbook"–an easy intervention for the granny syndrome: grandparents as a risk factor in unintentional pediatric exposures to pharmaceuticals. J Am Osteopath Assoc 2006;106:405–11.
19. Russo M, Pecker L, Wood J, et al. Grandparent involvement in exploratory pediatric poisonings: a hospital-based study [abstract]. Clin Toxicol 2013; 51:593.
20. Bronstein AC, Spyker DA, Cantilena LR Jr, et al. 2009 annual report of the American Association of Poison Control Centers' National Poison data system (NPDS): 27th annual report. Clin Toxicol 2010;48:979–1178.
21. Bronstein AC, Spyker DA, Cantilena LR Jr, et al. 2010 annual report of the American Association of Poison Control Centers' National Poison data system (NPDS): 28th annual report. Clin Toxicol 2011;49:910–41.
22. Bronstein AC, Spyker DA, Cantilena LR Jr, et al. 2011 annual report of the American Association of Poison Control Centers' National Poison data system (NPDS): 29th annual report. Clin Toxicol 2012;50:911–1164.
23. Litovitz T, Manoguerra A. Comparison of pediatric poisoning hazards: an analysis of 3.8 million exposure incidents. A report from the American Association of Poison Control Centers. Pediatrics 1992;89:999–1006.
24. Litovitz T, Whitaker N, Clark L, et al. Emerging battery-ingestion hazard: clinical implications. Pediatrics 2010;125:1168–77.
25. Walton WW. An evaluation of the Poison Prevention Packaging Act. Pediatrics 1982;69:363–70.
26. Bond GR, Woodward RW, Ho M. The growing impact of pediatric pharmaceutical poisoning. J Pediatr 2012;160:265–70.
27. Spiller HA, Buehler MC, Ryan ML, et al. Evaluation of changes in poisoning in young children: 2000–2010. Pediatr Emerg Care 2013;29:635–40.
28. Burghardt LC, Ayers JW, Brownstein JS, et al. Adult prescription use and pediatric medication exposures and poisonings. Pediatrics 2013;132:18–27.
29. Budnitz DS, Lovegrove MC. The last mile: taking the final steps in preventing pediatric pharmaceutical poisonings. J Pediatr 2012;160:190–2.
30. Yin S. Malicious use of pharmaceuticals in children. J Pediatr 2010;157:832–6.
31. Yin S. Malicious use of non-pharmaceuticals in children. Child Abuse Negl 2011; 35:924–9.

32. Wood JN, Pecker LH, Russo ME, et al. Evaluation and referral for child maltreatment in pediatric poisoning victims. Child Abuse Negl 2012;36:362–9.
33. Osterhoudt KC. A toddler with recurrent episodes of unconsciousness. Pediatr Emerg Care 2004;20:195–7.
34. Henretig FM, Paschall RT, Donaruma-Kwoh MM. Child abuse by poisoning. In: Reese RM, Christian CW, editors. Child abuse: medical diagnosis and management. Farmington Hills (MI): American Academy of Pediatrics; 2009. p. 549–99.
35. Fine JS. Pediatric principles. In: Nelson LS, Lewin NA, Howland MA, et al, editors. Goldfrank's toxicologic emergencies. 9th edition. New York: McGraw-Hill; 2011. p. 447–60.
36. Calello DP, Marcus SM, Lowry J. 2010 pediatric fatality review of the National Poison Center database: results and recommendations. Clin Toxicol 2012;50:25–6.
37. Fine JS, Calello DP, Marcus SM, et al. 2011 pediatric fatality review of the National Poison Data System [corrected]. Clin Toxicol 2012;50:872–4.
38. Wang GS, Tham E, Maes J, et al. Flecainide toxicity in a pediatric patient due to differences in pharmacy compounding. Int J Cardiol 2012;161:178–9.
39. Tzimenatos L, Bond GR, Pediatric Error Study Group. Severe injury or death in young children from therapeutic errors: a summary of 238 cases from the American Association of Poison Control Centers. Clin Toxicol 2009;47:348–54.
40. Risser DT, Rice MM, Salisbury ML, et al. The potential for improved teamwork to reduce medical errors in the emergency department. The MedTeams Research Consortium. Ann Emerg Med 1999;34:373–83.
41. Kaushal R, Barker KN, Bates DW. How can information technology improve patient safety and reduce medication errors in children's health care? Arch Pediatr Adolesc Med 2001;155:1002–7.
42. Funk RS, Brown JT, Abdel-Rahman SM. Pediatric pharmacokinetics: human development and drug disposition. Pediatr Clin North Am 2012;59:1001–16.
43. Mulla H. Understanding developmental pharmacodynamics: importance for drug development and clinical practice. Paediatr Drugs 2010;12:223–33.
44. Megarbane B, Alhaddad H. P-glycoprotein should be considered as an additional factor contributing to opioid-induced respiratory depression in paediatrics: the buprenorphine example. Br J Anaesth 2013;110:842–56.
45. Bamshad MJ, Wasserman GS. Pediatric clonidine intoxications. Vet Hum Toxicol 1990;32:220–3.
46. Kim HK, Smiddy M, Hoffman RS, et al. Buprenorphine may not be as safe as you think: a pediatric fatality from unintentional exposure. Pediatrics 2012;130: e1700–3.
47. McCarron MM, Challoner KR, Thompson GA. Diphenoxylate-atropine (Lomotil) overdose in children: an update (report of eight cases and review of the literature). Pediatrics 1991;87:694–700.
48. Tobin JR. Paradoxical effects of midazolam in the very young. Anesthesiology 2008;108:6–7.
49. Laer S, Elshoff JP, Meibohm B, et al. Development of a safe and effective pediatric dosing regimen for sotalol based on population pharmacokinetics and pharmacodynamics in children with supraventricular tachycardia. J Am Coll Cardiol 2005;46:1322–30.
50. Greene SL, Dargan PI, Jones AL. Acute poisoning: understanding 90% of cases in a nutshell. Postgrad Med J 2005;81:204–16.
51. Holstege CP, Dobmeier SG, Bechteel LK. Critical care toxicology. Emerg Med Clin North Am 2008;25:715–39.

52. Nelson LS, Lewin NA, Howland MA, et al. Initial evaluation of the patient: vital signs and toxic syndromes. In: Nelson LS, Lewin NA, Howland MA, et al, editors. Goldfrank's toxicologic emergencies. 9th edition. New York: McGraw-Hill; 2011. p. 33–6.

53. Nelson LS, Lewin NA, Howland MA, et al. Principles of managing the acutely poisoned or overdosed patient. In: Nelson LS, Lewin NA, Howland MA, et al, editors. Goldfrank's toxicologic emergencies. 9th edition. New York: McGraw-Hill; 2011. p. 37–44.

54. Liebelt EL, DeAngelis CD. Evolving trends and treatment advances in pediatric poisoning. JAMA 1999;282:1113–5.

55. Shannon M. Ingestion of toxic substances by children. N Engl J Med 2000;342: 186–91.

56. Eldridge DL, Van Eyk JV, Kornegay C. Pediatric toxicology. Emerg Med Clin North Am 2007;15:283–308.

57. Osterhoudt KC, Shannon M, Burns Ewald M, et al. Toxicologic emergencies. In: Fleisher GR, Ludwig S, editors. Textbook of pediatric emergency medicine. 6th edition. Philadelphia: Lippincott Williams & Wilkins; 2010. p. 1171–223.

58. Kleinman ME, Chameides L, Schexnayder SM, et al. Part 14: pediatric advanced life support: 2010 American Heart Association guidelines for cardiopulmonary resuscitation and emergency cardiovascular care. Circulation 2010; 122:S876–908.

59. Albertson TE, Dawson A, de Latorre F, et al. American Heart Association; International Liaison Committee on Resuscitation. TOX-ACLS: toxicologic-oriented advanced cardiac life support. Ann Emerg Med 2001;37:S78–90.

60. Vanden Hoek TL, Morrison LJ, Schuster M, et al. Part 12: cardiac arrest in special situations: 2010 American Heart Association guidelines for cardiopulmonary resuscitation and emergency cardiovascular care. Circulation 2010;122: S829–61.

61. Osterhoudt KC. No sympathy for a boy with obtundation. Pediatr Emerg Care 2004;20:403–6.

62. Shieh-Czaja A, Calello DP, Osterhoudt KC. Sick sisters. Pediatr Emerg Care 2005;21:400–2.

63. Walters D, Betensky M. An unresponsive 3-year old girl with an unusual whine. Pediatr Emerg Care 2012;28:943–6.

64. Osterhoudt KC, Mistry R. A boy with tremor, diaphoresis and altered behavior. Pediatr Emerg Care 2007;23:419–21.

65. Holstege CP, Borek HA. Toxidromes. Crit Care Clin 2012;28:479–98.

66. Mofenson HC, Greensher J. The unknown poison. Pediatrics 1974;54:336–42.

67. Kulig K. Initial management of ingestion of toxic substances. N Engl J Med 1992;326:1677–81.

68. Wiley JF II. Difficult diagnoses in toxicology: poisons not detected by the comprehensive drug screen. Pediatr Clin North Am 1991;38:725–37.

69. Gude AB, Hoegberg LCG. Techniques used to prevent gastrointestinal absorption. In: Nelson LS, Lewin NA, Howland MA, et al, editors. Goldfrank's toxicologic emergencies. 9th edition. New York: McGraw-Hill; 2011. p. 90–103.

70. Osterhoudt KC, Durbin D, Alpern ER, et al. Risk factors for emesis following therapeutic use of activated charcoal in the acutely poisoned child. Pediatrics 2004; 113:806–10.

71. Liebelt EL. Old antidotes, new antidotes, and a "universal " antidote: what should we be using for pediatric poisoning? Curr Opin Pediatr 2007;19: 199–200.

72. Rotenberg JS, Newmark J. Nerve agent attacks on children: diagnosis and management. Pediatrics 2003;112:648–58.
73. Henretig FM, Mechem C, Jew R. Potential use of autoinjector-packaged antidotes for treatment of pediatric nerve agent toxicity. Ann Emerg Med 2002;40: 405–8.
74. Amitai Y, Almog S, Singer R, et al. Atropine poisoning in children during the Persian Gulf crisis. A national survey in Israel. JAMA 1992;268:630–2.
75. Sung L, Simons JA, Dayneka NL. Dilution of IV N-acetylcysteine as a cause of hyponatremia. Pediatrics 1997;100:389–91.
76. Osterhoudt KC, Aplenc R, Calello D, et al. Medication error–overdose of intravenous N-acetylcysteine. Clin Toxicol 2006;44:767.
77. Bailey B, Blais R, Letarte A. Status epilepticus after a massive intravenous N-ace-tylcysteine overdose leading to intracranial hypertension and death. Ann Emerg Med 2004;44:401–6.
78. Brent J. Fomepizole for the treatment of pediatric ethylene and diethylene glycol, butoxyethanol, and methanol poisonings. Clin Toxicol (Phila) 2010;48:401–6.
79. Roy M, Bailey B, Chalut D, et al. What are the adverse effects of ethanol used as an antidote in the treatment of suspected methanol poisoning in children? J Toxicol Clin Toxicol 2003;41:155–61.
80. Geller RJ, Barthold C, Saiers JA, et al. Pediatric cyanide poisoning: causes, manifestations, management, and unmet needs. Pediatrics 2006;118:2146–58.
81. Berlin CM. The treatment of cyanide poisoning in children. Pediatrics 1970;46: 793–6.
82. Hall AH, Dart R, Bogdan G. Sodium thiosulfate or hydroxocobalamin for the empiric treatment of cyanide poisoning? Ann Emerg Med 2007;49:806–13.
83. Haouach H, Fortin JL, LaPostolle F. Prehospital use of hydroxocobalamin in children exposed to fire smoke [abstract]. Ann Emerg Med 2005;46:S30.
84. Sirianni AJ, Osterhoudt KC, Calello DP, et al. Use of lipid emulsion in the resuscitation of a patient with prolonged cardiovascular collapse after overdose of bupropion and lamotrigine. Ann Emerg Med 2008;51:412–5.e1.
85. Calello DP, Gosselin S. Resuscitative intravenous lipid emulsion therapy in pediatrics: is there a role? Clin Pediatr Emerg Med 2012;13:311–6.
86. Geib AJ, Liebelt E, Manini AF. Clinical experience with intravenous lipid emulsion for drug-induced cardiovascular collapse. J Med Toxicol 2011;8:10–4.
87. Levine M, Skolnick A, Levitan R, et al. Assessing the prevalence of pancreatitis following resuscitative use of intravenous lipid emulsion [abstract]. Clin Toxicol 2012;50:681.
88. Proudfoot AT, Krenzelok EP, Vale JA. Position paper on urine alkalinization. J Toxicol Clin Toxicol 2004;42:1–26.
89. Position statement and practice guidelines on the use of multi-dose activated charcoal in the treatment of acute poisoning. American Academy of Clinical Toxicology, European Association of Poisons Centres and Clinical Toxicologists. Clin Toxicol 1999;37:731–51.
90. Ghannoum M, Gosselin S. Enhanced poison elimination in critical care. Adv Chronic Kidney Dis 2013;20:94–101.
91. Donckerwolcke RA, Bunchman TE. Hemodialysis in infants and small children. Pediatr Nephrol 1994;8:103–6.
92. Liebelt EL, Shannon MW. Small doses, big problems: a selected review of highly toxic common medications. Pediatr Emerg Care 1993;9:292–7.
93. Michael JB, Sztajnkrycer MD. Deadly pediatric poisons: nine common agents that kill at low doses. Emerg Med Clin North Am 2004;22:1019–50.

94. Iyer SS, Haupt A, Henretig FM. Straight from the spring? Pediatr Emerg Care 2009;25:193–5.
95. Darracq MA, Daubert PG. A cyanotic toddler. Pediatr Emerg Care 2007;23: 195–8.
96. Mazzeo PA, Renny M, Osterhoudt KC. A toddler with curiosity and a cough. Pediatr Emerg Care 2010;26:232–5.
97. French LK, Campbell J, Hendrickson RG. A hypertensive child with irritability and a rash. Pediatr Emerg Care 2012;28:581–3.

Toxin-induced Coagulopathy

Peter Chai, MD, MMS[a], Kavita Babu, MD[b],*

KEYWORDS

- Oral anticoagulation • Prothrombin complex concentrates
- Direct thrombin inhibitors • Xa antagonists • Platelets

KEY POINTS

- New oral anticoagulation drugs now target specific components in the coagulation cascade.
- Vitamin K and fresh frozen plasma remain mainstays of treatment of minor bleeding from vitamin K antagonists.
- Prothrombin complex concentrates are available in 3- and 4-factor forms that have shown improved safety and efficacy when used to reverse bleeding from vitamin K antagonists and promise when used for the reversal of the new direct thrombin inhibitors and Xa inhibitors.

INTRODUCTION

Since their discovery in the early nineteenth century, anticoagulants have been a mainstay of treatment of venous thromboembolism (VTE) and pulmonary embolism (PE). Anticoagulation has also become a major arm of treatment for prevention of procoagulant states in patients with diseases ranging from atrial fibrillation to lupus to a myriad of genetic mutations that subject patients to clotting. Until recently, the choice of anticoagulation in patients who require it has remained relatively simple, because aspirin, heparins, and warfarin were the mainstay of treatment. In the early 2000s, new, potent anticoagulants were developed and brought to market. Increasingly, patients on the "new anticoagulants" are presenting to emergency departments (EDs) either with complications and toxicity from these new drugs, and it has become important for the emergency practitioners (EPs) to be aware of their potential complications. This article reviews the toxicity of anticoagulant drugs and suggests strategies for treating overdose and complications.

[a] Department of Emergency Medicine, Rhode Island Hospital, 593 Eddy Street, Claverick 274, Providence, RI 02903, USA; [b] Department of Emergency Medicine, University of Massachusetts Medical School, 55 Lake Avenue North, LA 166, Worcester, MA 01655, USA
* Corresponding author.
E-mail address: kavitambabu@gmail.com

Emerg Med Clin N Am 32 (2014) 53–78
http://dx.doi.org/10.1016/j.emc.2013.10.001
0733-8627/14/$ – see front matter © 2014 Elsevier Inc. All rights reserved.

emed.theclinics.com

BACKGROUND
The Coagulation Cascade

In the setting of injury or inflammation to blood vessels, the activation of the coagulation cascade attempts to achieve hemostasis and prevent bleeding. Injury to the endothelium of blood vessels exposes tissue factor and fibrinogen, which activate platelets in the primary hemostatic pathway.[1] Fibrinogen binds von Willebrand factor (vWF) on platelets and to induce aggregation. A myriad of other receptors on platelets contributes to this process, the most common of which is glycoprotein IIb/IIIa. Activated platelets bind to collagen exposed from endothelial damage.

Secondary hemostasis involves the three classic clotting cascades, the intrinsic, extrinsic, and common pathways.[1] The endpoint of coagulation is to convert soluble fibrinogen to fibrin, which provides the scaffolding for a platelet aggregate, allowing for a stable clot. The intrinsic pathway begins with binding of factor XII on exposed collagen from damaged tissue, in turn causing a cascade of activation of multiple other coagulation factors that drive the conversion of fibrinogen to fibrin. Simultaneously, the extrinsic clotting cascade is activated in the presence of tissue factor. Tissue factor attracts inactive factors X, V, and VII that are bound to cell membranes and activates them, converting prothrombin to thrombin. Thrombin provides positive feedback in the extrinsic pathway, activating more factors that in turn create more thrombin. The two pathways unite in the common pathway that will produce a strong fibrin clot with platelets that provides hemostasis. A variety of anticoagulation drugs take advantage of this cascade to target specific clotting factors, resulting in cessation of the coagulation cascade at specific points during the process (**Fig. 1**).

Measures of Anticoagulation

Simple laboratory tests can assess the activity of the intrinsic and extrinsic coagulation cascade. The activated partial thromboplastin time (aPTT) is a standard measurement of the intrinsic clotting cascade. Reference ranges depend on laboratories but typically are between 30 and 50 seconds. Activity of factors I, II, V, VIII, IX, X, XI, and XII must be present to have a normal aPTT. Notably, the presence of tissue factor is not included in this reaction and, as a result, the test is termed "partial." Deficiencies

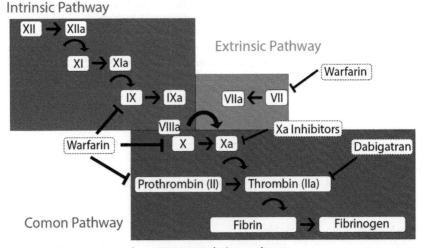

Fig. 1. Intrinsic, extrinsic, and common coagulation pathways.

in vWF may also portend slight abnormalities in the aPTT as it also serves as a carrier protein for factor VIII (**Table 1**).

The extrinsic clotting cascade is measured through the use of the prothrombin time (PT). PT is measured using blood plasma tissue factor. Because of laboratory variation in the measurement of aPTT and PT, the international normalized ratio (INR) was developed. The INR is a calculated number based on the PT in relation to the standardized correction factor, the international sensitivity index, of the machine used.

The final common pathway of coagulation involves the conversion of prothrombin to thrombin, forming a stable fibrin clot. Measurement of this phase is accomplished by the ecarin clotting time (ECT). A known amount of ecarin is added to blood plasma, which then cleaves prothrombin to meizothrombin, an unstable thrombin precursor. The direct thrombin inhibitors inhibit meizothrombin's thrombin-like activity and thus prolong the ECT; this correlates well with their activity.[2–6]

The thrombin time (TT) is another test that measures the conversion of fibrinogen to fibrin. As fibrinogen is the downstream thrombin activation target, the TT can provide a good measurement of thrombin activity. TT is readily available in most laboratories and has been proposed as a measurement target for assessment of dabigatran activity.[7,8]

Targeted Therapies

In 1916, second-year medical student Jay McLean at Johns Hopkins Medical School isolated a fat-soluble compound that functioned as a novel anticoagulant.[9] Together with physiologist Dr William Henry Howell they named the substance heparin from the Greek "hepar," or from the liver. In 1922, Howell introduced a protocol to isolate heparin at the American Physiological Society. Concomitantly, in the United States, cattle farmers were experiencing hemorrhagic deaths of herds of cattle grazing on the plains after rainstorms. Eventually, a bacteria-produced protein of the class coumarins was discovered to be the inciting factor and found to be a potent anticoagulant. Because the project was founded by the Wisconsin Alumni Research Foundation (WARF), the protein was named warfarin.[9,10]

Since its inception in the early 1950s, warfarin has been the mainstay drug of choice for oral anticoagulation and has remained so for the better half of a century. In the early

Table 1
Laboratory tests for measuring anticoagulation

Test	Measurement in Coagulation Cascade	Normal Parameters (s)	Commonly Monitored Medications
Activated partial thromboplastin time (aPTT)	Intrinsic pathway	30–50	Heparin
Anti-factor Xa	Factor Xa inhibition	N/A	Apixaban Heparin Rivaroxaban
Ecarin clotting time (ECT)	Prothrombin to thrombin activity	N/A	Dabigatran
International normalized ratio (INR)	Extrinsic and common pathway	0.8–1.2	Warfarin
Prothrombin time (PT)	Extrinsic pathway	10–12	Heparin
Thrombin time (TT)	Common pathway (thrombin activity)	12–14	Dabigatran

2000s, researchers began to exploit the clotting cascade and development of novel anticoagulants came to light (**Table 2**). The first of these was a direct thrombin inhibitor, ximelgatran, developed in 2006.[11] However, ximelgatran was found to cause significant hepatic injury during phase III clinical trials, and it never achieved United States marketing approval.[12,13] Despite the failure of ximelgatran, its development opened the doors for a multitude of anticoagulants to enter the market. In 2009, the RE-LY trial debuted another direct thrombin inhibitor, dabigatran etexilate, demonstrating its noninferiority to warfarin for anticoagulation in patients with atrial fibrillation.[14] Since its adoption, dabigatran has ushered in a new series of oral anticoagulants with new targets. As physicians gain comfort with their use, novel anticoagulants have begun to make their appearance in EDs.

TARGETED ANTICOAGULATION
Platelet Inhibitors

The search for an anticoagulant agent that mitigates the effect of endothelial damage, one of the first steps in triggering of the coagulation cascade, led scientists to focus on platelets. Platelets are fragments of large megakaryocytes that are produced in the bone marrow and circulate throughout the body. Their major action is to bind damaged endothelium through a multitude of receptors and function as part of the latticework of primary hemostasis.[1] The platelets' ADP receptors are integral to their ability to bind to each other and to activate.[15]

Clopidogrel

Clopidogrel (Plavix) is an oral antiplatelet agent that covalently binds platelet ADP receptors, preventing platelet aggregation and causing delay and prevention of primary hemostasis. It is administered orally in a prodrug that requires hepatic activation via the CYP2C19 system (and potentially others) and a second oxidative step for conversion into its active form. In vivo, clopidogrel irreversibly binds the $P2Y_{12}$ ADP receptor, resulting in the inability of platelets to group together and preventing clot formation.[15–17] The onset of action is rapid, with measurable activity within hours.

Table 2 Oral anticoagulants		
Drug	**Target**	**Potential Reversal**
Apixaban	Factor Xa (reversible inhibition)	PCC
Cangrelor[a]	Platelet $P2Y_{12}$ ADP receptor (reversible antagonism)	Platelets
Clopidogrel	Platelet $P2Y_{12}$ ADP receptor (irreversible antagonism)	Platelets
Dabigatran	Thrombin (competitive inhibition)	Hemodialysis, PCC
Edoxaban[a]	Factor Xa (reversible inhibition)	PCC
Prasugrel	Platelet $P2Y_{12}$ ADP receptor (irreversible antagonism)	Platelets
Rivaroxaban	Factor Xa (reversible inhibition)	PCC
Ticagrelor	Platelet $P2Y_{12}$ ADP receptor (reversible antagonism)	Platelets
Warfarin	Vitamin K epoxide reductase Vitamin K quinone reductase (irreversible inhibition)	Vitamin K, FFP, PCC

[a] These medications have not yet received US marketing approval.

Clopidogrel is orally administered as a prodrug and absorbed through the gastrointestinal mucosa. Approximately half of the drug is bioavailable in various active metabolites. Clopidogrel and its metabolites undergo hydrolysis and conjugation with carboxylic acid that converts clopidogrel into an inactive form, which is eventually excreted in the urine.[18] Typical oral dosing of 75 mg daily allows clopidogrel to reach steady state in the blood after a few hours. Alternatively, a loading dose of 300 mg once allows for rapid effect in the bloodstream. Clopidogrel is used primarily for prevention of recurrent thrombus and ischemic events in patients with vascular disease, acute coronary syndrome, and acute ST elevation myocardial infarction.

Prasugrel

Prasugrel (Effient) is a thienopyridine ADP receptor antagonist, similar to clopidogrel. It irreversibly binds the $P2Y_{12}$ on platelets, preventing aggregation and therefore preventing thrombus formation.[19–21] In comparison to its predecessor, clopidogrel, prasugrel is a simpler prodrug that requires fewer steps to convert into an active metabolite.[20] As a result, the time to adequate platelet inhibition when loaded with prasugrel is quicker than when loaded with clopidogrel. Taken orally, prasugrel is hepatically metabolized. In addition to its hepatic metabolism by the CYP-450 system, prasugrel is also converted via hydrolysis in the intestine and plasma into its active form, resulting in more rapid platelet inhibition.[19,20] Because of its multiple activation pathways, prasugrel is not as dependent on hepatic metabolism as clopidogrel and can be used as an alternative agent in patients who are clopidogrel nonresponders.[22]

In 2007, investigators from the TRITON-TIMI study published a large randomized trial comparing the use of prasugrel and clopidogrel in ACS looking at primary endpoints of cardiovascular death, myocardial infarction, and stroke.[23] The TRITON-TIMI study showed that prasugrel was associated with statistically significant reduction in primary endpoints as well as other study components, including cardiac stent rethrombosis and repeat ischemia three days after event.[22,23] Despite its benefit, prasugrel was associated with an increased rate of bleeding events in the elderly and in patients who weighed less than 60 kg. In 2009, the US Food and Drug Administration (FDA) approved prasugrel as an antiplatelet agent for ACS, with a "black box" warning for patients older than 75 years of age or those weighing less than 60 kg.[24]

Prasugrel is manufactured as 5-mg and 10-mg tablets for oral administration.[24] It is recommended that an initial loading dose of 60 mg be given at initiation of therapy. Afterward, maintenance therapy at 10 mg daily should be prescribed. In patients who weight less than 60 kg, the recommended daily dose is 5 mg daily, but the loading dose of 60 mg remains the same.

Ticagrelor

The thienopyridines, clopidogrel and prasugrel, are mainstays in the prevention of thrombosis in the setting of acute coronary syndromes. However, both drugs are prodrugs of an active ADP receptor antagonist that requires activation through intact hepatic metabolism.[18,22] Because of this, there is a delayed onset of action lasting approximately 3 hours.[15,18,25] Due to the delayed onset of action, it has been recommended to increase the loading dose of clopidogrel from 150 mg to 300 mg to allow for faster onset of action in acute scenarios, but as with other anticoagulants, the major complication with increased dosing remains bleeding. In addition, because of the irreversible nature of their binding to platelet ADP receptors, patients are at a higher risk of bleeding complications if they require emergent surgical revascularization.[26]

Because of the bleeding risk and irreversibility of clopidogrel, a new reversible $P2Y_{12}$ inhibitor was developed in 2006, ticagrelor (Brilinta).[27,28] Ticagrelor is orally administered in its active form and does not require activation. It binds directly to $P2Y_{12}$ platelet receptors to prevent platelet aggregation and coagulation. Ticagrelor is reversible and dissociates from platelets in a steady fashion after oral administration.[28,29] In 2009, the results of a multicenter, double-blind phase III trial, the platelet inhibition and patient outcomes (PLATO) trial, which evaluated the efficacy of ticagrelor versus clopidogrel in prevention of cardiovascular events in patients treated for acute coronary syndromes, were published.[30,31] PLATO demonstrated that patients treated with ticagrelor seemed to have improved survival, including decreased rates of cardiovascular related death and repeat myocardial infarction.

Ticagrelor is formulated in 90-mg tablets.[32] It is recommended that an initial loading dose of 180 mg be given to attain steady state. The recommended maintenance dosing is 90 mg twice daily. A "black box" warning recommends decreasing the daily dose of aspirin to 75 to 100 mg daily when taken with ticagrelor.

Heparin

Heparin and its low-molecular-weight derivatives are naturally occurring polysaccharides that have anticoagulant properties (**Table 3**). Heparin was isolated from liver tissue and found to cause excessive bleeding in animal studies.[10] After further refinement, heparin was commercialized and initially manufactured from beef liver. After successful animal studies showed its ability to prevent thrombosis in traumatized veins in dogs, researchers turned to the first human studies in 1935 to prevent PE after orthopedic surgery.[33,34] Heparin binds the enzyme antithrombin III (AT III) to cause a conformational change that results in activation of the enzyme. Activated AT III binds and inactivates a variety of enzymes including thrombin and, perhaps most notably, factor Xa, resulting in anticoagulation.[35,36] In addition to activation of AT III, heparin also binds to receptors on macrophages, and smooth muscle endothelium, prolonging its half-life.[36,37] It can also bind to vWF, causing some functional platelet inhibition.[37] Heparin is available as an unfractionated version as well as low-molecular-weight formulations. Low-molecular-weight heparin (LMWH) is replacing unfractionated heparin as the therapy of choice in many scenarios because it has a much more reliable pharmacologic profile and a slightly longer half-life.[37]

Heparin is not absorbed orally due to its negative charge and size, and as a result, it is administered parentally. It can also be administered subcutaneously or intramuscularly, although both methods pose risk of hematoma formation and intravenous is the preferred route. After administration, heparin is found in the bloodstream where it binds a variety of plasma proteins, most notably AT III. The heparin AT III complex

---

Table 3
Low-molecularweight heparinoids available in the United States

Drug	Description	Target	Potential Reversal
Dalteparin (Fragmin)	LMWH (MW$_a$ ~5000)	Factor Xa and IIa inhibition	Protamine
Fondaparinux (Arixtra)	Synthetic pentasaccharide (MW 1728)	Factor Xa inhibition	—
Enoxaparin (Lovenox)	LMWH (MW$_a$ ~4500)	Factor Xa and IIa inhibition	Protamine
Tinzaparin (Innohep)	LMWH (MW$_a$ ~5500–7500)	Factor Xa and IIa inhibition	Protamine

Abbreviations: MW, molecular weight; MWa, average molecular weight.

then proceeds to inactivate a variety of clotting factors. Because of its action on various clotting factors, heparin remains plasma bound and is not distributed to the surrounding tissues.[38] In addition to being a highly plasma protein bound, heparin is also found at variable doses to bind to vascular endothelium and receptors on macrophages.[36,37] This vascular sequestration of heparin may allow the endothelium and circulating cells to function as a reservoir to replace heparin as it is eliminated from the plasma.[38–41]

Heparin is absorbed by cells and degraded in a dose-dependent manner that makes up for its first-order elimination.[42] In addition, there is a dose-independent steady-state renal elimination of free heparin in the plasma.[37,42,43] Heparin follows predictable kinetics, with a dose-dependent biologic half-life ranging from 30 to 150 minutes.[37] Because of its short half-life, heparin must be maintained at a continuous intravenous infusion to sustain its anticoagulant properties. The dosing of intravenous heparin is based on actual weight and indication, with typical regimens starting with a bolus followed by a standard drip rate that is then titrated based on the PTT.[37]

Vitamin K Antagonists

Warfarin (coumadin) has been the mainstay of anticoagulation therapy over the past 70 years. Originally discovered in the 1940s, warfarin was first used as a potent rodenticide. The drug is a synthetic derivative of the naturally occurring compound dicoumarol, which is found in many different plants.[9,10] Its ability to prevent blood from clotting and oral administration gave warfarin an advantage over the only other anticoagulant at that time, heparin. Warfarin inhibits the enzyme vitamin K epoxide reductase in the liver, which is important in the recycling of oxidized vitamin K. Vitamin K is an important catalyst in the production of clotting factors X, IX, VII, and II. With inhibition of these factors, coagulopathy occurs. Because vitamin K epoxide reductase is also required for synthesis of protein C and S, patients may also have a brief period where they are paradoxically prone to thrombus formation. In contrast to heparin, warfarin takes a few days to achieve its effect, because inhibition of vitamin K-dependent clotting factors takes time to affect downstream thrombin. Clinically, warfarin is used as secondary prevention of thrombotic states or in the prevention of production of blood clots in patients who have a range of diseases from atrial fibrillation to antiphospholipid syndrome.

Warfarin is orally administered and absorbed through the gastrointestinal mucosa. It undergoes activation via the liver.[44] Warfarin is almost entirely eliminated via conjugation with the CPY2C9 enzyme complex in the liver, rendering it susceptible to multiple drug-drug and drug-food interactions.

Warfarin suffers from the need for careful and precise monitoring. Excess drug predisposes to spontaneous (and sometimes catastrophic) bleeding, whereas too little drug fails to achieve the desired anticoagulation. Multiple dosing regimens have been proposed, but each requires constant titration.[45,46] Typical dosing is initiated between 5 and 10 mg daily and changes according to the INR, which may need to be monitored weekly in the outpatient setting, with dosing adjustments depending on the results.[47] After the patient has remained stable at the desired goal INR for a period of time, the interval in between monitoring can be decreased. Patients who are on warfarin must be counseled to avoid vitamin K–rich foods.

Direct Thrombin (Factor II) Inhibitors

Because management of anticoagulation with warfarin can be cumbersome, there has been a push to develop new, easier to monitor and manage anticoagulants. Investigators began to search inhibitors downstream from warfarin and settled on the pathway of inhibition of prothrombin to thrombin. Inhibition of this step, the final common pathway of anticoagulation, would theoretically be a method to prevent thrombosis. A variety of compounds that could inhibit thrombin were developed and refined for human use.[48] As a result, in 2006, the first direct thrombin inhibitor, ximelagatran, was developed.[11] Ximelgatran was an oral drug that did not require monitoring of its anticoagulant properties. Initial trials showed noninferiority for ximelgatran to warfarin for prevention of a variety of conditions including VTE and atrial fibrillation.[49] In 2003, the SPORTIF II and III trials showed ximelgatran as an equally effective drug in comparison to warfarin for prevention of stroke and systemic embolism in patients in nonvalvular atrial fibrillation.[50,51] However, hepatotoxicity during clinical trials led to ximelgatran's withdrawal from the (non-US) markets where it had been approved.[12,13,52]

Dabigatran

Despite ximelgatran's failure, researchers continued to investigate thrombin inhibition as a target for anticoagulation. In 2003, the peptide dabigatran (Pradaxa) was developed for its potent inhibition of thrombin and its ability to anticoagulate blood in monkeys.[53,54] By early 2003 dabigatran entered phase IIb/III clinical trials for VTE, and in 2005, clinical trials for dabigatran for the prevention of embolism due to atrial fibrillation were initiated. In 2009, the RE-LY trial placed dabigatran at the forefront as a viable option for oral anticoagulation in patients with nonvalvular atrial fibrillation.[14]

Dabigatran offered potential advantages over warfarin. It had a stable pharmacologic profile that did not require routine monitoring (although some argued this was actually caused by the lack of a widespread, available routine monitoring mechanism such as the ECT), and it remains a standard-dose oral regimen. The Boehringer-Ingelheim Study in Thrombosis (BISTRO I) study in 2002 was the first major clinical trial that evaluated escalating doses of dabigatran in the treatment of VTE.[55] Subsequent trials have shown dabigatran to be noninferior to warfarin in the treatment of VTE and prevention of stroke in patients with atrial fibrillation, whereas bleeding complications remain the same or in some cases less in patients on dabigatran compared with warfarin.[56] Current trials are evaluating the use of dabigatran in acute coronary syndrome and as an alternative to heparin in VTE.[4] Dabigatran has been studied in patients with moderate liver failure and may be used with caution.[57]

Dabigatran is administered as a lipophilic prodrug, diabigatran etexilate, which is hepatically metabolized to the active form. Dabigatran requires an acidic environment for absorption, so it is compounded in a tartaric acid core that allows for an acidic microenvironment.[4,53,58,59] Dabigatran is highly selective for thrombin and binds and inactivates thrombin in a greater proportion to other proteins in the blood, such as factor Xa, or plasmin.[48] Steady state is achieved in plasma after approximately three days of therapy. Dabigatran undergoes conjugation with glucuronic acid and is 80% renally excreted.[54,58–61] This significant renal elimination excludes its use in patients with renal disease. Patients who present with bleeding complications on dabigatran are more likely to have renal disease.[56] Unlike other anticoagulants, there currently exists no reversal agent that has been shown to prevent bleeding effectively in the dabigatran-anticoagulated patient.[62–64] Because it is renally excreted, some small trials have suggested the use of hemodialysis (HD) to remove dabigatran in the setting of catastrophic hemorrhage, although concerns of emergent line placement and stability for dialysis remain a concern.[65,66] A direct antibody against dabigatran is also in development and has shown some success in animal trials.[67,68] Measuring the effect of reversal on the dabigatran-anticoagulated patient remains difficult. The ECT and TT seem to be effective measurements of dabigatran activity; however, these laboratory tests remain difficult to obtain in many centers.[7,59,68] The recommended dosing for dabigatran is 150 mg twice daily for the prevention of embolism in a variety of diseases, which included at the time of this writing, atrial fibrillation, deep vein thrombosis, and PE.[14,60,61,69] In patients with chronic kidney disease, the dose is adjusted by creatinine clearance. Dosing must also be decreased to 75 mg twice daily in patients who took P-glycoprotein (Pgp) inhibitors. In patients on Pgp inhibitors with a creatinine clearance less than 30 mL/min, dabigatran is contraindicated.[70]

Anti-Xa Inhibitors

Factor X plays a key role in the coagulation cascade, functioning as a "gatekeeper" for the common pathway. The extrinsic and intrinsic coagulation pathways merge to form the tenase complex, which acts as a serine protease in the activation of factor X to factor Xa. Factor Xa then proceeds to form a complex to create thrombin from prothrombin, resulting in effective coagulation (see **Fig. 1**). Because of factor Xa activity in the common coagulation pathway, it has been a target of directed anticoagulation research.[71–73] In 1987, Tuszynski discovered the first naturally occurring Xa inhibitor.[74] Since its discovery, a number of Xa inhibitors have emerged and are progressing through clinical trials.

Currently, three major factor Xa inhibitors, rivaroxaban, apixaban, and edoxaban, are used in the prevention of thrombus formation in patients with VTE or atrial fibrillation.[71] Another parenteral factor Xa inhibitor, otamixaban, is under development for cardiovascular surgery. These synthetic Xa inhibitors are highly specific for factor Xa, and as a result, bind a dose-dependent amount of factor Xa. Because of its tight pharmacologic profile, there is no requirement for routine monitoring for any of the current Xa inhibitors. At the time of this writing, only rivaroxaban (Xalrelto) and apixaban (Eliquis) were approved in the United States. Activity of Xa inhibitors is difficult to measure. Because of their inhibition of factor Xa, the PT will be elevated, although the correlation with amount of Xa inhibition is unclear.[5] An anti-factor Xa assay is available at select laboratories. This test combines serum with rivaroxaban-specific antibodies to determine activity of the inhibitor; however, the availability and ease of test make the assay difficult to use in the setting of acute bleeding in the ED.[75–77]

Rivaroxaban

Rivaroxaban was the first Xa inhibitor approved in the United States. Rivaroxaban was first approved for the prevention of PE in VTE and since 2011 has been used for stroke prevention in atrial fibrillation and other uses.[78,79] Rivaroxaban is typically administered once daily and comes in 10-mg tablets. Its peak onset of action is between 2 and 4 hours after administration.[71,80,81] Rivaroxaban is administered orally and is quickly absorbed through the gastrointestinal mucosa, with approximately 50% to 60% bioavailability.[82] Rivaroxaban is both renally and hepatically excreted, and as a result, the drug persists for a longer duration in patients with renal or liver disease.[80,83,84] Rivaroxaban is oxidized in the liver, and its metabolite is recirculated and eliminated in urine and feces.[82] Because the liver is responsible for metabolism before renal excretion, caution should be exercised in patients with liver disease.[82,85] Rivaroxaban is orally dosed from 10 to 20 mg once daily depending on indication. Patients taking rivaroxaban for deep venous thrombosis prophylaxis can start on a low dose of 10 mg daily, whereas patients on rivaroxaban for stroke prevention in nonvalvular atrial fibrillation typically start at the higher 20-mg daily dosing.[86]

Apixaban

Apixaban was approved in 2012 for use in the prevention of stroke and thrombus formation in patients with atrial fibrillation. It is the second factor Xa inhibitor to gain widespread use in the United States. Because of its affinity for factor Xa and strict pharmacologic profile, there is no need for routine monitoring.[73,87] Apixaban has proved in clinical trials to be noninferior to warfarin in the prevention of VTE and prevention of stroke in patients who have atrial fibrillation.[87,88] Apixaban is administered orally and absorbed through the gastrointestinal mucosa to reach peak concentrations within hours.[89] Apixaban is both hepatically and renally eliminated. Apixaban accumulates in the liver where it undergoes hydroxylation and sulfation. The sulfated metabolites are then excreted in bile.[89,90] In addition, recirculated apixaban metabolites are renally excreted, and this seems to be the major mechanism of elimination.[90] Because of the dual method of excretion, apixaban is considered safe in patients with chronic kidney disease or mild liver impairment. Apixaban is orally dosed at 5 mg once daily. In the United States, it is currently only FDA approved for stroke prevention in patients with nonvalvular atrial fibrillation. Care must be taken in patients who take other drugs that inhibit the CYP3A4 and Pgp enzymes, and in these cases, dosing is decreased to 2.5 mg once daily.[91]

REVERSAL STRATEGIES

The most concerning and perhaps devastating toxicity from the oral anticoagulants is bleeding. Bleeding risk is highly variable and depends on patient comorbidities, the presence of monitoring, the risk of trauma, and patient compliance. In 2001, several authors proposed a standardized definition of bleeding complications to aid in the reversal of anticoagulant-mediated bleeding by defining fatal, major, and minor bleeding emergencies.[92,93] More recently, the Bleeding Academic Research Consortium proposed a unified definition of bleeding to address heterogeneity across clinical trials (**Box 1**).[94] In the ED, practitioners frequently encounter patients on anticoagulants who are suffering from major gastrointestinal hemorrhage, spontaneous intracerebral bleeding, or traumatic injuries with associated significant bleeding. All of these patients require rapid and efficient reversal of their anticoagulation to control potentially life-threatening bleeding. The bleeding risk of the newer anticoagulants, direct thrombin inhibitors, and factor Xa inhibitors, are evaluated in comparison to the gold standard of warfarin. Although warfarin has been in use for many years, studies disagree on the incidence of major bleeding, partially because the definition of major or catastrophic bleeding varies from study to study.[95] Despite, this, it seems that approximately 10% to 17% of patients on warfarin will have a bleeding event annually, while the risk of major bleeding ranges from 2% to 5% per year and fatal bleeding from 0.5% to 1% per year.[95–98]

Multiple risk factors account for bleeding events in patients who are on oral anticoagulants. Among these, perhaps the most important risk factor is age. Some studies have pointed to an increased risk of major and catastrophic bleeding in patients older than 80 that is nearly twice that of a similar, but younger cohort.[96,98–100] Female gender is also thought to be a risk factor for bleeding, although no clear studies have shown a significant effect. Elevated INR, especially INR greater than 4.5, has also long been known to be a poor prognostic factor.[101] In addition, it seems that patients who initiate anticoagulation therapy are at higher risk of bleeding in the first 90 days of therapy.[98,102–104]

When assessing the bleeding patient on anticoagulants, it is important to determine the severity or projected severity of bleeding, type of anticoagulant agent they are taking, their indication for anticoagulation, and potential comorbidities that may impact the type of reversal agent chosen. For minor bleeding, oozing, or superficial ecchymosis, there may be no reversal required, or simple maneuvers such as holding

> **Box 1**
> **Classification of major and minor bleeding events on anticoagulation**
>
> Type 0: No bleeding
>
> Type 1: Nonactionable bleeding that does not cause patient to seek medical care, additional studies, or hospitalization
>
> Type 2: Mild bleeding (not type 3–5) that requires either health care nonsurgical intervention or hospitalization
>
> Type 3: Major bleeding
>
> Type 3a: Drop in hemoglobin 3–5 g, or any bleeding requiring transfusion
>
> Type 3b: >5 g drop in hemoglobin, or cardiac tamponade, bleeding requiring vasopressor agents, bleeding requiring surgical intervention (not hemorrhoid/dental/skin/epistaxis)
>
> Type 3c: Intracranial hemorrhage or intraocular hemorrhage causing visual impairment
>
> Type 4: Coronary artery bypass grafting related bleeding, including perioperative intracranial hemorrhage, bleeding requiring reoperation, transfusion >5 units of blood products in 48 hours, or chest tube output >2 L in 24 hours
>
> Type 5: Fatal bleeding
>
> Type 5a: Clinical suspicion of fatal hemorrhage without autopsy or imaging evidence
>
> Type 5b: Definite fatal hemorrhage confirmed via autopsy or imaging
>
> *Adapted from* Mehran R, Rao SV, Bhatt DL, et al. Standardized bleeding definitions for cardiovascular clinical trials: a consensus report from the bleeding academic research consortium. Circulation 2011;123:2736–47.

the anticoagulant agent may be sufficient. The emergence of the new anticoagulants, direct thrombin inhibitors and factor Xa inhibitors, pose a new quandary for EPs. No clear guidelines exist for reversal of these new agents, and there are no definitive antidotes that are readily available for patients who experience catastrophic bleeding. In addition, the typical long half-life of the new oral anticoagulants places patients at risk when emergent diagnostic or therapeutic procedures, central venous access, lumbar puncture, or surgical interventions, are required.

Protamine Sulfate

Protamine sulfate is a polypeptide originally isolated from salmon sperm in the 1930s that was found to be able to reverse the anticoagulation effects of heparin in a dose-dependent manner.[105] Because protamine is a positively charged cation, it is able to bind the negatively charged heparin and inactivate its activity. The protamine-bound heparin complexes are rapidly cleared mostly via phagocytosis through the reticuloendothelial system.[105,106] In addition to binding heparin, the administration of protamine induces a significant histamine release that can cause hypotension and anaphylaxis.[106] Protamine itself appears to be an anticoagulant through inhibition of platelet ADP binding sites, and when excess protamine is added to heparin anticoagulated blood, there seems to be a paradoxic increase in anticoagulation.[107–109] As a result, care must be given when administering protamine to reverse heparin-induced anticoagulation.

Because heparin has such a short half-life, typically stopping heparin use or in the case of continuous infusion, stopping the infusion, will prevent further bleeding. However, when there is catastrophic bleeding from heparin, protamine is a viable antidote. In 2012, the American College of Chest Physicians released guidelines for reversal of heparins using protamine.[37] One milligram of protamine sulfate is able to neutralize 100 units of heparin. It is recommended that a single intravenous bolus of protamine appropriate to the dose of heparin be given to the patient to neutralize the heparin. The half-life of protamine is approximately seven minutes, whereas the half-life of heparin is 60 minutes, so protamine may need to be readministered. In the case of a continuous infusion, the amount of protamine should be calculated based on the total amount of heparin infused over the past 60 minutes.[37,106,109] In the case of subcutaneous heparin, protamine may need to be provided as a continuous infusion.

Patients who are on LMWH present a difficult challenge in reversal. Because protamine requires a large sulfate group on heparin to bind, it is unable to bind most LMWH strongly, resulting in persistent bleeding.[108] The clinical significance of the incomplete reversal of LMWH is unclear. A single small case study in 1986 on patients undergoing cardiac bypass surgery showed persistent bleeding in patients on enoxaparin that required repeat protamine dosing.[110] However, more recent animal models have failed to show any clinical significance of this incomplete reversal of LMWH.[111] As a result, protamine is still recommended for reversal of major bleeding from LMWH, typically at 1 mg protamine for every 100 anti-Xa IU provided, which may require repetition at one-half this dose for persistent anticoagulation.

Phytonadione

Vitamin K (phytonadione) is a naturally occurring fat-soluble vitamin that plays an important role in the synthesis of certain coagulation factors. The most common anticoagulant used, warfarin, blocks the activity of vitamin K to produce its anticoagulant effect. As a result, vitamin K has become one of the most common reversal agents in patients who experience bleeding from warfarin. In 2003, The American College of Cardiology recommended that in addition to stopping warfarin therapy on patients with elevated INR, the second modality of treatment includes administration of vitamin K.[47] The goal of vitamin K administration is to decrease the INR to between 2 and 3 to decrease the risk of bleeding complications.[47,102,112,113] Holding warfarin therapy may reverse the INR to a safe range, between 2 and 3, in approximately 4 to 5 days, depending on the initial INR, whereas administration of vitamin K dramatically reduces the time to correction to approximately 24 hours or less.[47,93,113,114] Multiple professional organizations have recommended vitamin K therapy for urgent reversal of warfarin anticoagulation. However, vitamin K is not indicated for reversal of direct thrombin inhibitors or factor Xa inhibitors.

Vitamin K can be administered as an oral, intravenous, intramuscular, or subcutaneous injection, and comes in 5-mg and 10-mg doses. For uncomplicated, elevated INR without active signs of bleeding, the practitioner can administer a single oral dose of vitamin K to decrease the INR. Even with mild bleeding and an elevated INR, a single oral dose of vitamin K in addition to cessation of warfarin therapy may be sufficient to reverse hemorrhage.[47,93,114] In the event of major bleeding, intravenous vitamin K is preferred. When compared with subcutaneous or oral dosing, a single dose of intravenous vitamin K is able to reverse the INR within 8 hours, while subcutaneous or oral dosing takes 24 hours for its effect to be seen[93,115,116] and can be confounded by poor subcutaneous tissue absorption or poor gut absorption due to hemorrhage, ischemia, or comorbid conditions in the patient experiencing major complications of warfarin therapy.[47,93,114,116,117] The bioavailability of vitamin K after intravenous administration is reliable and allows for faster normalization of the INR. Complications of vitamin K administration include thrombosis as the patient's anticoagulated state is reversed. There is a small risk of anaphylactoid reaction when vitamin K is given intravenously and, as a result, it is recommended that it is administered over 20 to 30 minutes to 1 hour.

Platelets

With the increasing use of antiplatelet agents, emergency medicine providers should expect to see increasing amounts of patients who present with bleeding complications who are taking these agents. After the TRITON study, it became clear that with the new antiplatelet agent, prasugrel, in the market, there may be a higher incidence of bleeding complications.[23] It was originally postulated that platelet transfusion in a patient who is on antiplatelet agents may help mitigate the effects of hemorrhage in patients who present with bleeding.[118] Multiple studies, albeit retrospective in nature, have shown that platelet transfusion in itself is effective in raising the platelet count in patients who are bleeding from antiplatelet agents.[119,120] However, there is evidence that despite the increase in platelet count, the antiplatelet agent present in the bloodstream merely inactivates transfused platelets, resulting in persistent hemorrhage.[121] In 2009, investigators performed the first retrospective review of patients presenting to the ED on antiplatelet agents with intracranial hemorrhage.[122] From this study, it was clear that antiplatelet agents alone increased mortality in the event of hemorrhage. Further retrospective studies have shown that in both traumatic and spontaneous intracranial hemorrhage, platelet transfusions do not impact hematoma expansion or mortality.[122,123]

Platelet transfusion in itself is not a benign process. Like other blood products, there is a risk of transmissible disease, as well as complications from volume expansion and antibody reactions. In addition to fresh frozen plasma (FFP), platelet transfusions may result in transfusion-related acute lung injury.[124,125] Currently, there is no definitive evidence to support platelet transfusion in patients on antiplatelet agents presenting with acute hemorrhage.[121,126]

FFP

FFP is the centrifuged effluent of a unit of human blood that contains variable concentrations of coagulation factors, fats, carbohydrates, and plasma proteins. A single unit of FFP is typically between 200 and 250 mL. FFP has been used since the early 1940s, initially as a fluid for volume expansion, and since the discovery of warfarin, for reversal of anticoagulation.[9,127] FFP is frozen and must be thawed before use, and infusion must be completed by 6 hours.[128] Since the advent of warfarin, the use of FFP has risen dramatically as a reversal agent for anticoagulation-induced bleeding.[127–129]

Because the INR is a logarithmic scale, escalating doses of FFP must be administered to reverse anticoagulation effectively. The typical dose of FFP is between 10 and 20 mL/kg to achieve a 20% to 30% decrease in the INR.[62,64,128,130] Once the INR approaches 1.7, there is virtually no effect with continued transfusion of FFP.[127,131] Currently, the use of FFP is recommended for reversal of warfarin-induced anticoagulation in the context of severe bleeding. FFP should not be used for an elevated INR absent signs of hemorrhage.[47,127,132] In the United States, FFP is also recommended as an adjunct with PCC in the reversal of direct thrombin inhibitors and factor Xa inhibitors.

FFP possesses several disadvantages when used as a reversal agent for anticoagulant-induced bleeding. As a plasma product, there is an inherent risk of transfusion reactions and infectious disease. Allergic reaction to FFP is not uncommon during administration, occurring in up to 1 in 100 transfusions.[133] To treat the INR adequately, a large volume of FFP must be used, which patients may not tolerate. In the population of patients who are anticoagulated with warfarin for atrial fibrillation, artificial heart valves, or cardiomyopathy, the amount of FFP commonly needed to reverse bleeding complications may induce heart failure and pulmonary edema. As a result, FFP administration is typically dosed inadequately and may not achieve the desired effect.[93,129,131]

Prothrombin Complex Concentrate

Prothrombin complex concentrates (PCCs) are human-derived lyophilized powder that contains variable amounts of factors II, IX, VII, X, protein C, and protein S. PCCs are manufactured from large pools of plasma concentrate and are standardized in regard to the content of factor IX. PCC products undergo manufacturer-specific viral inactivation and reduction steps before use.[134] As lyophilized powders, they must be reconstituted before administration. Historically, PCCs have been used for major bleeding events in patients with hemophilia, but have recently been expanded for use in major bleeding and intracranial hemorrhage in patients on oral anticoagulation.[113,134–136]

In the United States, PCCs are produced in 3-factor (Profilnine, Bebulin) and 4-factor forms (Kcentra). Three-factor PCC does contain small amounts of factor VII: ≤ 0.35 IU factor VII per IU factor IX (Profilnine) and ≤ 0.20 IU factor VII per IU factor IX (Bebulin). PCC formulations may also contain small amounts of antithrombotic proteins C and S or heparin. Only Kcentra carries a specific FDA indication for reversal of vitamin K antagonists such as warfarin in the setting of major bleeding. Although the cost of PCCs is substantially higher than FFP, several advantages exist. Because of viral inactivation processes, the risk of disease transmission by PCCs is diminished compared with FFP. In addition, their lyophilized form makes it easier to access. PCC does not need to be cross-matched or thawed like FFP, although it does require careful reconstitution. An additional advantage of PCC is the ability to deliver large doses in small volumes, avoiding the risk of pulmonary edema, as it is reconstituted at time of use. PCC can be administered via rapid infusion over 10 minutes, whereas typical FFP administration can take hours to complete.[134,135,137] Given the ease of reversal, smaller volume, and potentially fewer side effects, it may be efficacious to use PCC in the context of catastrophic bleeding from anticoagulants.[138]

PCCs are able to reduce the INR much more rapidly when compared with FFP. One study showed that 3-factor PCC dosed at 50 IU/kg was able to reverse the INR in patients with intracranial hemorrhage within 30 minutes.[139] A retrospective study of PCC reversal of warfarin-induced bleeding showed similar reversal times of the INR and significant decrease in heart failure with a single 1000 to 1500 IU dose.[140] In vitro studies demonstrate PCCs' ability to generate increased thrombin, leading to improved coagulation, a process completed much more efficaciously when compared with FFP.[141] PCC is currently indicated for severe bleeding on patients on warfarin, with limited evidence showing some benefit in reversal of direct thrombin inhibitors and factor Xa inhibitors.

PCC dosing in the setting of anticoagulant-induced bleeding remains controversial, although most experts suggest a weight-based dosing regimen. Most experience with PCC dosing is based on its use in hemophilia patients; however, a similar dosing regimen has been tested on warfarin-induced bleeding.[134,135] Most authorities suggest using 25 to 50 IU/kg of PCC in cases of persistent and severe bleeding from warfarin.[47,113,132,134,135,139,142] However, there is evidence that this dosing regimen may be excessive, or in the case of 3-factor PCC, insufficient, and each case should be considered individually and bleeding parameters monitored. Patients who have higher INR or more severe bleeding may require higher initial PCC dosing.[135,139,141,143]

Special consideration must be used when dosing PCC for reversal of anticoagulation in the United States. A higher dose of 3-factor PCC may be required to reverse bleeding.[139,143] Because 3-factor PCC lacks factor VII, there is relatively less activation of the extrinsic coagulation cascade. In the context of warfarin reversal, there is also a lack of factor VII because of warfarin's inhibition of vitamin K epoxide reductase. Because of these issues, it has been suggested to coadminister one to two units of FFP in conjunction with 3-factor PCC for adequate reversal of anticoagulation.[135,139,143] The approved dose of 4-factor PCC (Kcentra) in units of factor IX per kilogram is 25 units/kg, 35 units/kg, and 50 units/kg, for INRs of 2 to less than 4, 4 to 6, and greater than 6, respectively. The maximum dose should not exceed 2500, 3500, and 5000 units for these respective categories.

Although there is evidence to suggest that PCC is useful and likely more efficacious in reversal of bleeding in patients on warfarin, there is limited and equivocal evidence in the use of PCCs in patients bleeding from direct thrombin inhibitors and factor Xa inhibitors. Multiple case reports have demonstrated either benefit or equivocal effect of PCC in reversal of patients on dabigatran used in conjunction with factor VII, and FFP.[144–146] A rabbit model has also shown the potential benefit of 4-factor PCC in reversal of dabigatran.[147] Perhaps the clearest evidence comes from two randomized crossover studies that studied the effect of PCC alone in reversal of dabigatran and rivaroxaban.[148,149] Ten healthy male subjects were randomized to dabigatran 150 mg once daily or rivaroxaban 20 mg twice daily. Patients were provided either a single 50 unit/kg bolus of PCC, which is the recommended dose for warfarin reversal, or normal saline. The study investigators found that PCC reversed the PTT in patients on rivaroxaban, but was ineffective in reversal of the ECT or TT in patients taking dabigatran.[149] A similar study using either PCC or factor VIIa to reverse dabigatran or rivaroxaban showed potential reversal activity of low-dose PCC.[148] Both of these trials, although the first to objective study PCC in the context of the new anticoagulants, were done with healthy male volunteers without renal impairment. In addition, both studies used once-daily dabigatran dosing, while typical dosing is twice daily. Although there are minimal data on use of PCC in the setting of bleeding from the new anticoagulants, in patients with severe, life-threatening bleeding, use of PCC has been recommended.[62,64,68,134,135,142,150,151]

Factor VIIa

Factor VII is a vital player in the extrinsic coagulation cascade. It is activated by tissue factor and in turn activates factor X, which directly activates prothrombin to thrombin, resulting in clot formation. Recombinant factor VIIa (rVIIa) has been in use for years in the treatment of bleeding in hemophiliacs, and recently in acute trauma with massive coagulopathy.[152,153] A Cochrane review in 2009 found rVIIa to have no survival benefit in trauma patients and to be harmful in the elderly, with increased severe arterial thrombotic events.[154,155]

Although the use of rVIIa is only recommended as compassionate therapy in trauma, its use in reversal of the new anticoagulants and warfarin remains equivocal.[156] Some small studies have shown the ability of rVIIa to reverse the INR within minutes in patients with intracranial hemorrhage as a result of warfarin.[157,158] These same studies also cautioned about the use of rVIIa in patients with previous myocardial infarction, stroke, or mechanical valves, given the elevated risk of arterial and venous thromboses in these patients. Although rVIIa is able to reverse the INR quickly, it is unclear whether this offers any improvement in cessation of bleeding compared with PCCs. Two rat studies with head-to-head comparison of a 50 IU/kg of PCC versus 100 μg/kg of rVIIa found that while rVIIa was able to substantially reduce the PT, PCC was able to restore normal thrombin generation effectively in the context of warfarin.[159,160] There are no clear guidelines for the dosing of rVIIa whether in the reversal of warfarin or the new anticoagulants. Although the FDA-approved dosing for hemophilia can range as high as 100 μg/kg, studies have varied dosing from 15 to 100 μg/kg.[154,156] In one study rVIIa doses ranging from 5 μg/kg to 320 μg/kg in healthy male volunteers on vitamin K antagonists found that even a low 5 μg/kg dose was able to normalize the INR for 12 hours.[161]

There is even less evidence to suggest the benefit or use of rVIIa in the context of the new anticoagulants. In a randomized crossover trial, healthy human subjects were given dabigatran or rivaroxaban and their serum was treated with PCC, rVIIa, or a combination of PCC and rVIIa.[62,68,148] rVIIa was found to reverse the PT in these patients; however, it is unclear whether this would correlate to an increase in thrombin generation. A single rat and primate study in 2013 evaluated the use of rVIIa or PCC to reverse rivaroxaban-poisoned rats and baboons.[162] Both rVIIa and PCC were able to reverse the PT; however, only PCC was able to restore thrombin generation, suggesting that rVIIa may not be as useful in the reversal of bleeding in the novel anticoagulants.

HD

HD has been used as an antidote in poisonings involving drugs that are highly plasma bound or renally cleared. HD can be used as an adjunct to augment the renal clearance of drugs or in the context of renally cleared drugs in the setting of acute renal failure.[163] Of the oral anticoagulants, only dabigatran is highly renally eliminated and thus potentially amenable to HD. Apixaban and rivaroxaban are highly plasma protein bound and are not candidates for HD.[62] Case reports of successful HD to remove dabigatran in the incidence of acute bleeding have been described, although rebound may occur.[65,66,164–166] In a single phase I clinical trial of HD for removal of dabigatran, a single 4-hour high-flow, large-surface-area HD session could remove up to 50% of blood dabigatran, and this decrease was correlated with improved thrombosis.[167] However, this study was done in patients with end-stage renal disease, and all patients who received dialysis had pre-existing AV fistulas, not the typical patient in the ED that presents with dabigatran-associated bleeding. Nevertheless, multiple factors must come into play when considering the use of HD in dabigatran-associated hemorrhage. Augmented anticoagulation in this case suggests difficulty in placing a dialysis catheter, and patients who require such therapy may be unstable with intracranial hemorrhage or gastrointestinal hemorrhage and difficult to dialyze.[65,164]

SUMMARY

Anticoagulation has changed greatly with the introduction of new oral antiplatelet agents and factor-specific anticoagulants. The lack of required hematologic monitoring while on dabigatran and its efficacy in patients with nonvalvular atrial fibrillation made it an attractive alterative to warfarin, along with the subsequent market additions of rivaroxaban and apixaban. The inception of these drugs has led EPs with a quandary in the reversal of these agents. Traditional measures of vitamin K and FFP that have been long studied in warfarin reversal do not have much, if any, effect on the new anticoagulants.[62,64]

Complications associated with oral anticoagulation generally focus on the risk of bleeding. Although studies have shown that the risk of bleeding on the new anticoagulants generally is similar to that of warfarin, there remain multiple controversies in regard to management of acute and especially life-threatening bleeding on the new anticoagulants. PCCs have emerged as potential therapies for bleeding associated with direct thrombin inhibitors and factor Xa inhibitors, although there is much to discover in this field.[62,64,144,148,162,168]

Reversal of dabigatran, the only direct thrombin inhibitor available, has been particularly difficult, because it inhibits the last step in hemostasis, the generation of thrombin from prothrombin. Although there is little effect from PCC, anecdotal evidence suggests that PCC may have a role in dabigatran reversal in the life-threatening bleeding case.[64,142,144,145,148] In addition, because dabigatran is largely renally cleared, HD has emerged as a potential therapy in the case of bleeding, although patients must be relatively stable to tolerate the hours of dialysis, insertion of a temporary dialysis catheter, and dabigatran rebound.[65,66,164–167]

Promising antidotes on the horizon for both direct thrombin inhibitors and factor Xa inhibitors include antibodies to dabigatran and potential antidotes to both Xa inhibitors.[67,169] An antibody to dabigatran, anti-Dabi-fab, functions as a thrombin analogue and is highly specific for dabigatran, allowing it to bind to the antibody instead of thrombin. It has been shown in rats to reverse anticoagulation with improvement in TT and PTT.[67] Similarly, a synthetic factor Xa analogue with high affinity for factor Xa inhibitors has been shown to reverse anticoagulation in a rabbit model given rivaroxaban.[169]

Perhaps the best treatment of bleeding complications on the new anticoagulants is withdrawal of the drug and supportive care. As dabigatran and the factor Xa inhibitors have relatively short half-lives, holding the drug may be enough to mitigate bleeding.[62,68] However, patients presenting with severe bleeding in the ED may need more timely reversal and/or blood products. Currently, PCC has been recommended for emergent reversal of warfarin, dabigatran, and factor Xa inhibitors. One to two units of FFP are provided with 3-factor PCC forms if the intent is to reverse major bleeding, due to their minimal factor VII activity. The 4-factor PCC obviates this requirement. Because of these subtle differences between 3- and 4-factor PCC, it is important to understand local hospital pharmacy formularies to tailor the dosing and expected effect of PCC. rVIIa has been used in conjunction with PCC in reversal of the new anticoagulants, but it appears that although rVIIa is able to reverse the PT, thrombin generation is still limited, and PCC alone may be a better option in these patients.

REFERENCES

1. Hoffman R, Benz EJ, Silberstein L, et al. Hematology: basic principles and practice. 6th edition. Philadelphia: Churchill Livingstone; 2012.
2. Moser M, Ruef J, Peter K, et al. Ecarin clotting time but not aPTT correlates with PEG-hirudin plasma activity. J Thromb Thrombolysis 2001;12:165–9.
3. Nowak G. The ecarin clotting time, a universal method to quantify direct thrombin inhibitors. Pathophysiol Haemost Thromb 2003;33:173–83.
4. Metha R. Novel oral anticoagulants. Part II: direct thrombin inhibitors. Expert Rev Hematol 2010;3:351–61.
5. Favaloro EJ, Bonar R, Butler J, et al. Laboratory testing for the new oral anticoagulants: a review of current practice. Pathology 2013;45:435–7.
6. Nowak G. Clinical monitoring of hirudin and direct thrombin inhibitors. Semin Thromb Hemost 2001;27:537–41.
7. Tripodi A. The laboratory and the direct oral anticoagulants. Blood 2013;121: 4032–5.
8. Douxfils J, Mullier F, Robert S, et al. Impact of dabigatran on a large panel of routine or specific coagulation assays. Laboratory recommendations for monitoring of dabigatran etexilate. Thromb Haemost 2012;107:985–97.
9. Wardrop D, Keeling D. The story of the discovery of heparin and warfarin. Br J Haematol 2008;141:757–63.

10. Gomez-Outes A, Suarez-Gea M, Calvo-Rojas G, et al. Discovery of anticoagulant drugs: a historical perspective. Curr Drug Discov Technol 2012;9:83–104.
11. Ho SJ, Brighton TA. Ximelagatran: direct thrombin inhibitor. Vasc Health Risk Manag 2006;2:49–58.
12. Lee WM, Larrey D, Olsson R, et al. Hepatic findings in long-term clinical trials of ximelagatran. Drug Saf 2005;28:351–70.
13. Keisu M, Andersson TB. Drug-induced liver injury in humans: the case of ximelagatran. Handb Exp Pharmacol 2010;(196):407–18.
14. Connolly SJ, Ezekowitz MD, Yusuf S, et al. Dabigatran versus Warfarin in patients with atrial fibrillation. N Engl J Med 2009;361:1139–51.
15. Savi P, Nurden P, Nurden AT, et al. Clopidogrel: a review of its mechanism of action. Platelets 1998;9:251–5.
16. Herbert JM, Savi P. P2Y12, a new platelet ADP receptor, target of clopidogrel. Semin Vasc Med 2003;3:113–22.
17. Savi P, Zachayus J, Delesque-touchard N, et al. The active metabolite of Clopidogrel disrupts P2Y12 receptor oligomers and partitions. Proc Natl Acad Sci U S A 2006;103:11069–74.
18. Caplain H, Donat F, Gaud C, et al. Pharmacokinetics of clopidogrel. Semin Thromb Hemost 1999;25(Suppl 2):25–8.
19. Jakubowski JA, Winters KJ, Naganuma H, et al. Prasugrel: a novel thienopyridine antiplatelet agent. A review of preclinical and clinical studies and the mechanistic basis for its distinct antiplatelet profile. Cardiovasc Drug Rev 2007;25:357–74.
20. Shan J, Sun H. The discovery and development of prasugrel. Expert Opin Drug Discov 2013;8:897–905.
21. Freeman MK. Thienopyridine antiplatelet agents: focus on prasugrel. Consult Pharm 2010;25:241–57.
22. Norgard NB, Dinicolantonio JJ. Clopidogrel, prasugrel, or ticagrelor? A practical guide to use of antiplatelet agents in patients with acute coronary syndromes. Postgrad Med 2013;125:91–102.
23. Wiviott SD, Braunwald E, McCabe CH, et al. Prasugrel versus clopidogrel in patients with acute coronary syndromes. N Engl J Med 2007;357:2001–15.
24. Eli Lilly and Company. Effient (prasugrel) tablets [prescribing information]. Indianapolis (IN): Eli Lilly and Company; 2009.
25. Savi P, Herbert JM. Clopidogrel and ticlopidine: P2Y12 adenosine diphosphate-receptor antagonists for the prevention of atherothrombosis. Semin Thromb Hemost 2005;31:174–83.
26. Fox KA, Mehta SR, Peters R, et al. Benefits and risks of the combination of clopidogrel and aspirin in patients undergoing surgical revascularization for non-ST-elevation acute coronary syndrome: the Clopidogrel in Unstable angina to prevent Recurrent ischemic Events (CURE) Trial. Circulation 2004;110:1202–8.
27. Husted S, Emanuelsson H, Heptinstall S, et al. Pharmacodynamics, pharmacokinetics, and safety of the oral reversible P2Y12 antagonist AZD6140 with aspirin in patients with atherosclerosis: a double-blind comparison to clopidogrel with aspirin. Eur Heart J 2006;27:1038–47.
28. Abergel E, Nikolsky E. Ticagrelor: an investigational oral antiplatelet treatment for reduction of major adverse cardiac events in patients with acute coronary syndrome. Vasc Health Risk Manag 2010;6:963–77.
29. Cheng JW. Ticagrelor: oral reversible P2Y(12) receptor antagonist for the management of acute coronary syndromes. Clin Ther 2012;34:1209–20.

30. James S, Akerblom A, Cannon CP, et al. Comparison of ticagrelor, the first reversible oral P2Y(12) receptor antagonist, with clopidogrel in patients with acute coronary syndromes: rationale, design, and baseline characteristics of the PLATelet inhibition and patient Outcomes (PLATO) trial. Am Heart J 2009; 157:599–605.
31. Wallentin L, Becker RC, Budaj A, et al. Ticagrelor versus clopidogrel in patients with acute coronary syndromes. N Engl J Med 2009;361:1045–57.
32. AstraZeneca LP. Brilinta (ticagrelor) tablets, for oral use [prescribing information]. Wilmington (DE): AstraZeneca LP; 2011.
33. Murray DW, Jaques LB, Perrett TS, et al. Heparin and vascular occlusion. Can Med Assoc J 1936;35:621–2.
34. Murray GD, Best CH. The use of heparin in thrombosis. Ann Surg 1938;108: 163–77.
35. Björk I, Lindahl U. Mechanism of the anticoagulant action of heparin. Mol Cell Biochem 1982;48:161–82.
36. Chuang YJ, Swanson R, Raja SM, et al. Heparin enhances the specificity of antithrombin for thrombin and factor Xa independent of the reactive center loop sequence. Evidence for an exosite determinant of factor Xa specificity in heparin-activated antithrombin. J Biol Chem 2001;276:14961–71.
37. Garcia DA, Baglin TP, Weitz JI, et al. Parenteral anticoagulants: antithrombotic therapy and prevention of thrombosis, 9th ed: American college of chest physicians evidence-based clinical practice guidelines. Chest 2012;141:e24S–43S.
38. Mahadoo J, Heibert L, Jaques LB. Vascular sequestration of heparin. Thromb Res 1978;12:79–90.
39. Hiebert LM, Jaques LB. The observation of heparin on endothelium after injection. Thromb Res 1976;8:195–204.
40. Hiebert LM, Wice SM, McDuffie NM, et al. The heparin target organ–the endothelium. Studies in a rat model. Q J Med 1993;86:341–8.
41. Dawes J. Interactions of heparins in the vascular environment. Haemostasis 1993;23(Suppl 1):212–9.
42. Olsson P, Lagergren H, Ek S. The elimination from plasma of intravenous heparin. An experimental study on dogs and humans. Acta Med Scand 1963;173: 619–30.
43. De Swart CA, Nijmeyer B, Roelofs JM, et al. Kinetics of intravenously administered heparin in normal humans. Blood 1982;60:1251–8.
44. Reilly BR, Aggeler PM, Leong LS. Studies on the coumarin anticoagulant drugs: the pharmacodynamics of warfarin in man. J Clin Invest 1963;42:1542–51.
45. Kovacs MJ, Rodger M, Anderson DR, et al. Comparison of 10-mg and 5-mg warfarin initiation nomograms together with low-molecular-weight heparin for outpatient treatment of acute venous thromboembolism. A randomized, double-blind, controlled trial. Ann Intern Med 2003;138:714–9.
46. Tait RC, Sefcick A. A warfarin induction regimen for out-patient anticoagulation in patients with atrial fibrillation. Br J Haematol 1998;101:450–4.
47. Hirsh J, Fuster V, Ansell J, et al. American Heart Association/American college of cardiology foundation guide to warfarin therapy. J Am Coll Cardiol 2003;41: 1633–52.
48. Hauel NH, Nar H, Priepke H, et al. Structure-based design of novel potent nonpeptide thrombin inhibitors. J Med Chem 2002;45:1757–66.
49. Fiessinger J, Huisman M, Davidson B, et al. Ximelagatran vs low-molecular-weight heparin and warfarin for the treatment of deep vein thrombosis. JAMA 2013;293:681–9.

50. Olsson SB. Stroke prevention with the oral direct thrombin inhibitor ximelagatran compared with warfarin in patients with non-valvular atrial fibrillation (SPORTIF III): randomised controlled trial. Lancet 2003;362:1691–8.
51. Petersen P, Grind M, Adler J. Ximelagatran versus warfarin for stroke prevention in patients with nonvalvular atrial fibrillation. SPORTIF II: a dose-guiding, tolerability, and safety study. J Am Coll Cardiol 2003;41:1445–51.
52. Gurewich V. Ximelagatran — promises and concerns. JAMA 2013;293:9–12.
53. Van Ryn J, Goss A, Hauel N, et al. The discovery of dabigatran etexilate. Front Pharmacol 2013;4:12.
54. Wienen W, Stassen JM, Priepke H, et al. In-vitro profile and ex-vivo anticoagulant activity of the direct thrombin inhibitor dabigatran and its orally active prodrug, dabigatran etexilate. Thromb Haemost 2007;98:155–62.
55. Eriksson BI, Dahl OE, Ahnfelt L, et al. Dose escalating safety study of a new oral direct thrombin inhibitor, dabigatran etexilate, in patients undergoing total hip replacement: BISTRO I. J Thromb Haemost 2004;2:1573–80.
56. Berger R, Salhanick SD, Chase M, et al. Hemorrhagic complications in emergency department patients who are receiving dabigatran compared with warfarin. Ann Emerg Med 2013;61:475–9.
57. Graff J, Harder S. Anticoagulant therapy with the oral direct factor Xa inhibitors rivaroxaban, apixaban and edoxaban and the thrombin inhibitor dabigatran etexilate in patients with hepatic impairment. Clin Pharm 2013;52:243–54.
58. Cabral KP. Pharmacology of the new target-specific oral anticoagulants. J Thromb Haemost 2013;36:133–40.
59. Van Ryn J, Stangier J, Haertter S, et al. Dabigatran etexilate–a novel, reversible, oral direct thrombin inhibitor: interpretation of coagulation assays and reversal of anticoagulant activity. Thromb Haemost 2010;103:1116–27.
60. Baetz BE, Spinler SA. Dabigatran etexilate: an oral direct thrombin inhibitor for prophylaxis and treatment of thromboembolic diseases. Pharmacotherapy 2008;28:1354–73.
61. Eisert WG, Hauel N, Stangier J, et al. Dabigatran: an oral novel potent reversible nonpeptide inhibitor of thrombin. Arterioscler Thromb Vasc Biol 2010;30:1885–9.
62. Thigpen JL, Limdi NA. Reversal of oral anticoagulation. Pharmacotherapy 2013. [Epub ahead of print].
63. Ma TK, Yan BP, Lam YY. Dabigatran etexilate versus warfarin as the oral anticoagulant of choice? A review of clinical data. Pharmacol Ther 2011;129:185–94.
64. Kaatz S, Crowther M. Reversal of target-specific oral anticoagulants. J Thromb Thrombolysis 2013;36:195–202.
65. Chang DN, Dager WE, Chin AI. Removal of dabigatran by hemodialysis. Am J Kidney Dis 2013;61:487–9.
66. Esnault P, Gaillard PE, Cotte J, et al. Haemodialysis before emergency surgery in a patient treated with dabigatran. Br J Anaesth 2013;111:776–7.
67. Schiele F, van Ryn J, Canada K, et al. A specific antidote for dabigatran: functional and structural characterization. Blood 2013;121:3554–62.
68. Siegal DM, Cuker A. Reversal of novel oral anticoagulants in patients with major bleeding. J Thromb Thrombolysis 2013;35:391–8.
69. Rudd KM, Phillips EL. New oral anticoagulants in the treatment of pulmonary embolism: efficacy, bleeding risk, and monitoring. Thrombosis 2013;2013: 973710.
70. Boehringer Ingelheim Pharmaceuticals, Inc. Pradaxa (dabigatran etexilate mesylate) capsules for oral use [prescribing information]. Ridgefield (CT): Boehringer Ingelheim Pharmaceuticals, Inc; 2013.

71. Yeh CH, Fredenburgh JC, Weitz JI. Oral direct factor Xa inhibitors. Circ Res 2012;111:1069–78.
72. Chi L, Rogers KL, Uprichard AC, et al. The therapeutic potential of novel anticoagulants. Expert Opin Investig Drugs 1997;6:1591–605.
73. Walenga JM, Jeske WP, Hoppensteadt D, et al. Factor Xa inhibitors. Methods Mol Med 2004;93:95–117.
74. Tuszynski GP, Gasic TB, Gasic GJ. Isolation and characterization of antistasin. An inhibitor of metastasis and coagulation. J Biol Chem 1987;262:9718–23.
75. Harris LF, Rainey P, Castro-López V, et al. A microfluidic anti-Factor Xa assay device for point of care monitoring of anticoagulation therapy. Analyst 2013; 138:4769–76.
76. Lindhoff-Last E, Samama MM, Ortel TL, et al. Assays for measuring rivaroxaban: their suitability and limitations. Ther Drug Monit 2010;32:673–9.
77. Barrett YC, Wang Z, Frost C, et al. Clinical laboratory measurement of direct factor Xa inhibitors: anti-Xa assay is preferable to prothrombin time assay. Thromb Haemost 2010;104:1263–71.
78. Lassen MR, Gent M, Kakkar AK, et al. The effects of rivaroxaban on the complications of surgery after total hip or knee replacement: results from the RECORD programme. J Bone Joint Surg Br 2012;94:1573–8.
79. Turun S, Banghua L, Yuan Y, et al. A systematic review of rivaroxaban versus enoxaparin in the prevention of venous thromboembolism after hip or knee replacement. Thromb Res 2011;127:525–34.
80. Sarich TC, Peters G, Berkowitz SD, et al. Rivaroxaban: a novel oral anticoagulant for the prevention and treatment of several thrombosis-mediated conditions. Ann N Y Acad Sci 2013;1291:1–14.
81. Kubitza D, Becka M, Roth A, et al. The influence of age and gender on the pharmacokinetics and pharmacodynamics of rivaroxaban–an oral, direct Factor Xa inhibitor. J Clin Pharmacol 2013;53:249–55.
82. Weinz C, Schwarz T, Kubitza D, et al. Metabolism and excretion of rivaroxaban, an oral, direct factor Xa inhibitor, in rats, dogs, and humans. Drug Metab Dispos 2009;37:1056–64.
83. Kubitza D, Roth A, Becka M, et al. Effect of hepatic impairment on the pharmacokinetics and pharmacodynamics of a single dose of rivaroxaban - an oral, direct Factor Xa inhibitor. Br J Clin Pharmacol 2013;76:89–98.
84. Kubitza D, Becka M, Mueck W, et al. Effects of renal impairment on the pharmacokinetics, pharmacodynamics and safety of rivaroxaban, an oral, direct Factor Xa inhibitor. Br J Clin Pharmacol 2010;70:703–12.
85. Kubitza D, Becka M, Wensing G, et al. Safety, pharmacodynamics, and pharmacokinetics of BAY 59-7939–an oral, direct Factor Xa inhibitor–after multiple dosing in healthy male subjects. Eur J Clin Pharmacol 2005;61:873–80.
86. Janssen Pharmaceuticals, Inc. Xarelto (rivaroxaban) tablets, for oral use [Prescribing information]. Titusville (NJ): Janssen Pharmaceuticals, Inc; 2013.
87. Alquwaizani M, Buckley L, Adams C, et al. Anticoagulants: a review of the pharmacology, dosing, and complications. Curr Emerg Hosp Med Rep 2013;1: 83–97.
88. Keating GM. Apixaban: a review of its use for reducing the risk of stroke and systemic embolism in patients with nonvalvular atrial fibrillation. Drugs 2013; 73:825–43.
89. Frost C, Wang J, Nepal S, et al. Apixaban, an oral, direct factor Xa inhibitor: single dose safety, pharmacokinetics, pharmacodynamics and food effect in healthy subjects. Br J Clin Pharmacol 2013;75:476–87.

90. Raghavan N, Frost CE, Yu Z, et al. Apixaban metabolism and pharmacokinetics after oral administration to humans. Drug Metab Dispos 2009;37:74–81.

91. Bristol-Myers Squibb Company. ELIQUIS (apixaban) tablets for oral use [prescribing information]. Princeton (NJ): Bristol-Myers Squibb Company; 2012.

92. Makris M, Watson H. The management of coumarin-induced over-anticoagulation. Br J Haematol 2001;114:271–80.

93. Hanley JP. Warfarin reversal. J Clin Pathol 2004;57:1132–9.

94. Mehran R, Rao SV, Bhatt DL, et al. Standardized bleeding definitions for cardiovascular clinical trials: a consensus report from the Bleeding Academic Research Consortium. Circulation 2011;123:2736–47.

95. Schulman S, Kearon C. Definition of major bleeding in clinical investigations of antihemostatic medicinal products in non-surgical patients. J Thromb Haemost 2005;3:692–4.

96. Rubboli A, Becattini C, Verheugt FW. Incidence, clinical impact and risk of bleeding during oral anticoagulation therapy. World J Cardiol 2011;3:351–8.

97. Stehle S, Kirchheiner J, Lazar A, et al. Pharmacogenetics of oral anticoagulants: a basis for dose individualization. Clin Pharmacokinet 2008;47:565–94.

98. Choudhry NK, Anderson GM, Laupacis A, et al. Impact of adverse events on prescribing warfarin in patients with atrial fibrillation: matched pair analysis. BMJ 2006;332:141–5.

99. Connolly SJ, Wallentin L, Ezekowitz MD, et al. The long term multi-center observational study of dabigatran treatment in patients with atrial fibrillation: (RELY-ABLE) study. Circulation 2013;128:237–43.

100. Chiong JR, Cheung RJ. Long-term anticoagulation in the extreme elderly with the newer antithrombotics: safe or sorry? Korean Circ J 2013;43:287–92.

101. Fihn SD, Mcdonell M, Martin D, et al. Risk factors for complications of chronic anticoagulation a multicenter study. Ann Intern Med 1993;118:511–20.

102. Palareti G, Leali N, Coccheri S, et al. Hemorrhagic complications of oral anticoagulant therapy: results of a prospective multicenter study ISCOAT (Italian Study on Complications of Oral Anticoagulant Therapy). G Ital Cardiol 1997; 27:231–43 [in Italian].

103. Fang MC, Chang Y, Hylek EM, et al. Advanced age, anticoagulation intensity, and risk for intracranial hemorrhage among patients taking warfarin for atrial fibrillation. Ann Intern Med 2004;141:745–52.

104. Hylek EM, Evans-Molina C, Shea C, et al. Major hemorrhage and tolerability of warfarin in the first year of therapy among elderly patients with atrial fibrillation. Circulation 2007;115:2689–96.

105. Jacques L. Protamine - antagonist to heparin. Can Med Assoc J 1973;108: 1291–3.

106. Carr JA, Silverman N. The heparin-protamine interaction. A review. J Cardiovasc Surg (Torino) 1999;40:659–66.

107. Mochizuki T, Olson PJ, Szlam F, et al. Protamine reversal of heparin affects platelet aggregation and activated clotting time after cardiopulmonary bypass. Anesth Analg 1998;87:781–5.

108. Crowther MA, Berry LR, Monagle PT, et al. Mechanisms responsible for the failure of protamine to inactivate low-molecular-weight heparin. Br J Haematol 2002;116:178–86.

109. Ni Ainle F, Preston RJ, Jenkins PV, et al. Protamine sulfate down-regulates thrombin generation by inhibiting factor V activation. Blood 2009;114:1658–65.

110. Massonnet-Castel S, Pelissier E, Bara L, et al. Partial reversal of low molecular weight heparin (PK 10169) anti-Xa activity by protamine sulfate: in vitro and

in vivo study during cardiac surgery with extracorporeal circulation. Haemostasis 1986;16:139–46.

111. Van Ryn-McKenna J, Cai L, Ofosu FA, et al. Neutralization of enoxaparine-induced bleeding by protamine sulfate. Thromb Haemost 1990;63:271–4.

112. Hull R, Hirsh J, Jay R, et al. Different intensities of oral anticoagulant therapy in the treatment of proximal-vein thrombosis. N Engl J Med 1982;307:1676–81.

113. Baker RI, Coughlin PB, Gallus AS, et al. Warfarin reversal: consensus guidelines, on behalf of the Australasian Society of Thrombosis and Haemostasis. Med J Aust 2004;181:492–7.

114. Schulman S, Beyth RJ, Kearon C, et al. Hemorrhagic complications of anticoagulant and thrombolytic treatment: American College of Chest physicians evidence-based clinical practice guidelines (8th edition). Chest 2008;133: 257S–98S.

115. Watson HG, Baglin T, Laidlaw SL, et al. A comparison of the efficacy and rate of response to oral and intravenous Vitamin K in reversal of over-anticoagulation with warfarin. Br J Haematol 2001;115:145–9.

116. Raj G, Kumar R, McKinney P. Time course of reversal of anticoagulant effect of Warfarin by intravenous and subcutaneous phytonadione. Arch Intern Med 1999;159:2721–5.

117. Lubetsky A, Yonath H, Olchovsky D, et al. Comparison of oral vs intravenous phytonadione (Vitamin K 1) in patients with excessive anticoagulation. Arch Intern Med 2003;163:2469–73.

118. McMillian WD, Rogers FB. Management of prehospital antiplatelet and anticoagulant therapy in traumatic head injury: a review. J Trauma 2009;66:942–50.

119. Naidech AM, Bernstein RA, Levasseur K, et al. Platelet activity and outcome after intracerebral hemorrhage. Ann Neurol 2009;65:352–6.

120. Naidech AM, Rosenberg NF, Bernstein RA, et al. Aspirin use or reduced platelet activity predicts craniotomy after intracerebral hemorrhage. Neurocrit Care 2011;15:442–6.

121. Washington CW, Schuerer DJ, Grubb RL. Platelet transfusion: an unnecessary risk for mild traumatic brain injury patients on antiplatelet therapy. J Trauma 2011;71:358–63.

122. Ivascu FA, Howells GA, Junn FS, et al. Predictors of mortality in trauma patients with intracranial hemorrhage on preinjury aspirin or clopidogrel. J Trauma 2008; 65:785–8.

123. Creutzfeldt CJ, Weinstein JR, Longstreth WT, et al. Prior antiplatelet therapy, platelet infusion therapy, and outcome after intracerebral hemorrhage. J Stroke Cerebrovasc Dis 2010;18:221–8.

124. Spiess BD. Platelet transfusions: the science behind safety, risks and appropriate applications. Best Pract Res Clin Anaesthesiol 2010;24:65–83.

125. Caudrillier A, Kessenbrock K, Gilliss BM, et al. Platelets induce neutrophil extracellular traps in transfusion-related acute lung injury. J Clin Invest 2012;122: 2661–71.

126. Nishijima DK, Zehtabchi S, Berrong J, et al. Utility of platelet transfusion in adult patients with traumatic intracranial hemorrhage and preinjury antiplatelet use: a systematic review. J Trauma Acute Care Surg 2012;72:1658–63.

127. O'Shaughnessy DF, Atterbury C, Bolton Maggs P, et al. Guidelines for the use of fresh-frozen plasma, cryoprecipitate and cryosupernatant. Br J Haematol 2004; 126:11–28.

128. DomBourian M, Holland L. Optimal use of fresh frozen plasma. J Infus Nurs 2012;35:28–32.

129. Tavares M, DiQuattro P, Nolette N, et al. Reduction in plasma transfusion after enforcement of transfusion guidelines. Transfusion 2011;51:754–61.
130. Abdel-Wahab OI, Healy B, Dzik WH. Effect of fresh-frozen plasma transfusion on prothrombin time and bleeding in patients with mild coagulation abnormalities. Transfusion 2006;46:1279–85.
131. Holland LL, Brooks JP. Toward rational fresh frozen plasma transfusion the effect of plasma transfusion on coagulation test results. Am J Clin Pathol 2006;126: 133–9.
132. Keeling D, Baglin T, Tait C, et al. Guidelines on oral anticoagulation with warfarin - fourth edition. Br J Haematol 2011;154:311–24.
133. Reutter JC, Sanders KF, Brecher ME, et al. Incidence of allergic reactions with fresh frozen plasma or cryo-supernatant plasma in the treatment of thrombotic thrombocytopenic purpura. J Clin Apher 2001;16:134–8.
134. Franchini M, Lippi G. Prothrombin complex concentrates: an update. Blood Transfus 2010;8:149–54.
135. Patanwala AE, Acquisto NM, Erstad BL. Prothrombin complex concentrate for critical bleeding. Ann Pharmacother 2011;45:990–9.
136. Ferreira J, Delossantos M. The clinical use of prothrombin complex concentrate. J Emerg Med 2013;44:1201–10.
137. Toth P, Van Veen JJ, Robinson K, et al. Real world usage of PCC to "rapidly" correct warfarin induced coagulopathy. Blood Transfus 2012. [Epub ahead of print].
138. Khorsand N, Giepmans L, Meijer K, et al. A low fixed dose of prothrombin complex concentrate is cost effective in emergency reversal of vitamin K antagonists. Haematologica 2013;98(6):65–7.
139. Imberti D, Magnacavallo A, Dentali F, et al. Emergency reversal of anticoagulation with vitamin K antagonists with 3-factor prothrombin complex concentrates in patients with major bleeding. J Thromb Thrombolysis 2013;36:102–8.
140. Hickey M, Gatien M, Taljaard M, et al. Outcomes of urgent warfarin reversal using fresh frozen plasma versus prothrombin complex concentrate in the emergency department. Circulation 2013;128:360–4.
141. Ogawa S, Szlam F, Ohnishi T, et al. A comparative study of prothrombin complex concentrates and fresh-frozen plasma for warfarin reversal under static and flow conditions. Thromb Haemost 2011;106:1215–23.
142. Kalus JS. Pharmacologic interventions for reversing the effects of oral anticoagulants. Am J Health Syst Pharm 2013;70:S12–21.
143. Baggs JH, Patanwala AE, Williams EM, et al. Dosing of 3-factor prothrombin complex concentrate for international normalized ratio reversal. Ann Pharmacother 2012;46:51–6.
144. Dumkow LE, Voss JR, Peters M, et al. Reversal of dabigatran-induced bleeding with a prothrombin complex concentrate and fresh frozen plasma. Am J Health Syst Pharm 2012;69:1646–50.
145. Wychowski MK, Kouides PA. Dabigatran-induced gastrointestinal bleeding in an elderly patient with moderate renal impairment. Ann Pharmacother 2012; 46:e10.
146. Truumees E, Gaudu T, Dieterichs C, et al. Epidural hematoma and intraoperative hemorrhage in a spine trauma patient on Pradaxa (dabigatran). Spine (Phila Pa 1976) 2012;37:E863–5.
147. Pragst I, Zeitler SH, Doerr B, et al. Reversal of dabigatran anticoagulation by prothrombin complex concentrate (Beriplex P/N) in a rabbit model. J Thromb Haemost 2012;10:1841–8.

148. Marlu R, Hodaj E, Paris A, et al. Effect of non-specific reversal agents on antico-agulant activity of dabigatran and rivaroxaban: a randomised crossover ex vivo study in healthy volunteers. Thromb Haemost 2012;108:217–24.
149. Eerenberg ES, Kamphuisen PW, Sijpkens MK, et al. Reversal of rivaroxaban and dabigatran by prothrombin complex concentrate: a randomized, placebo-controlled, crossover study in healthy subjects. Circulation 2011;124:1573–9.
150. Dichgans M, Ell C, Endres M, et al. Recommendations for the emergency man-agement of complications associated with the new direct oral anticoagulants (DOACs), apixaban, dabigatran and rivaroxaban. Clin Res Cardiol 2013;102: 399–412.
151. Kaatz S, Kouides PA, Garcia DA, et al. Guidance on the emergent reversal of oral thrombin and factor Xa inhibitors. Am J Hematol 2012;87(Suppl 1):S141–5.
152. Neal MD, Marsh A, Marino R, et al. Massive transfusion. Arch Surg 2013;147: 563–71.
153. Mamtani R, Nascimento B, Rizoli S, et al. The utility of recombinant factor VIIa as a last resort in trauma. World J Emerg Surg 2012;7(Suppl 1):S7.
154. Lin Y, Stanworth S, Birchall J, et al. Recombinant factor VIIa for the prevention and treatment of bleeding in patients without haemophilia. Cochrane Database Syst Rev 2011;(2):CD005011.
155. Levi M, Levy JH, Andersen HF, et al. Safety of recombinant activated factor VII in randomized clinical trials. N Engl J Med 2010;363:1791–800.
156. Silva IR, Provencio JJ. Intracerebral hemorrhage in patients receiving oral anti-coagulation therapy. J Intensive Care Med 2013. [Epub ahead of print].
157. Freeman WD, Brott TG, Barrett KM, et al. Recombinant factor VIIa for rapid reversal of warfarin anticoagulation in acute intracranial hemorrhage. Mayo Clin Proc 2004;79:1495–500.
158. Sørensen B, Johansen P, Nielsen GL, et al. Reversal of the international normal-ized ratio with recombinant activated factor VII in central nervous system bleeding during warfarin thromboprophylaxis: clinical and biochemical aspects. Blood Coagul Fibrinolysis 2003;14:469–77.
159. Dickneite G. Prothrombin complex concentrate versus recombinant factor VIIa for reversal of coumarin anticoagulation. Thromb Res 2007;119:643–51.
160. Tanaka KA, Szlam F, Dickneite G, et al. Effects of prothrombin complex concen-trate and recombinant activated factor VII on vitamin K antagonist induced anticoagulation. Thromb Res 2008;122:117–23.
161. Erhardtsen E, Nony P, Dechavanne M, et al. The effect of recombinant factor VIIa (NovoSeven) in healthy volunteers receiving acenocoumarol to an Interna-tional Normalized Ratio above 2.0. Blood Coagul Fibrinolysis 1998;9:741–8.
162. Perzborn E, Gruber A, Tinel H, et al. Reversal of rivaroxaban anticoagulation by haemostatic agents in rats and primates. Thromb Haemost 2013;110:162–72.
163. Bayliss G. Dialysis in the poisoned patient. Hemodial Int 2010;14:158–67.
164. McLellan AJ, Schlaich M. Dabigatran elimination: is haemodialysis effective? Thromb Haemost 2013;4:580–1.
165. Chen BC, Sheth NR, Dadzie KA, et al. Hemodialysis for the treatment of pulmo-nary hemorrhage from dabigatran overdose. Am J Kidney Dis 2013;62:591–4.
166. Liesenfeld KH, Staab A, Härtter S, et al. Pharmacometric characterization of dabigatran hemodialysis. Clin Pharmacokinet 2013;52:453–62.
167. Khadzhynov D, Wagner F, Formella S, et al. Effective elimination of dabigatran by haemodialysis. A phase I single-centre study in patients with end-stage renal disease. Thromb Haemost 2013;109:596–605.

168. Lazo-Langner A, Lang ES, Douketis J. Clinical review: clinical management of new oral anticoagulants: a structured review with emphasis on the reversal of bleeding complications. Crit Care 2013;17:230.
169. Lu G, DeGuzman FR, Hollenbach SJ, et al. A specific antidote for reversal of anticoagulation by direct and indirect inhibitors of coagulation factor Xa. Nat Med 2013;19:446–51.

Toxin-Induced Cardiovascular Failure

David H. Jang, MD, MSc[a],*, Meghan B. Spyres, MD[b],
Lindsay Fox, MD[c], Alex F. Manini, MD, MS[d]

KEYWORDS

- β-blocker • Cardiac arrest • Cardiac injury • Calcium channel blocker • Digoxin
- Dysrhythmia • Overdose

KEY POINTS

- Adverse cardiovascular events represent an immediate life threat in the setting of acute drug overdose and poisoning.
- Drugs of abuse, amphetamine-like substances, dietary supplements, and weight-reduction agents are common causes of toxicologic tachycardia.
- Cardioactive steroids, β-adrenergic antagonists, and calcium channel blockers are important causes of toxicologic bradycardia to consider.
- High-dose insulin euglycemia should be instituted in all cases of severe β-adrenergic antagonist and calcium channel blocker poisoning.
- In cases of cardiac arrest from a suspected poisoning, consider administration of intravenous lipid emulsion during the resuscitation.

INTRODUCTION: NATURE OF THE PROBLEM

Patients involved with poisoning or drug overdose, compared with cardiac clinical trial patients, are typically younger with less cardiovascular burden. Despite this, adverse cardiovascular events (ACVE) comprise a large portion of the morbidity and mortality in drug overdose emergencies reported in the American Association of Poison Control Centers National Poisoning Data System (NPDS).[1] In 2011, among over 2.7 million poisonings reported in NPDS, cardiovascular drugs were involved in 3.7% of exposures,

[a] Division of Medical Toxicology, Department of Emergency Medicine, School of Medicine, New York University, 462 First Avenue, 27th Street, Room A340, New York, NY 10016, USA; [b] Emergency Medicine Residency, School of Medicine, New York University, 462 First Avenue, 27th Street, Room A340, New York, NY 10016, USA; [c] Emergency Medicine Residency, Icahn School of Medicine at Mount Sinai, One Gustave L. Levy Place, New York, NY 10029-657, USA; [d] Division of Medical Toxicology, Department of Emergency Medicine, Elmhurst Hospital Center, Icahn School of Medicine at Mount Sinai, One Gustave L. Levy Place, New York, NY 10029-657, USA
* Corresponding author.
E-mail address: kiteboarder.dj@gmail.com

Emerg Med Clin N Am 32 (2014) 79–102
http://dx.doi.org/10.1016/j.emc.2013.10.003
0733-8627/14/$ – see front matter © 2014 Elsevier Inc. All rights reserved.

yet accounted for a disproportionate 10.8% of all reported poisoning fatalities, and were among the top three substance categories with most rapidly increasing exposures. Drug-related ACVEs include the following: myocardial injury (by biomarker or electrocardiogram [ECG] evidence); shock (hypotension or hypoperfusion requiring vasopressors); ventricular dysrhythmias (ventricular tachycardia/fibrillation, torsades des pointes); or cardiac arrest (loss of pulse requiring cardiopulmonary resuscitation).[2,3] Recently, the incidence of ACVE from hospitalized drug overdose patients was estimated to be as high as 16.9%.[4] This high morbidity implies that emergency practitioners should be particularly adept at caring for these potentially critical patients.

ADVERSE CARDIOVASCULAR EVENTS

Based on the revised clinical classification of myocardial infarction, mechanisms and pathophysiology of drug-induced myocardial injury are outlined in **Table 1**.[4,5] Drugs may cause myocardial injury through a variety of mechanisms. Myocardial injury is the most common ACVE that occurs in overdose.[4] Serum cardiac troponin I is released into the bloodstream after myocardial cell necrosis or injury.[6] Drug-induced shock is the second most common ACVE that occurs because of drug overdose.[4] A conceptual model of how drug overdose may lead to shock is illustrated in **Fig. 1**, which may manifest as cardiogenic, distributive, or hypovolemic shock.

Sudden cardiac death in a young healthy population is statistically most likely to be drug-related.[7,8] Ventricular dysrhythmia is the third most common ACVE that occurs in drug overdose.[4] Mechanisms and pathophysiology of overdose-related dysrhythmia are outlined in **Table 1**. Ventricular fibrillation is the final common pathway of most sudden cardiac deaths, but rhythm disturbances may begin with monomorphic or polymorphic ventricular tachycardia (VT) and torsades des pointes (TdP), a form of polymorphic VT that is identified characteristically on the ECG.[9] Poisoning is an infrequent cause of cardiac arrest in elderly patients, but is the leading cause of cardiac arrest in patients younger than 40 years of age.[1,10,11]

Table 1		
Mechanisms and pathophysiology of ACVEs after drug overdose		
ACVE	**Mechanism**	**Pathophysiology**
Myocardial injury	Decreased myocardial O_2 supply	Coronary artery vasospasm Decreased O_2 carrying capacity
	Increased myocardial O_2 demand	Hyperthermia, agitation Tachycardia, hypertension
	Myocardial cell death	Inhibition of oxidative phosphorylation
Shock	Decreased intravascular volume	Fluid losses Gastrointestinal hemorrhage
	Decreased SVR	Vasodilation
	Diminished myocardial contractility	β-Adrenergic antagonism Ca^{2+}/Na^+ channel blockade
Ventricular dysrhythmia	Myocardial sensitization	QT prolongation/dispersion K^+ channel blockade
	Triggered beats	Premature contractions Intracellular Ca^{2+} release

Abbreviations: ACVE, adverse cardiovascular events; SVR, systemic vascular resistance.

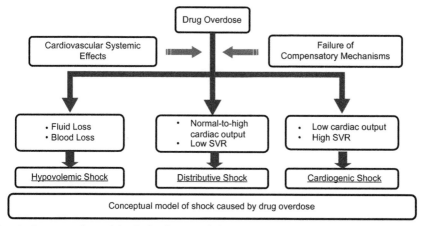

Fig. 1. Conceptual model of shock caused by drug overdose. SVR, systemic vascular resistance.

TOXICOLOGIC TACHYCARDIA

Under normal circumstances, the sinoatrial (SA) node is the most rapidly firing cardiac pacemaker. However, some drugs can speed the rate of rise during phase 4 of the action potential. Alternatively, drugs may inappropriately increase the firing rate of extrinsic pacemakers. The resultant toxicologic tachycardia may prove either disastrous or life-saving, depending on the clinical circumstances. In addition, physiologic causes of tachycardia may result from drug toxicity, such as anxiety, dehydration, pain, or hyperthermia. The most significant toxicologic causes of tachycardia include cyclic antidepressants (CA), sympathomimetics, anticholinergics, methylxanthines, and other agents that may open cardiac sodium channels.

In CA overdose, sodium channel blockade is also accompanied by antimuscarinic effects and α-adrenoceptor antagonism. The result is a rhythm with a wide QRS complex that may resemble VT. The duration of the QRS has also been studied as a marker of prognosis. A landmark prospective study in CA poisoned patients demonstrated that a QRS duration less than 100 milliseconds was an indicator of good prognosis, whereas a QRS greater than 100 milliseconds was associated with increased risk of seizures, and greater than 160 milliseconds was associated with increased risk of ventricular dysrhythmia.[12] CAs seem to preferentially antagonize the right-sided intraventricular conductive system. Delayed depolarization of the right ventricle results in several ECG findings that are specific to the CA poisoning, which include a right axis deviation between 130 and 270 degrees, and a terminal 40 milliseconds R-wave in aVR.[13] While later studies found varying degrees of sensitivity and specificity for these markers in CA poisoning, they remain valuable indicators to actively seek out and address. Additional ECG manifestations of right ventricular depolarization delay include the Brugada pattern and right bundle branch block.[14]

Sympathomimetics encompass drugs of abuse (eg, cocaine, amphetamines, "bath salts"), and amphetamine-like substances, which include decongestants (eg, pseudoephedrine), dietary supplements (eg, ephedra, ma huang), and weight-reduction agents (eg, phentermine and fenfluramine ["phen-fen"], phenylpropanolamine). Increased central nervous system (CNS) synaptic terminal output of norepinephrine leads to α- and β-adrenoceptor agonism at the postsynaptic receptor, which clinically results in tachycardia and hypertension. Additionally, ST segment changes may result from coronary artery vasoconstriction leading to myocardial injury. Sympathomimetics may generate early after depolarizations, which can lead to malignant cardiac dysrhythmias.

Anticholinergic toxicity results in tachycardia by reducing the baseline suppressive vagal tone on the SA node. Common anticholinergic toxins include such drugs as diphenhydramine and CAs, and such plants as *Datura stramonium* (Jimson weed). Clinical hallmarks of anticholinergic toxicity include skin flushing, drying of sweat glands and mucous membranes, mild hyperthermia, decreased bowel sounds, urinary retention, and altered mental status. Management includes supportive care and antidotal administration of physostigmine (contraindications include cardiac conduction abnormalities, such as a prolonged QRS or PR interval in severe cases of central and peripheral toxicity).

Methylxanthines are plant-derived alkaloids from tea leaves, coffee beans, and cacao beans. Commonly encountered methylxanthines include caffeine, theophylline, and theobromine. Structurally, they are all variants of the compound xanthine and similar to adenosine, an inhibitory CNS neurotransmitter. The mechanism of toxicity includes adenosine receptor antagonism, release of endogenous epinephrine from the adrenals, histamine release in the respiratory smooth muscle, and phosphodiesterase inhibition. Antagonism of adenosine receptors in the CNS results in agitation and seizures. Endogenous epinephrine release causes cardiac and CNS excitation along with gastrointestinal (eg, vomiting) and metabolic (eg, hypokalemia, hyperthermia) effects. Histaminergic effects in respiratory smooth muscle results in bronchodilation. Phosphodiesterase inhibition results in elevated intracellular cAMP, which enhances adrenergic effects (ie, cardiac stimulation, CNS excitation). Cardiovascular manifestations of methylxanthine toxicity include tachycardia, palpitations, premature ventricular contractions, and rarely dysrhythmias. Additionally, severe hypokalemia may complicate the clinical presentation with associated ECG changes. Sinus tachycardia is the most common ECG finding, followed by multifocal atrial tachycardia, and rarely myocardial injury. Cardiac complications are the main cause of death in methylxanthine poisoning; thus, management of cardiovascular toxicity should be aggressive. Gastrointestinal decontamination often includes multidose activated charcoal (MDAC). Supraventricular tachycardia is managed with calcium channel blockers (CCBs) or β-adrenergic antagonists (BAAs, β-blockers). Ventricular dysrhythmias should be treated with lidocaine or β-blockers. Supportive care should include blood pressure support and correction of electrolyte anomalies. Severe toxicity warrants extracorporeal removal with hemodialysis or hemoperfusion (if available).

Sodium channel activators or openers, such as aconitine or monkshood, are popular in Asian herbal medicine. These agents have severe cardiovascular manifestations in overdose. Aconite, the active alkaloid in *Aconitum* spp., may cause cardiac arrest at doses as low as 2 mg.[15] The mechanism of toxicity is sodium channel opening, resulting in prolonged myocardial sodium current influx and slowed repolarization. Initial bradycardia caused by central parasympathetic stimulation causes vulnerability to subsequent early after depolarizations leading to VT, ventricular fibrillation, or torsades des pointes. Supportive management should include aggressive measures, such as orogastric lavage, atropine for bradycardia, and cardiac pacing. Cardiac arrest may require prolonged cardiopulmonary resuscitation with consideration of cardiac bypass or placement of a balloon pump until toxicity resolves.

TOXICOLOGIC BRADYCARDIA

Bradycardia is defined as a ventricular rate of less than 60 beats per minute. Although this can be a normal variant in well-conditioned subjects, bradycardia usually arises from two basic disturbances. The first disturbance is from depression of the dominant pacemaker, typically the sinus node, causing sinus bradycardia. The other disturbance is a block in the conduction system where impulses are incompletely carried to the atrioventricular (AV) node and the ventricular tissues. The causes of bradycardia are diverse and can include hypothermia, myocardial infarction, and pharmacologic agents.

Medications that can cause significant bradycardia include the agents in **Box 1**. Most of the drugs causing bradycardia are from the cardiovascular drug class. Although many of the medications are safe when dosed appropriately, there are a few types within the cardiovascular drug class associated with significant morbidity and mortality in the overdose setting that is important for the clinician to be aware of. The two major classes of importance are the BAAs or β-blockers and the calcium channel antagonist or CCBs. Although other agents such as cardioactive steroids (ie, digoxin) and α_2-adrenergic agents (ie, clonidine, tizanidine) are associated with toxicity, BAAs and CCBs are responsible for most of the reported deaths related to cardioactive medication poisoning.

A brief discussion of the cardiac cycle is critical to understand the mechanism of β-blockers and CCBs along with the various treatment modalities discussed in this article. The normal cardiac cycle consists of a complex series of ion movements that result in myocyte depolarization and repolarization. In normal conditions the heart rate is determined by the SA node. Pacemaker cell depolarization is caused by either rhythmic release of calcium from the sarcoplasmic reticulum or inward cation current. During systole, voltage sensitive L-type calcium channels located on the membrane myocyte open. This allows calcium to flow down its concentration gradient into the myocyte. The local increase in calcium concentration triggers the ryanodine receptors to release more calcium that results in binding with troponin C and allows actin-myosin interaction with subsequent myocyte contraction. During diastole, several pumps actively remove calcium from the cytosol that results in dissociation of calcium from troponin with relaxation.

β-adrenergic receptors are divided into β_1, β_2, and β_3 subtypes. In normal individuals, about 80% of all cardiac β-receptors are β_1 and 20% are β_2, with a very small number of β_3 receptors.[16] β_1 adrenergic receptors mediate increased inotropy involving cAMP and various protein kinases. Stimulation of this receptor subtype also increases chronotrophy. Acute β-adrenergic stimulation improves cardiac function but chronic stimulation results in several detrimental effects, such as dysrhythmias and impaired contraction. BAAs competitively antagonize the effects of catecholamines at the β-receptors to blunt the chronotropic and inotropic response to catecholamines. β_2-adrenergic receptors mediate smooth muscle relaxation in various

Box 1
Agents causing bradycardia
α_2-Adrenergic agonists (eg, clonidine, tizanidine)
β-Adrenergic antagonists
Calcium channel blockers
Cardioactive steroids (eg, digoxin, foxglove, yellow oleander)
Cholinergic agents (eg, organophosphates, carbamates, sarin)
Ergot alkaloids
Opioids

tissues, such as the lung and peripheral vascular tissue, so stimulation of this receptor subtype leads to bronchodilation and peripheral vasodilation. β_3-adrenergic receptor mediates lipolysis in adipose tissue and thermogenesis in skeletal muscles.

BAAs are commonly used to treat hypertension, tachydysrhythmias, and coronary artery disease. Other indications include congestive heart failure, migraine headaches, anxiety, and hyperthyroidism. Within this diverse class of medications are certain BAAs that contain additional properties that are important for clinician to be aware (**Table 2**). Propranolol is the very lipid-soluble and considered the most toxic of the BAAs. Propranolol has membrane-stabilizing effects that result in inhibition of fast sodium channels similar to what is seen with tricyclic antidepressants, resulting in seizures and dysrhythmias.[17,18] Sotalol is another BAA with additional potassium channel blocking, resulting in QT prolongation and an additional TdP liability.

CCBs are a commonly used cardiovascular drug class. The primary action of all CCBs available in the United States is antagonism of the L-type voltage-gated calcium channels.[19] Although CCBs are often structurally classified into three groups (**Box 2**), it is often more logical to classify them into two groups based on their mechanism of action: nondihydropyridine and dihydropyridine CCBs. The former includes verapamil and diltiazem, whereas the latter includes such drugs as nifedipine and amlodipine. Each group binds a slightly different region of the α_{1c} subunit of the calcium channel and thus has different affinities for the various L-type calcium channels, both in the myocardium and the vascular smooth muscle. Verapamil and diltiazem have inhibitory effects at the SA and AV nodal tissue and are commonly used to achieve rate control in atrial flutter and atrial fibrillation and abolishing supraventricular reentrant tachycardias. The dihydropyridines have little effect on the myocardium at therapeutic doses and act primarily at the peripheral vascular tissue to produce resulting in dilatation. They are often used for various conditions with increased vascular tone, such as hypertension, migraine headaches, and postintracranial bleed vasospasm.

The clinical hallmarks of BAA and CCB poisoning are primarily an extension of their therapeutic effects and include hypotension and bradycardia from the combination of myocardial depression and peripheral vasodilation. A variety of myocardial conduction abnormalities may also occur with significant poisonings (idioventricular rhythms, complete heart block, and junctional escape rhythms).[20,21] Certain BAAs, such as sotalol,

Table 2		
Selected β-adrenergic antagonists		
Selective β$_1$-Antagonists	**Nonselective β$_1$- and β$_2$-Antagonists**	**β$_1$- and β$_2$-Antagonists with α$_1$-Antagonism**
Acebutolol[a,b]	Carteolol[b,c]	Carvedilol[a]
Atenolol	Levobunolol[c]	Labetalol[a,b]
Betaxolol[a,c]	Metipranol[c]	
Bisoprolol	Naldolol	
Esmolol	Oxprenolol[a,b]	
Metoprolol[a]	Penbutolol[b]	
	Pindolol[a,b]	
	Propanolol[a]	
	Sotalol[d]	
	Timolol[c]	

[a] Membrane stabilizing (sodium channel blocking) activity.
[b] Intrinsic sympathomimetic (agonist) activity.
[c] Available as an antiglaucoma formulation.
[d] Potassium channel blocking activity.

Box 2
Calcium channel blockers
Benzothiazepine
Diltiazem[a]
Dihydropyridines
First generation
Nicardipine
Nifedipine
Second generation
Felodipine
Isradipine
Nimodipine
Nisoldipine
Third generation
Amlodipine
Clevidipine
Phenylalkylamine
Verapamil[a]
[a] Sodium channel inhibition.

block the potassium rectifier channel, which can lead to QT prolongation, resulting in torsades de pointes.[22] The negative inotropic effects may be so profound, particularly with verapamil, that ventricular contraction may be completely ablated. Dihydropyridines, particularly amlodipine, may increase nitric oxide (NO) release, contributing to toxicity. Early symptoms may include dizziness and lightheadedness. Patients with severe poisoning may manifest syncope, altered mental status, coma, and sudden death.[23,24] Patients may also present asymptomatic with early ingestions but deteriorate rapidly into severe cardiogenic shock, especially with large ingestions of sustained-release preparations.

Although BAA and CCB poisoning are indistinguishable in many cases, there are some features that may aid in separating the two drug classes. CCB poisoning may cause hyperglycemia, caused by the blockage of pancreatic L-type calcium channels in the pancreas resulting in decreased insulin secretion.[25] This is in contrast to BAAs, which can cause hypoglycemia, although this is a less reliable presentation in toxicity. Another feature that may be seen in isolated CCB poisoning is preservation of mental status. BAA poisoning is commonly associated with lethargy and depressed mental status. The mechanism for this difference is not entirely clear, but research points to calcium channel–mediated apoptosis, and CCBs may preserve CNS function. Distinguishing between the two classes is not essential and management should be initiated based on the premise that either or both drug classes may be involved.

TOXICOLOGIC VASOCONSTRICTION

Toxicologic vasoconstriction can result from exposure to numerous substances, including drugs of abuse, such cocaine and amphetamines, and dieting drugs and antimigraine medications. Toxicologic vasoconstriction often occurs through direct stimulation of α-adrenergic receptors, although it can also occur indirectly by actions on other receptors causing release of endogenous catecholamines or inhibition of vasodilatory neuropeptides. It is often seen as part of a sympathomimetic toxidrome consisting of hypertension; tachycardia (or sometimes reflex bradycardia); hyperthermia; agitation; diaphoresis; and seizures. Toxicologic vasoconstriction may directly cause end-organ damage by local ischemia or infarction of nearly any part of the body, or it may cause damage by the effects of severe hypertension.

Cocaine is a tropane alkaloid derived from the leaves of the coca plant with anesthetic and sympathomimetic activity. Cocaine is a schedule II substance sometimes used as a local anesthetic and vasoconstrictive agent, particularly in otolaryngologic procedures. It is more commonly encountered as a drug of abuse that can be nasally insufflated, smoked, ingested, or injected. In 2011, a national survey found that 14.3% of Americans over the age of 12 had used cocaine in their lifetime.[26] Cocaine was related to 488,101 emergency department visits in 2010.[27] Cocaine blocks the reuptake of dopamine, epinephrine, norepinephrine, and serotonin, and produces a sympathomimetic toxidrome with profound vasospasm. The vasoconstrictive effects of cocaine have been shown to produce deleterious effects in nearly every organ system. The danger of cocaine's vasoactive effects is heightened by associated hypercoagulability, impaired thrombolysis, and accelerated atherosclerosis. In particular, the hypertension, tachycardia, and increased oxygen demand, combined with vasoconstriction, atherosclerosis, and a hypercoagulable state create a particular significant cardiovascular threat. Cocaine can cause myocardial ischemia and infarction even in young adults, and may be responsible for 25% of myocardial infarctions in adults younger than 45 years.[28] Cocaine has been associated with ischemia and infarction of the brain, eyes, nasal septum, heart, lungs, intestines, colon, spleen, kidney, limbs, and skin. In pregnant women cocaine use is associated with intrauterine growth restriction by vasoconstriction of fetal blood supply.[29] The hypertension resulting from vasoconstriction can also cause nontraumatic hemorrhage. This is particularly dangerous in the CNS, where cocaine has been noted to precipitate subarachnoid, intraventricular, and intraparenchymal bleeding.[30]

Amphetamines refer to the class of substances structurally related to phenylethylamine. This class includes the well-known drugs of abuse methamphetamine and methylenedioxymethamphetamine, hundreds of structurally similar designer amphetamines, and synthetic cathinones, or "bath salts." Synthetic cathinones in particular have experienced an explosion in popularity in recent years.[31] Illicit use of amphetamines was estimated to be related to 159,783 emergency department visits in 2010.[27] This class also includes the prescription medications methylphenidate, pemoline, phentermine, phendimetrazine, amphetamine, dextroamphetamine, and methamphetamine, which have historically been prescribed for a variety of indications but currently are limited to treatment of attention-deficit/hyperactivity disorder, narcolepsy, and short-term weight reduction. Prescriptions for amphetamines are increasing; in the 5 years between 1996 and 2000, total US amphetamine prescriptions increased from 1.3 million to nearly 8 million.[32] Misuse of prescription amphetamines was related to 15,416 emergency department visits in 2010.[27] The primary mechanism of action of amphetamines is the release of catecholamines, particularly dopamine and norepinephrine, from the presynaptic terminals. Some amphetamines, such as methylenedioxymethamphetamine, have increased serotonergic effects. The catecholamine release results in the stimulation of peripheral α- and β-adrenergic receptors causing a sympathomimetic toxidrome. Similar to cocaine, vasospasm combined with hypertension and tachycardia can cause cerebral ischemia, infarction, or hemorrhage; myocardial ischemia or infarction; ischemic colitis; aortic dissection; and obstetric complications. In addition, case reports are emerging of compartment syndrome associated with synthetic cathinone use, possibly caused by a combination of agitation, vasospasm, and muscle reperfusion.[33]

There are several dieting agents that have demonstrated vasoconstrictive toxic effects, including phenylpropanolamine, ephedrine, phentermine, fenfluramine, and dexfenfluramine. Phenylpropanolamine is a sympathomimetic amine that directly stimulates α-adrenergic receptors, and also causes norepinephrine release. It can cause severe hypertension, and was withdrawn after it was noted to cause hemorrhagic stroke in women.[34] Ephedrine is another sympathomimetic amine used in dieting agents. Ephedrine is the primary alkaloid in the ephedra plant (ma huang), which also contains several other ephedra alkaloids. Ephedra was formerly used as a dieting agent, but was banned because of the risk of adverse events including hypertension, myocardial infarction, cardiac arrest, and stroke.[35] It can still be found in traditional Chinese medicine preparations for asthma and colds. Phentermine is an amphetamine-like substance that was previously sold in combination with fenfluramine ("phen-fen"), and is still available by prescription as an anorectic; it has been associated with stroke.[36] Fenfluramine and dexfenfluramine are serotonergic agents available as dieting aids. Both drugs were associated with primary pulmonary hypertension, and have since been withdrawn.[37]

Ergot alkaloids are substances largely derived from the fungus *Claviceps purpurea*, including ergotamine, dihydroergotamine, ergonvine, methylergonovine, methsergide, and bromocriptine. They are most commonly used to treat vascular headaches, but may also be used in obstetrics and Parkinson disease, among other clinical uses. Ergot alkaloids act centrally and peripherally on serotonergic, dopaminergic, and α-adrenergic receptors.[38] The bioavailability of ergot alkaloids is highly variable, as is the dose at which toxicity occurs. The classic toxicologic syndrome of ergotism from epidemic outbreaks of fungal grain infections includes gangrene; nausea and vomiting; abnormal sensations, such as burning, formications, and pruritis; and CNS manifestations, such as hallucinations, seizure, and coma. However, in modern times ergot toxicity tends to be related to use of pharmacologic products and to be more exclusively vascular in nature.[39] Vascular complications most frequently involve the peripheral vasculature of the lower extremities, but may also be seen in coronary, cerebral, mesenteric, and renal vascular beds.[39–43]

Triptans are antimigraine medications that produce vasoconstrictive effects through interaction with 5-HT$_{1B}$ and 5-HT$_{1D}$ receptors. They include sumatriptan, naratriptan, zolmitriptan, rizatriptan, eletriptan, almotriptan, and frovatriptan, and may be administered orally, sublingually, or subcutaneously. They have been observed to have toxic vasoconstrictive effects at therapeutic and supratherapeutic doses. The desired effects of triptans occur through vasoconstriction in the CNS; however, they have also been known to cause adverse neurologic events including transient ischemic attack, stroke, and spinal cord infarction.[44–46] Additionally, sumatriptan can cause chest pressure or pain in up to 15% of users, which may or may not reflect ischemia of coronary vessels.[47] Sumatriptan has been associated with myocardial ischemia and infarction in several cases.[48–50] Triptans have also been associated with splenic infarct, renal infarct, and ischemic colitis.[38,51,52]

DIGOXIN AND CARDIOACTIVE STEROID TOXICITY

Digoxin is a prototypical cardioactive steroids used in medicine for many years. Today, digoxin is used to treat patients with congestive heart failure and/or rate control of rapid ventricular response caused by atrial fibrillation or flutter. Digoxin was originally procured from foxglove plant (*Digitalis lanata*), and there are several other naturally occurring sources that may cause severe toxicity in humans.[53] **Table 3** lists various sources. It is important for the emergency providers to recognize that these cardioactive steroids may be incorporated into several readily available legal and illegally prepared products. Severe toxicity from cardioactive steroids has been documented in products sold for increased sexual performance and male enhancement, herbal colon cleansing, and as rodenticides.[53]

Clinically there is a combination of increased ventricular automaticity and increased vagal effects resulting AV nodal blocking. This lethal combination can produce almost any type of dysrthymias, except for a rapidly conducted supraventricular tachycardia. **Box 3** provides common ECG findings associated with cardioactive steroid poisoning.[54]

The noncardiac clinical manifestations may vary with acute or chronic exposure. Acute toxicity presents with nausea and vomiting, and may be accompanied by lethargy, confusion, and weakness. Before the introduction of specific antidotal therapy, a potassium level greater than 5.5 mEq/L in the setting of acute digitoxin overdose was associated with 100% mortality.[55] Although hyperkalemia is a key prognostic feature and manifestation of acute toxicity, it is rarely high enough to cause clinical toxicity. Lethal dysrhythmias lead to demise. Chronic digoxin toxicity may produce vague clinical presentations. A more insidious symptom spectrum may include gastrointestinal upset, drowsiness, headache, visual disturbances, and delirium.[56] **Box 4** indicates several risk factors that may lead to chronic digoxin toxicity. In addition to acute toxicity, chronic toxicity is also associated with hyperkalemia, which seems to increase mortality and antidote requirements.[57]

Table 3 Selected cardioactive steroids	
Origin	**Source**
Pharmaceutical preparations	Deslanoside C (desacetyl lanatoside C)[a] Digoxin Digitoxin[a] Gitalin[a] Lanatoside C[a] Ouabain[a]
Animals	Bufo toads (*Bufo* spp.) Fireflies (*Photius* spp.) Milkweed butterflies (*Danainae* spp.)
Plants	Bushman's poison (*Carissa acokanthera*) Crown flower (*Calotropis gigantea*) Dogbane (*Apocynum cannabinum*) Foxglove (*Digitalis* spp) Lily of the valley (*Convallaria mejalis*) Milkweed (*Asclepias* spp) Oleander (*Nerium oleander*) Ordeal tree (*Tanghinia venenifera*) Red squill (sea onion, *Urginea maritime*) Rubber vine (*Cryptostegia grandifolia*) Sea mango (*Cerbera manghas*) Wintersweet (*Carissa spectabilis*) Woody liana (*Strophanthus gratus*) Yellow oleander (*Thevetia peruviana*)

[a] Not commercially available in the United States.

Box 3
ECG findings in cardioactive steroids

Atrial fibrillation or flutter with slow ventricular response

Atrial tachycardia with high-grade atrioventricular block

Bidirectional ventricular tachycardia (rare, but pathognomonic)

Premature ventricular contractions (most common)

"Scooped" T waves (marker of therapeutic use, not necessarily overdose)

Sinus bradycardia

Ventricular fibrillation

Ventricular tachycardia

Cardioactive steroid toxicity should be considered when patients present with unexplained bradycardia, nausea and vomiting, history of congestive heart failure or atrial fibrillation and flutter, ECG findings in **Box 3**, and in patients who are prescribed digoxin with risk factors in **Box 4**.

GENERAL MANAGEMENT APPROACH

Aggressive attention to airway, breathing, and circulation is mandatory. Intravenous access should be obtained, with appropriate laboratory evaluations as described below. All patients with suspected cardiovascular poisoning should undergo prompt evaluation and be placed on a monitor even when the initial vital signs are normal. Early gastrointestinal decontamination and pharmacologic therapies should be considered before patients become unstable. This is particularly important in the setting of ingestions of sustained-release formulations. All patients who become hypotensive should receive a fluid bolus of 10 to 20 mL/kg of crystalloid, repeated as needed. Caution for aggressive fluid resuscitation should be given to patients with congestive heart failure, acute lung injury, or renal failure.

Diagnostic Testing

Any patients with suspected cardiovascular poisoning should be evaluated for potential hemodynamic compromise. All patients should be placed on continuous cardiopulmonary monitoring, and a 12-lead ECG performed to evaluate for potential QRS or QT interval widening. Bedside glucometry may suggest BAA or CCB toxicity, as previously described. A chest radiograph, pulse oximetry, and serum chemistry should also be obtained in the setting of hypotension. The most specific biomarker

---

Box 4
Risk factors leading to chronic digoxin toxicity

Change in kidney function (often unrecognized)

Dehydration

Dose unadjusted for renal insufficiency

Drug interactions (amiodarone, quinidine, verapamil, others)

Macrolide use (decreased gut flora that normally metabolizes digoxin)

for end-organ injury in drug-induced shock is serum lactate.[58] Cardioactive steroids should be a consideration in the setting of bradycardia with hyperkalemia and normal renal function, in which case a serum digoxin concentration may be useful. Most hospitals are able to process emergent digoxin assays, but in patients with significant toxicity, empiric therapy may be required.

In patients with exposure to an agent that may cause toxic vasoconstriction, focal neurologic deficits should prompt investigation with imaging, usually noncontrast brain computed tomography. Chest pain should be taken seriously even in young patients, and should involve routine evaluations, such as an ECG, cardiac enzymes, and chest radiography. The potential for acute coronary syndromes, aortic/arterial dissections, pulmonary infarction, and pulmonary hypertension should be contemplated and evaluated where appropriate. Abdominal pain and bloody stools should prompt consideration of mesenteric ischemia and ischemic colitis. Renal and splenic infarct may also occur. Limb ischemia, rhabdomyolysis, and compartment syndrome should be included in the differential of muscular pain. Creatinine kinase testing should be considered in any patient with a sympathomimetic toxidrome.

Gastrointestinal Decontamination

Gastrointestinal decontamination should strongly be considered in all patients who present with a significant ingestion of a cardiotoxic agent, such as BAA or CCB, given their morbidity in severe poisoning. Patients who present early with minimal or no symptoms may have delayed cardiovascular toxicity that can be profound and refractory to conventional treatment, making early gastrointestinal decontamination a cornerstone in management. Ipecac was once commonly used in all cases of suspected ingestions to induce emesis to help prevent gastrointestinal absorption, thus potentially limiting significant toxicity. Significant complications including aspiration, perforation, and the potential for rapid deterioration in patients with BAA or CCB poisoning do not warrant its use. The efficacy of orogastric lavage has not been evaluated with BAA or CCB poisoning, but because of significant morbidity, this technique should be considered by capable practitioners for all patients who present early after large ingestions and for patients who are critically ill. When performing this technique it is important to use a large-caliber tube, because the pills may be large and/or poorly soluble. Because lavage may increase vagal tone, exacerbating any bradydysrhythmias, atropine may be required as a pretreatment.[59]

The use of activated charcoal should be considered in all patients with ingestions of BAAs of CCBs. Awake patients should receive 1 g/kg of activated charcoal orally. Activated charcoal should be withheld in patients who have altered mental status or where a sudden decline in mental status is expected (ie, tricyclic antidepressant ingestion) because of concern for aspiration, unless the airway is definitively protected. MDAC (0.5 g/kg) without a cathartic should be administered to nearly all patients with either sustained-release pill ingestions or signs of continuing absorption.[60] The effect of MDAC may be a result of the continuous presence of activated charcoal throughout the gastrointestinal tract, which may continue to absorb drugs that are extended-release. MDAC should not be administered to a patient with inadequate gastrointestinal function. Whole-bowel irrigation (WBI) with polyethylene glycol-electrolyte lavage solution (PEG-ELS, 1–2 L/h orally or by nasogastric tube in adults, up to 500 mL/h in children) should be considered for patients who ingest sustained-release products. WBI should be withheld in patients who have immediate-release ingestion because of concern for enhancing absorption by the dissolution of pill fragments. Administration is continued until the rectal effluent is clear.[61]

Management of Toxicologic Vasoconstriction

The principles for management of toxicologic vasoconstriction are generally similar regardless of substance. Testing to identify the offending substance is rarely of use in medical decision-making. Diagnosis and reversal of toxic vasoconstrictive effects and treatment of the accompanying symptoms of a sympathomimetic toxidrome are critical actions. Management of associated hyperthermia is of utmost importance and should be treated aggressively with cooling. Agitation and seizures should be treated with benzodiazepines, which may in some cases obviate the need for antihypertensive agents. Local vasoconstriction and systemic hypertension can be controlled with direct-acting vasodilators, such as nitroglycerin or nitroprusside; α-adrenergic antagonists, such as phentolamine; or titratable CCBs.[38,62] β-blockade is contraindicated in toxic ingestions with α-adrenergic effects, particularly cocaine, because of the risk of unopposed α activity.[62] Aspirin and heparin or low-molecular-weight heparin are recommended for myocardial ischemia, but the indication for revascularization with thrombolysis or cardiac catheterization is less clear, and should be decided based on the clinical situation.[38,62,63] The management of toxicologic vasoconstriction should prioritize treatment of a sympathomimetic toxidrome with benzodiazepines, cooling, and intravenous fluids, and should focus on identifying end-organ damage of vasoconstriction and treating this damage with vasodilators, α-adrenergic antagonists, CCBs, aspirin, and heparin as clinically indicated.

Management of Toxicologic Bradycardia

Patients often require pharmacologic intervention in significant ingestions. The use of agents should focus on maintaining the cardiac output and peripheral tone. Various agents, such as atropine, dopamine, and phosphodiesterase inhibitors, have been used with success; no single intervention as been shown to consistently treat severe poisoning. Although patients with unintentional or small ingestions often respond well to crystalloids and atropine, significant ingestions often require more aggressive management and multiple pharmacologic agents.

Although it would be ideal to initiate each therapy individually and monitor the patient's hemodynamic response to each treatment, in the most critically ill patients, multiple therapies may be administered simultaneously. The following is a description of recommended treatment modalities and agents.

Atropine

Atropine competitively antagonizes the muscarinic acetylcholine receptor. It is commonly used as a first-line agent in the treatment of symptomatic bradycardia from toxicologic causes that include organophosphorus compounds, cardioactive steroids, BAAs, and CCBs. Although atropine has been shown experimentally to improve heart rate and cardiac output, it is often ineffective in the setting of severe poisoning.[64] Atropine dosing for drug-induced bradycardia is similar to that dose used in advanced cardiac life support. Dosing should begin with 0.5 to 1 mg (0.02 mg/kg in children, with a minimum of 0.1 mg) intravenously every 2 or 3 minutes up to a maximum dose of 3 mg in all patients with symptomatic bradycardia.

Atropine is relatively safe when dosed appropriately. However, treatment failures should be anticipated in severely poisoned patients. In patients with suspected ingestions of extended-release formulations where in WBI or MDAC will be used, the use of atropine must be carefully considered, weighing the potential benefits of improved hemodynamics against the potential decreased gastrointestinal motility from atropine's antimuscarinic effects.

Calcium

Calcium is often used for CCB poisoning or other causes of toxicologic hypotension. The exact mechanism is not clear, but is most likely from an increase in extracellular calcium concentration with an increase in transmembrane concentration gradient. Pretreatment with intravenous Ca^{2+} prevents hypotension without diminishing the antidysrhythmic efficacy before verapamil use in the therapeutic setting.[65] This also is observed with CCB poisoning where Ca^{2+} tends to improve blood pressure more than heart rate. Experimental models have also demonstrated the utility of calcium salts with CCC poisoning. In verapamil-poisoned dogs, improvement in inotropy and blood pressure was demonstrated after increasing the serum Ca^{2+} concentration by 2 mEq/L with an intravenous infusion of 10% calcium chloride ($CaCl_2$) at 3 mg/kg/min.[66]

Clinical experiences demonstrate that calcium ions reverse the negative inotropy, impaired conduction, and hypotension in humans poisoned by CCBs.[60,67] Unfortunately, this effect is often short lived and more severely poisoned patients may not improve significantly with Ca^{2+} administration. Although some authors believe that these failures might represent inadequate dosing, optimal effective dosing of Ca^{2+} is unclear and they recommend repeat doses of calcium salts to increase the serum ionized calcium to very high concentrations.[68] Caution in the administration of Ca^{2+} should be exercised in patients who may have suspected acute cardioactive steroid poisoning as a cause of their bradycardia. The use of Ca^{2+} in the setting of cardioactive steroid poisoning may result in cardiac complications, such as asystole.[69]

Reasonable recommendations for poisoned adults include an initial intravenous infusion of approximately 10 to 20 mL of 10% calcium chloride or 30 to 60 mL of 10% calcium gluconate, followed by either repeat boluses every 15 to 20 minutes for up to three to four doses or a continuous infusion. Careful selection and attention to the type of calcium salt used is critical for dosing. Although there is no difference in efficacy of calcium chloride or calcium gluconate, 1 g of calcium chloride contains 13.4 mEq of Ca^{2+}, which is more than three times the 4.3 mEq found in 1 g of calcium gluconate. Consequently, to administer equimolar doses of Ca^{2+}, three times the volume of calcium gluconate compared with that of calcium chloride is required.

The main limitation of using calcium chloride, however, is the significant potential for tissue injury if extravasated. Administration should ideally be by central venous access. If repeat dosing or continuous infusions are necessary serum Ca^{2+} and PO_4^{-3} concentrations should be closely monitored to detect developing hypercalcemia or hypophosphatemia. Caution should be exercised with aggressive calcium salt use because there are reports of fatality with the use of infusions. Other adverse effects of intravenous Ca^{2+} include nausea, vomiting, flushing, constipation, confusion, and angina.

Cardioactive steroid poisoning and digoxin-specific antibody fragments

Cardioactive steroid poisoning should be considered in patients presenting with increased ventricular automaticity and a high-degree AV block. Patients who are unstable with acute life-threatening dysrthymias warrant emergent empiric treatment with digoxin-specific antibody fragments (Digibind, Digifab).[70] **Box 5** provides indications to treat with digoxin immune antibody fragments. These antibodies bind free serum digoxin, and also reach interstitial sites to bind digoxin at such sites as the myocardial cell. The digoxin-antibody complex is renally eliminated.[70] Some patients may demonstrate reversal of ventricular dysrthymias within 2 minutes and most have resolution of all dysrthymias within 30 minutes.[71]

The ECG should guide diagnosis and management because serum concentrations do not correlate well with toxicity. **Table 4** describes the dosing regimens for

---

Box 5
Indications for digoxin-specific antibody fragments

Any potential cardioactive steroid dysrhythmia

Bradydysrhythmia refractory to atropine

Chronic poisoning with end-organ manifestations (eg, altered mental status, gastrointestinal distress, renal impairment)

Digoxin ingestion of 10 mg or more in an adult (4 mg in a child)

Digoxin concentration[a] equal to or exceeding 15 ng/mL at anytime or ≥10 ng/mL beyond 6 hours postingestion

Nondigoxin cardioactive steroid poisoning

Potassium exceeding 5 mEq/L in acute digoxin toxicity

Shock or hemodynamic instability

[a] Some laboratories report digoxin concentrations in mmol/L. To convert mmol/L to ng/mL, multiply by 0.78.

---

digoxin-specific antibody fragments. Because it makes several assumptions about the volume of distribution and bioavailability, the clinical picture should guide the potential need for administration of additional vials. It should also be noted that once digoxin immune antibody fragments are provided, routine hospital assays for digoxin are useless, and will likely be falsely elevated, because they measure free digoxin and digoxin bound to antibodies.

Acute cardioactive steroid poisoning may present with elevated serum potassium, which is a poor prognostic marker but rarely the cause of toxicity. If therapy for hyperkalemia is required, sodium bicarbonate and insulin and glucose can be used safely. Concurrent calcium therapy for the treatment of hyperkalemia is to be avoided when cardioactive steroid poisoning is suspected or confirmed. Intracellular calcium is already elevated, and administration of calcium salts is believed to cause tetanic myocardial contractions or "stone heart" that was reported to be fatal in the 1930s.[69] The administration of digoxin-specific antibody fragments lowers serum potassium.[70] This and other potential complications of therapy are provided in **Box 6**.

It is critical to understand in patients poisoned with nondigoxin cardioactive steroids that the cross-reactivity in the serum assays and the digoxin-specific antibody

---

Table 4
Dosing of digoxin-specific antibody fragments[a]

Clinical Scenario	Dose
Empiric dosing, acute toxicity	10–20 vials (adult or pediatric)
Empiric dosing, chronic toxicity	3–6 vials (adult) 1–2 vials (child)
Known ingested digoxin dose	$\text{Vials} = \dfrac{\text{Amount ingested (mg)} \times 0.8}{0.5 \text{ mg}}$
Known serum digoxin concentration[b]	$\text{Vials} = \dfrac{[\text{digoxin concentration (ng/mL)}] \times [\text{weight (kg)}]}{100}$

[a] Each vial binds ~0.5 mg digoxin.
[b] Some laboratories report digoxin concentrations in mmol/L. To use this equation, to convert mmol/L to ng/mL, multiply by 0.78.

fragments is incomplete. Patients may have negative or "therapeutic" serum digoxin concentrations even with severe acute life-threatening poisoning. They may also require very large amounts of digoxin-specific antibody fragments; 35 vials of digoxin-specific antibody fragment were insufficient to save one patient who ingested a cardioactive steroid–containing compound derived from a bufo toad.[72,73]

Glucagon

Glucagon is an endogenous polypeptide hormone secreted by the pancreatic α cells used for its inotropic and chronotropic effects for BAA poisoning (off label). Thus, glucagon is unique in that it is functionally a "pure" β_1 agonist, with no peripheral vasodilatory effects.[74] However, in CCB poisoning, because the cellular lesion is downstream from adenylate cyclase, glucagon may have limited effect is this setting. There are reports of successes and failures of glucagon in CCB-poisoned patients who failed to respond to fluids, calcium salts, or dopamine and dobutamine.[75,76] There is also experimental evidence that illustrates the failure of glucagon with severe CCB poisoning compared with other preferred treatments, such as high-insulin therapy.[77] Dosing for glucagon is not well established. An initial dose of 3 to 5 mg intravenously, slowly over 1 to 2 minutes, is reasonable in adults, and if no hemodynamic improvement occurs within 5 minutes, retreatment with a dose of 4 to 10 mg may be effective. The initial pediatric dose is 50 µg/kg. Because of glucagon's short half-life, repeat doses may be useful. A maintenance infusion should be initiated once a desired effect is achieved. Common adverse effects include vomiting and hyperglycemia, particularly in diabetics or during continuous infusion. Patients who receive repeat administration of glucagon may exhibit tachyphylaxis, which is an acute decrease in response to a drug after repeated administration.

High-dose insulin euglycemia therapy

CCB poisoning often results in metabolic derangements resembling diabetes including acidemia, hyperglycemia, and insulin deficiency. Supportive care and traditional treatment detailed previously are not always sufficient in severe poisonings. Insulin, however, has been used historically to augment cardiac function and when administered in high doses can ameliorate many of the previously mentioned abnormalities. In recent years high-dose insulin euglycemia (HIE) therapy for CCB and BAA poisoning has been shown to have a greater effect on hemodynamics than conventional measures, such as vasopressors. HIE which is an off label therapy, has now emerged as the treatment of choice for severe cases of CCB and BAA poisonings.

In addition to impairment in myocardial function and vascular tone induced by calcium channel inhibition, CCB and BAA poisoning cause metabolic derangements, which further compromise cardiac function. Under conditions of stress like those induced by cardiotoxic drug poisoning, the heart's energy source shifts away from preferred free fatty acids toward carbohydrates, which require insulin for uptake into myocardial cells.[78] Simultaneously, CCBs and BAAs inhibit calcium-dependent insulin release from the β-islet cells of the pancreas and induce insulin resistance. Glucose uptake into myocardium then relies on concentration gradients rather than insulin-mediated active transport, and use of the heart's primary energy source is impaired. HIE exerts its therapeutic effect through two pathways: increased inotropy and vascular dilation. Insulin improves inotropy through the PI3K pathways and through augmented glucose uptake into myocardial cells, improving energy supply and use. Insulin-mediated induction of endothelial nitric oxide synthase vasodilates coronary, pulmonary, and systemic vasculature thus improving perfusion and increasing cardiac output independent of increased inotropy.[76]

Animal studies have established HIE as superior to conventional treatment across multiple hemodynamic parameters including improved coronary artery blood flow, contractility, cardiac output, and overall survival. On the contrary, vasopressors increase systemic vascular resistance, increasing afterload and decreasing cardiac output, and have been repeatedly shown to be less effective than HIE in cardiotoxic drug poisoning. Clinical studies of HIE are limited to case reports and case series but consistently show beneficial effects of HIE in cardiotoxic drug poisonings.[79] In a review of 78 cases of CCB and BAA poisonings that received HIE after conventional therapy, survival was 88%. In the few cases of HIE treatment failure, insufficient dosing, concomitant vasopressor use, and delayed treatment have been cited.[76]

Although the dose of insulin is not definitively established, most clinicians recommend a bolus of 1 U/kg of regular human insulin along with 0.5 g/kg of dextrose. If blood glucose is greater than 300–400 mg/dL (16.6–22.2 mmol/L), the dextrose bolus is withheld. An infusion of regular insulin should follow the bolus, starting at 1 U/kg/h and titrated up to 2 U/kg/h or higher if no improvement is evident after 15 to 30 minutes. A continuous dextrose infusion beginning at 0.5 g/kg/h should also be started. D25W or D50W administered by a central venous catheter may be used to avoid large fluid volumes required with more dilute dextrose solutions. Some authors advocate the use of even higher doses (10 U/kg) of insulin, and case reports of doses more than 10 U/kg have not been associated with clinically significant adverse events.[80] Glucose should be monitored every half hour for the first 4 hours and titrated to maintain euglycemia. Potassium concentrations should also be monitored closely because insulin shifts potassium intracellularly. The response to insulin is typically delayed for 15 to 60 minutes. This necessitates early consideration for HIE if severe poisoning is suspected or with evidence of myocardial dysfunction. There are no studies evaluating the best way to discontinue HIE after cardiac function improves. A taper and abrupt cessation have been used but glucose and potassium should be monitored after HIE discontinuation for prolonged hypoglycemia and hypokalemia as insulin clears. The primary complications of HIE include hypoglycemia and electrolyte imbalances, particularly hypokalemia from intracellular potassium shifts. It is important to impress on the clinical team caring for these patients that HIE is safe and effective. Clinical human experiences support the lack of clinically relevant episodes of hypoglycemia or hypokalemia.[81]

Intravenous lipid emulsion

Intravenous lipid emulsion (ILE), also referred to in the literature as intravenous fat emulsion (IFE), is a 20% free fatty acid mixture used to deliver parenteral calories to patients unable to take oral nutrition.[82] After its unintentional discovery in the early 1990s as an antidote to bupivacaine toxicity,[83,84] ILE has since been widely studied in bupivacaine and other local anesthetics and is now firmly established in the anesthesia literature as an antidote to local-anesthetic systemic toxicity. The first nonlocal anesthetic use of ILE was published in 2008 describing an adolescent with a buprop-rion and lamotrigine overdose who survived cardiovascular collapse after an anesthe-siologist suggested giving ILE when maximal therapy had failed.[49] ILE is now emerging as a potential off label rescue therapy for other cardiotoxic lipophilic drugs including CCBs and BAAs.[85]

There are three proposed mechanisms of action for ILE in the treatment of cardiovas-cular toxicity. First, ILE provides a myocardial energy substrate in the form of free fatty acids, the preferred energy source of the heart. Provision of free fatty acids is particu-larly important in CCB toxicity because induced insulin deficiency limits the heart's abil-ity to use carbohydrates. Second, ILE increases myocardial calcium as a result of triglyceride activity on calcium channels. This may have specific benefit in CCB and BAA toxicity by improving function of antagonized ion channels. Third and perhaps the prevailing theory is the lipid sink model where lipid-soluble drugs can be extracted and contained, thus limiting the drug's ability to exert toxic effects on tissues.

An important property of medications that may determine the effectiveness of IFE is the lipophilicity of a drug. Lipophilicity is the tendency of a drug to partition between lipophilic phase and the aqueous phase, and value of lipophilicity most commonly refers to logarithm of partition coefficient P (log P) between these two phases. For ionizable compounds, the partition is changed as a function of pH; this relationship fol-lows a distribution constant (log D). Drugs that are highly lipophillic may benefit more from the use of IFE in severe poisoning. Based on a favorable (positive) Log D/Log P, CCBs and BAAs that might be particularly amenable to ILE include amlodipine, bepri-dil, diltiazem, felodipine, isradipine nicardipine, nimodipine, verapamil, acebutolol, betaxolol, carvedilol, labetalol, levobunolol, penbutolol, and propranolol.

Animal data demonstrate improved hemodynamics and survival after ILE adminis-tration, and case reports show survival in patients with severe cardiotoxicity receiving ILE after failure of standard therapy.[86] A retrospective chart review showed a 55% sur-vival to discharge in patients with cardiovascular collapse and extremely poor pre-dicted outcome after receiving ILE for cardiotoxic drug ingestions.[85]

Dosing strategies are based on animal data and case reports. Expert opinion rec-ommends an initial bolus of 1.5 mg/kg ideal body weight of 20% ILE to be infused over 1 minute followed by an infusion of 0.25 mL/kg/min. The bolus dose can be repeated up to two times for refractory cardiovascular collapse and the infusion dose can be doubled to 0.5 mL/kg/min for persistent hypotension. The infusion should be continued for 10 minutes after stabilization of hemodynamics. The maximum dose should not exceed 10 mL/kg over the first 30 minutes.[87] The data supporting dosing regimens are extremely limited and the necessity of an infusion is debated among experts. One small review found no improvement in survival for patients receiving in-fusions or multiple boluses compared with those receiving a single bolus.[88]

Concern exists over possible adverse effects of ILE, primarily lipid embolic com-plications seen when administering lipid in high doses or rapid infusions. No such pulmonary complications have been reported for ILE when used as an antidote. Hyper-amylasemia without subsequent pancreatitis has been reported. Lipemia subsequent to ILE infusion can potentially alter interpretation of laboratory values. There exists one case report of this complication, occurring after a massive ILE overdose.[89] Currently, ILE as rescue therapy is considered reasonable for refractory cardiovascular collapse after ingestion of cardiotoxic drugs.

Adjunctive Hemodynamic Support

The most severely cardiovascular-poisoned patients may not respond to any pharma-cologic intervention. Transthoracic or intravenous cardiac pacing may be required to improve heart rate, as several case reports demonstrate. However, in a prospective cohort of CCB poisonings, two of four patients with significant bradycardia requiring electrical pacing failed electrical capture. In addition, even if electrical pacing is effective in increasing the heart rate, blood pressure often remains unchanged due to persistent impaired inotropy.[21] More invasive measures may be considered as bridge therapies while awaiting toxin elimination. Intra-aortic balloon counterpulsation is one such supportive option to be considered in cardiovascular poisoning refractory to pharmacologic therapy. Intra-aortic balloon counterpulsation was used successfully to improve cardiac output and blood pressure in a patient with a mixed verapamil and atenolol overdose. Severely cardiovascular-poisoned patients have also been supported for days and subsequently recovered fully with the more invasive and technologically demanding extracorporeal membrane oxygenation and emergent open and percutaneous cardiopulmonary bypass. The major limitation of all these technologies, however, is that they are available only at tertiary care facilities.[90]

The use of albumin dialysis with molecular adsorbents recirculating system therapy has also been reported because of its unique ability to selectively remove from circulation protein-bound toxins (and potentially drugs) that are not cleared by conventional hemodialysis. The use of molecular adsorbents recirculating system (MARS) therapy is under current investigation with *Amanita* poisoning, but reportedly was successfully used in three patients with severe CCB poisoning.[91]

Urgent consultation with a medical toxicologist or regional poison control center is recommended in cases of cardiotoxicity, because standard guidelines for non–drug-related emergency cardiovascular care may not apply to the management of acute overdose.[92,93] Rather, administering an atypical life-saving antidote or specific continuous monitoring may be deciding factors for whether or not a patient survives a severe overdose. Unfortunately, many recommendations for emergency care of drug-related cardiovascular events lack firm scientific foundation, and further research is needed.[94]

Disposition

Patients who manifest any signs or symptoms of BAA or CCB toxicity should be admitted to an intensive care setting. Because of the potential for delayed toxicity, patients ingesting sustained-release products should be admitted for 24 hours to a monitored setting, even if asymptomatic. This is particularly important for toddlers and small children in whom even one or a few tablets may produce significant toxicity. Activated charcoal and WBI should be strongly considered in those with a history of sustained-release product ingestion.

SUMMARY

The hallmarks of BAA and CCB toxicity include bradydysrhythmias, hypotension, and shock, which are an extension of the pharmacologic effects of these agents. Most patients with immediate-release ingestions develop symptoms of hypoperfusion, such as lightheadedness, nausea, or fatigue, within hours of a significant ingestion; while sustained-release formulations may result in significant delays to hemodynamic consequences and prolonged toxicity. Aggressive decontamination of patients with exposures to sustained-release products should begin as soon as possible and should not be delayed by waiting for signs of toxicity. The use of high-dose insulin therapy should be instituted early due to the temporal delay in its efficacy. In cases of severe toxicity, the use of ILE therapy should be considered. Patients who fail to respond to all pharmaceutical interventions should be considered for extracorporeal mechanical support whenever available.

REFERENCES

1. Bronstein AC, Spyker DA, Cantilena LR Jr, et al. 2011 Annual report of the American Association of Poison Control Centers' National Poison Data System (NPDS): 29th Annual Report. Clin Toxicol (Phila) 2012;50:911–1164.
2. Albertson TE, Dawson A, de Latorre F, et al, American Heart Association; International Liaison Committee on Resuscitation. TOX-ACLS: toxicologic-oriented advanced cardiac life support. Ann Emerg Med 2001;37(Suppl 4):S78–90.
3. Manini AF, Nelson LS, Skolnick AH, et al. Electrocardiographic predictors of adverse cardiovascular events in suspected poisoning. J Med Toxicol 2010;6: 106–15.
4. Manini AF, Nelson LS, Stimmel B, et al. Incidence of adverse cardiovascular events in adults following drug overdose. Acad Emerg Med 2012;19(7):843–9.
5. Thygesen K, Alpert JS, Jaffe AS, et al, The writing group on behalf of the joint ESC/ACCF/AHA/WHF task force for the universal definition of myocardial infarction. Third universal definition of myocardial infarction. J Am Coll Cardiol 2012; 60(12):1581–98.
6. Gaze DC, Collinson PO. Cardiac troponins as biomarkers of drug- and toxin-induced cardiac toxicity and cardiac protection. Expert Opin Drug Metab Toxicol 2005;1:715–25.
7. Huikuri HV, Castellanos A, Myerburg RJ. Sudden death due to cardiac arrhythmias. N Engl J Med 2001;345:1473–82.
8. Roden D, Woosley R, Primm R. Incidence and clinical features of the quinidine-associated long QT syndrome: implications for patient care. Am Heart J 1986; 111:1088–93.
9. Viskin S. Long QT syndromes and torsades de pointes. Lancet 1999;354: 1625–33.
10. McCaig LF, Burt CW. Poisoning-related visits to emergency departments in the USA, 1993-1996. J Toxicol Clin Toxicol 1999;37:817–26.
11. Paulozzi L, Crosby A, Ryan G. Increases in age-group-specific injury mortality— USA, 1999-2004. MMWR Morb Mortal Wkly Rep 2007;56(49):1281–4.
12. Liebelt EL, Ulrich A, Francis PD, et al. Serial electrocardiogram changes in acute tricyclic antidepressant overdoses. Crit Care Med 1997;25:1721–6.
13. Niemann JT, Bessen HA, Rothstein RJ, et al. Electrocardiographic criteria for tricyclic antidepressant cardiotoxicity. Am J Cardiol 1986;57:1154–9.
14. Bebarta VS, Phillips S, Eberhardt A, et al. Incidence of Brugada electrocardiographic pattern and outcomes of these patients after intentional tricyclic antidepressant ingestion. Am J Cardiol 2007;100(4):656–60.
15. Dickens P, Tai YT, But PP, et al. Fatal accidental aconitine poisoning following ingestion of Chinese herbal medicine: a report of two cases. Forensic Sci Int 1994;67(1):55–8.
16. Wallukat G. The beta-adrenergic receptors. Herz 2002;27:683–90.
17. Hurwitz MD, Kallenbach JM, Pincus PS. Massive propranolol overdose. Am J Med 1986;81:1118.
18. Jovic-Stosic J, Gligic B, Putic V, et al. Severe propranolol and ethanol overdose with wide complex tachycardia treated with intravenous lipid emulsion: a case report. Clin Toxicol (Phila) 2011;49:426–30.
19. Abernethy DR, Schwartz JB. Calcium-antagonist drugs. N Engl J Med 1999; 341:1447–57.
20. Connolly DL, Nettleton MA, Bastow MD. Massive diltiazem overdose. Am J Cardiol 1993;72:742–3.

21. Ramoska EA, Spiller HA, Winter M, et al. A one-year evaluation of calcium chan-nel blocker overdoses: toxicity and treatment. Ann Emerg Med 1993;22: 196–200.
22. Assimes TL, Malcolm I. Torsade de pointes with sotalol overdose treated suc-cessfully with lidocaine. Can J Cardiol 1998;14:753–6.
23. Barrow PM, Houston PL, Wong DT. Overdose of sustained-release verapamil. Br J Anaesth 1994;72:361–5.
24. Benaim ME. Asystole after verapamil. Br Med J 1972;2:169–70.
25. Bechtel LK, Haverstick DM, Holstege CP. Verapamil toxicity dysregulates the phosphatidylinositol 3-kinase pathway. Acad Emerg Med 2008;15:368–74.
26. Substance Abuse and Mental Health Services Administration. Results from the 2011 National Survey on Drug Use and Health. Available at: http://www. drugabuse.gov/national-survey-drug-use-health. Accessed on May 1, 2013.
27. Substance Abuse and Mental Health Services Administration. Drug Abuse Warning Network, 2010: national estimates of drug-related emergency depart-ment visits. HHS Publication No. (SMA) 12–4733, DAWN Series D-38. Rockville (MD): Substance Abuse and Mental Health Services Administration; 2012.
28. Qureshi AI, Suri MF, Guterman LR, et al. Cocaine use and the likelihood of nonfatal myocardial infarction and stroke: data from the third national health and nutrition examination survey. Circulation 2001;103:502–6.
29. Fajemirokun-Odudeyi O, Lindow SW. Obstetric implications of cocaine use in pregnancy: a literature review. Eur J Obstet Gynecol Reprod Biol 2004; 112:2–8.
30. Prosser JM, Hoffman RS. Cocaine. In: Nelson LS, Lewin NA, Howland MA, et al, editors. Goldfrank's toxicologic emergencies. 9th edition. New York: McGraw-Hill; 2011. p. 1091–102.
31. Prosser JM, Nelson LS. The toxicology of bath salts: a review of synthetic cath-inones. J Med Toxicol 2012;8:33–42.
32. Lin SJ, Crawford SY, Patricia L. Trend and area variation in amphetamine pre-scription usage among children and adolescents in Michigan. Soc Sci Med 2005;60(3):617–26.
33. Levine M, Levitan R, Skolnik A. Compartment syndrome after "bath salts" use: a case series. Ann Emerg Med 2013;61(4):480–3.
34. Kernan WN, Viscoli CM, Brass LM, et al. Phenylpropanolamine and the risk of hemorrhagic stroke. N Engl J Med 2000;343:1826–32.
35. Haller CA, Benowitz NL. Adverse cardiovascular and central nervous system events associated with dietary supplements containing ephedra alkaloids. N Engl J Med 2000;343:1833–8.
36. Kokkinos J, Levine SR. Possible association of ischemic stroke with phenter-mine. Stroke 1993;24:310–3.
37. Abenhaim L, Moride Y, Brenot F, et al. Appetite-suppressant drugs and the risk of primary pulmonary hypertension. International Primary Pulmonary Hyperten-sion Study Group. N Engl J Med 1996;335(9):609–16.
38. Chu J. Antimigraine medications. In: Nelson LS, Lewin NA, Howland MA, et al, ed-itors. Goldfrank's toxicologic emergencies. 9th edition. New York: McGraw-Hill; 2011. p. 763–9.
39. Harrison TE. Ergotaminism. JACEP 1978;7:162–9.
40. de Labriolle A, Genée O, Heggs LM, et al. Acute myocardial infarction following oral methyl-ergometrine intake. Cardiovasc Toxicol 2009;9(1):46–8.
41. Senter HJ, Lieverman AN, Pinto R. Cerebral manifestations of ergotism. Report of a case and review of the literature. Stroke 1976;7:88–92.

42. Rogers DA, Mansberger JA. Gastrointestinal vascular ischemia caused by ergotamine. South Med J 1989;82:1058–9.
43. Webb J. Renal failure associated with ergot poisoning. Br Med J 1977;2(6098): 1355.
44. Meschia JF, Malkoff MD, Biller J. Reversible segmental cerebral arterial vasospasm and cerebral infarction: possible association with excessive use of sumatriptan and Midrin. Arch Neurol 1998;55:712–4.
45. Jayamaha JE, Street MK. Fatal cerebellar infarction in a migraine sufferer whilst receiving sumatriptan. Intensive Care Med 1995;21:82–3.
46. Vijayan N, Peacock JH. Spinal cord infarction during use of zolmitriptan: a case report. Headache 2000;40:57–60.
47. Deleu D, Hanssens Y. Current and emerging second-generation triptans in acute migraine therapy: a comparative review. J Clin Pharmacol 2000;40: 687–700.
48. Abbrescia VD, Pearlstein L, Kotler M. Sumatriptan-associated myocardial infarction: report of case with attention to potential risk factors. J Am Osteopath Assoc 1997;97:162–4.
49. Main ML, Ramaswamy K, Andrews TC. Cardiac arrest and myocardial infarction immediately after sumatriptan injection. Ann Intern Med 1998;128:874.
50. Ottervanger JP, Paalman HJ, Boxma GL, et al. Transmural myocardial infarction with sumatriptan. Lancet 1993;341:861–2.
51. Arora A, Arora S. Spontaneous splenic infarction associated with sumatriptan use. J Headache Pain 2006;7:214–6.
52. Knudsen JF, Friedman B, Chen M, et al. Ischemic colitis and sumatriptan use. Arch Intern Med 1998;158:1946–8.
53. Barrueto F, Jortani S, Valdes R, et al. Cardioactive steroid poisoning from an herbal cleansing preparation. Ann Emerg Med 2003;41:396–9.
54. Ma G, Brady WJ, Pollack M, et al. Electrocardiographic manifestations: digitalis toxicity. J Emerg Med 2001;20:145–52.
55. Bismuth C, Gaultier M, Conso F, et al. Hyperkalemia in acute digitalis poisoning: prognostic significance and therapeutic implications. Clin Toxicol 1973;6: 153–62.
56. Lindenbaum J, Rund DG, Butler VP, et al. Inactivation of digoxin by the gut flora: reversal by antibiotic therapy. N Engl J Med 1981;305:789–94.
57. Manini AF, Nelson LS, Hoffman RS. Prognostic utility of serum potassium in chronic digoxin toxicity: a case-control study. Am J Cardiovasc Drugs 2011; 11(3):173–8.
58. Manini AF, Kumar A, Olsen D, et al. Utility of serum lactate to predict drug-overdose fatality. Clin Toxicol (Phila) 2010;48(7):730–6.
59. Thompson AM, Robins JB, Prescott LF. Changes in cardiorespiratory function during gastric lavage for drug overdose. Hum Toxicol 1987;6:215–8.
60. Roberts D, Honcharik N, Sitar DS, et al. Diltiazem overdose: pharmacokinetics of diltiazem and its metabolites and effect of multiple dose charcoal therapy. J Toxicol Clin Toxicol 1991;29:45–52.
61. Buckley N, Dawson AH, Howarth D, et al. Slow-release verapamil poisoning. Use of polyethylene glycol whole-bowel lavage and high-dose calcium. Med J Aust 1993;158:202–4.
62. Chiang WK. Amphetamines. In: Nelson LS, Lewin NA, Howland MA, et al, editors. Goldfrank's toxicologic emergencies. 9th edition. New York: McGraw-Hill; 2011.
63. McCord J, Jneid H, Hollander JE, et al. Management of cocaine-associated chest pain and myocardial infarction. A scientific statement from the American

Heart Association Acute Cardiac Care Committee of the Council on Clinical Cardiology. Circulation 2008;117:1897–907.

64. Proano L, Chiang WK, Wang RY. Calcium channel blocker overdose. Am J Emerg Med 1995;13:444–50.

65. Dolan DL. Intravenous calcium before verapamil to prevent hypotension. Ann Emerg Med 1991;20:588–9.

66. Hariman RJ, Mangiardi LM, McAllister RG Jr, et al. Reversal of the cardiovascular effects of verapamil by calcium and sodium: differences between electrophysiologic and hemodynamic responses. Circulation 1979;59:797–804.

67. Luscher TF, Noll G, Sturmer T, et al. Calcium gluconate in severe verapamil intoxication. N Engl J Med 1994;330:718–20.

68. Howarth DM, Dawson AH, Smith AJ, et al. Calcium channel blocking drug overdose: an Australian series. Hum Exp Toxicol 1994;13:161–6. p. 1078–90.

69. Bower JO, Mengle H. The additive effects of calcium and digitalis: a warning with a report of two deaths. JAMA 1936;106:1151–3.

70. Antman EM, Wenger TL, Butler VP, et al. Treatment of 150 cases of life-threatening digitalis intoxication with digoxin-specific Fab antibody fragments. Final report of a multicenter study. Circulation 1990;81:1744–52.

71. Flanagan R, Jones A. Fab antibody fragments: some applications in clinical toxicology. Drug Saf 2004;27:1115–33.

72. Shumaik GM, Wu AW, Ping AC. Oleander poisoning: treatment with digoxin-specific Fab antibody fragments. Ann Emerg Med 1988;17:732–5.

73. Soghoian S, Nelson LS, Hoffman RS. Death after ingestion of a topical aphrodisiac containing toad venom. Abstracts of the XXIX International Congress of the European Association of Poison Centres and Clinical Toxicologists. Stockholm (Sweden): 47:436–510. 2009.

74. Yagami T. Differential coupling of glucagon and beta-adrenergic receptors with the small and large forms of the stimulatory G protein. Mol Pharmacol 1995;48: 849–54.

75. Agarwal A, Yu SW, Rehman A, et al. Hyperinsulinemia euglycemia therapy for calcium channel blocker overdose: a case report. Tex Heart Inst J 2012;39:575–8.

76. Engebretsen KM, Kaczmarek KM, Morgan J, et al. High-dose insulin therapy in beta-blocker and calcium channel-blocker poisoning. Clin Toxicol (Phila) 2011; 49:277–83.

77. Kline JA, Tomaszewski CA, Schroeder JD, et al. Insulin is a superior antidote for cardiovascular toxicity induced by verapamil in the anesthetized canine. J Pharmacol Exp Ther 1993;267:744–50.

78. Kline JA, Raymond RM, Leonova ED, et al. Insulin improves heart function and metabolism during non-ischemic cardiogenic shock in awake canines. Cardiovasc Res 1997;34:289–98.

79. Holger JS, Stellpflug SJ, Cole JB, et al. High-dose insulin: a consecutive case series in toxin-induced cardiogenic shock. Clin Toxicol (Phila) 2011;49:653–8.

80. Holger JS, Engebretsen KM, Marini JJ. High dose insulin in toxic cardiogenic shock. Clin Toxicol (Phila) 2009;47:303–7.

81. Greene SL, Gawarammana I, Wood DM, et al. Relative safety of hyperinsulinaemia/euglycaemia therapy in the management of calcium channel blocker overdose: a prospective observational study. Intensive Care Med 2007;33:2019–24.

82. Driscoll DF. Lipid injectable emulsions: pharmacopeial and safety issues. Pharm Res 2006;23:1959–69.

83. Foxall G, McCahon R, Lamb J, et al. Levobupivacaine-induced seizures and cardiovascular collapse treated with Intralipid. Anaesthesia 2007;62:516–8.

84. Warren JA, Thoma RB, Georgescu A, et al. Intravenous lipid infusion in the successful resuscitation of local anesthetic-induced cardiovascular collapse after supraclavicular brachial plexus block. Anesth Analg 2008;106:1578–80 [table of contents].

85. Geib AJ, Liebelt E, Manini AF. Clinical experience with intravenous lipid emulsion for drug-induced cardiovascular collapse. J Med Toxicol 2012;8:10–4.

86. Bania TC, Chu J, Perez E, et al. Hemodynamic effects of intravenous fat emulsion in an animal model of severe verapamil toxicity resuscitated with atropine, calcium, and saline. Acad Emerg Med 2007;14:105–11.

87. Markowitz S, Neal JM. Immediate lipid emulsion therapy in the successful treatment of bupivacaine systemic toxicity. Reg Anesth Pain Med 2009;34:276.

88. Cave G, Harvey M, Graudins A. Intravenous lipid emulsion as antidote: a summary of published human experience. Emerg Med Australas 2011;23:123–41.

89. West PL, McKeown NJ, Hendrickson RG. Iatrogenic lipid emulsion overdose in a case of amlodipine poisoning. Clin Toxicol (Phila) 2010;48:393–6.

90. Holzer M, Sterz F, Schoerkhuber W, et al. Successful resuscitation of a verapamil-intoxicated patient with percutaneous cardiopulmonary bypass. Crit Care Med 1999;27:2818–23.

91. Pichon N, Dugard A, Clavel M, et al. Extracorporeal albumin dialysis in three cases of acute calcium channel blocker poisoning with life-threatening refractory cardiogenic shock. Ann Emerg Med 2012;59:540–4.

92. Facility assessment guidelines for regional toxicology treatment centers. American Academy of Clinical Toxicology. J Toxicol Clin Toxicol 1993;31:211–7.

93. Poison information and treatment systems. American College of Emergency Physicians. Ann Emerg Med 1996;28:384.

94. Sayre MR, Koster RW, Botha M, Adult Basic Life Support Chapter Collaborators. Part 5: adult basic life support: 2010 International Consensus on Cardiopulmonary Resuscitation and Emergency Cardiovascular Care Science With Treatment Recommendations. Circulation 2010;122(Suppl 2):S298–324.

Toxin-Induced Hepatic Injury

Annette M. Lopez, MD[a,b,]*, Robert G. Hendrickson, MD[a,b,c]

KEYWORDS

- Toxin • Liver injury • Management • Acetaminophen • Valproic acid • Amanita
- Ethanol • Statins

KEY POINTS

- Toxins such as pharmaceuticals, herbals, foods, and supplements may lead to hepatic damage that presents as nonspecific symptoms in the setting of liver test abnormalities.
- Most cases of toxin-induced damage are caused by acetaminophen, which is treated with N-acetylcysteine.
- The most important step in the patient evaluation is to gather an extensive history that includes toxin exposure and excludes common causes of liver dysfunction.
- Patients with acute liver failure benefit from transfer to a transplant service for further management.
- The mainstay in management for most exposures is cessation of the offending agent.

EPIDEMIOLOGY

Nature and Scope of the Problem

Toxin-induced hepatic injury may be defined as damage to the liver caused by a xenobiotic or toxin that leads to abnormalities of liver-related blood tests or liver function.[1,2] Toxin-induced hepatic injury may range from a mild increase in aminotransferase concentrations to fulminant liver failure and may manifest as acute hepatic necrosis, cholestasis, steatosis, cirrhosis, or asymptomatic increased aminotransferase concentration. Hepatic injury is a common diagnostic and treatment dilemma for the emergency physician, and a comprehensive understanding of the causes, evaluation, and treatment are essential.

Disclosures: None.
[a] Department of Emergency Medicine, Oregon Health and Science University, 3181 South West, Sam Jackson Park Road, CSB-550, Portland, OR 97239, USA; [b] Medical Toxicology, Oregon Health and Science University, 3181 South West Sam Jackson Park Road, CSB-550, Portland, OR 97239, USA; [c] Oregon Poison Center, 3181 South West, Sam Jackson Park Road, CSB 550, Portland, OR 97239, USA
* Corresponding author. Department of Emergency Medicine, Oregon Health and Science University, 3181 South West, Sam Jackson Park Road, CSB-550, Portland, OR 97239.
E-mail address: lopezan@ohsu.edu

Incidence

It is difficult to assess the true frequency and incidence of toxin-induced hepatic injury because of difficulties establishing the cause, the retrospective nature of studies, and the intrinsic selection bias of many studies performed in liver transplant centers.[1] To date, one prospective study was restricted to pharmaceuticals and demonstrated an incidence of drug-induced liver injury of 14 cases per 100,000 inhabitants.[1–3] Retrospective studies in Sweden and the United Kingdom have noted incidences of 2 to 3 cases per 1000,000 inhabitants; in Spain, the annual incidence is reported at 1 per 100,000 inhabitants.[1,3] With regard to nonpharmaceutical herbs and dietary supplements, there are few studies available. In one study, 10 of the 20 patients with acute liver failure who were referred for liver transplantation had used an herb or dietary supplement with potential hepatotoxicity.[4,5] The incidence of toxin-mediated hepatic injury may be dynamic, particularly with the increasing use of pharmaceuticals, supplements, and herbals.[6]

Overdose of acetaminophen is common, due to its ready availability over the counter and in prescribed combination products in the United States and the developed world. Acetaminophen has an estimated annual incidence of 21 overdoses per 100,000 people in the United States.[7] In 2011, there were 85,069 intentional and unintentional exposures to acetaminophen reported to US poison centers.[8]

Other drugs such as antibacterials, nonsteroidal antiinflammatory agents, and anticonvulsants accounted for 4% to 10% of cases of jaundice admitted to inpatient hospitals.[3,9,10] Of those drugs, amoxicillin/clavulanic acid is the most common compound leading to hepatic injury. Hepatotoxin incidence may also vary by region. In western countries, herbals account for less than 10% of reported cases of toxicity; however in Asia, these agents account for a much higher proportion.[10]

An individual's risk of hepatotoxicity may also vary based on identified factors that are independently associated with worse prognosis, including advanced age, female sex, and increased aspartate aminotransferase (AST) concentrations.[3,10] Both chronic disease (diabetes, hepatitis B and C, psoriasis, obesity) and xenobiotic dose have been associated with higher risk of toxin-induced heptatotoxicity.[2,3,11] Several risk factors have been identified for specific types of hepatotoxicity as well:[10]

African Americans are at an increased risk of anticonvulsant hepatotoxicity.
Younger patients are at increased risk for hepatotoxicity from valproic acid and salicylates.
Younger patients are also more likely to develop drug-induced hepatocellular injury.
Older age increases the risk of developing cholestatic injury.
Females may be at higher risk of drug-induced hepatotoxicity, particularly autoimmune hepatic injuries.
Alcohol (ethanol) use may increase toxicity in patients with repeated supratherapeutic ingestion of acetaminophen, methotrexate overdose, and toxicity from antituberculosis medications.

Morbidity

The morbidity of toxin-related hepatic injury varies widely from patients with asymptomatic increased aminotransferase concentrations to those with acute liver failure. The short-term morbidity of patients with asymptomatic increased aminotransferase concentrations in the emergency department (ED) is likely low. Most of these ED patients have mild transient increases in aminotransferase concentrations and many have chronic increased aminotransferase concentrations from repeated ethanol use. However, care must be taken to avoid missing cases with reversible causes that lead to high morbidity, such as acetaminophen toxicity, toxin-related acute hepatic necrosis, cholestasis, and so forth.

To determine the prognosis for toxin-induced acute liver failure, it is best to separate exposures into two groups: acetaminophen and non-acetaminophen. Within the non-acetaminophen group, there is a poor probability of recovery from acute liver failure without liver transplantation.[7] Risk factors for a poor prognosis include duration of symptoms greater than seven days, high bilirubin concentration, and severe hypoprothrombinemia. The overall morbidity from acetaminophen toxicity is low. However, a small percentage develop acute liver failure and significant morbidity. Those who survive, however, experience complete resolution of their hepatotoxicity without long-term morbidity.

Mortality

Mortality from hepatotoxicity ranges from very low to exceedingly high, depending on the toxin, the dose, and host factors. Mortality after acetaminophen overdose varies greatly; overall mortality is less than 1% for all overdoses, but is as high as 80% to 90% for those who develop acute liver failure and meet transplant criteria.

Once a patient develops acute liver failure, the leading causes of mortality are infection, cerebral edema, and refractory hypotension with multiorgan failure.[7]

PHYSIOLOGY
Liver Structure

The liver, the largest organ of the body, is found in the right upper quadrant of the abdomen where it is held in place by multiple ligaments to surrounding structures. Its dual blood supply arises from the hepatic artery, which provides oxygen-rich blood and accounts for 20% of the blood flow, and the nutrient-rich portal vein, which drains the upper gastrointestinal tract.[12]

The bulk of the liver is made up of hepatocytes, cells responsible for the functions typically ascribed to the liver. The remainder is comprised of Kupffer cells (resident macrophages), stellate cells (fat-storing cells), endothelial cells, bile ductular cells, and supporting structures. The morphology of the liver can be best described by two models: structural and functional (**Fig. 1**). In the structural model, the liver is organized into lobules composed of the portal vein in the periphery and the central vein within the center. In the functional model, the liver is organized into acini. Within the

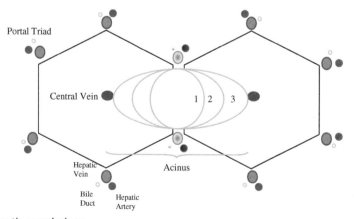

Fig. 1. Hepatic morphology.

acini, there are three zones of importance. Zone 1 spans the portal area that contains the blood flow coming from the hepatic artery and the portal vein. Blood continues to flow through the sinusoids of the hepatocytes (zone 2) on its way to the central hepatic veins. In contrast, bile drainage occurs in the opposite direction of blood flow.[12] Zone 3, the centrilobular area, has the lowest oxygen content.

Bile originates within the hepatocytes and from the ductular epithelium of the liver. The flow of the bile out of the liver is modulated by osmotic flow. Hepatocyte-generated bile contains bile salts, bilirubin, cholesterol, phospholipids, and drug metabolites. Xenobiotics and bile salts are passed into the bile cannalicula across the biliary endothelium mostly via active transporters. The ductular cells are responsible for the secretion of water and the electrolyte component to bile.[13]

Liver Function

The liver is the body's primary organ responsible for the metabolism (detoxification) of pharmaceuticals and toxins.[4] Ingested compounds are absorbed by the gastrointestinal tract and transported to the liver via the portal circulation.[14] Most human toxins are lipophilic. Thus, to be excreted through urine or bile, they require enzymatic modification within the hepatocytes to become water soluble.[15]

Pathophysiology

There are multiple mechanisms responsible for the development of toxin-induced liver dysfunction. The toxin itself can inhibit metabolism, leading to accumulation of endogenous agents. Some toxins can covalently bind to proteins, leading to cell membrane disruption and eventual cell death. Covalent bonding can lead to the formation of adducts, which can act as immune targets and/or initiate an immunologic response. Toxins may also be responsible for the disruption of transporters and pumps responsible for bile flow, causing cholestasis and cell injury. They may also inhibit mitochondrial activity, resulting in the formation of reactive oxygen species, lipid peroxidation, and the accumulation of fat, energy failure, and cell death.[2,4]

Forms of Hepatotoxicity

Acute necrosis

Acute hepatic necrosis may occur when large numbers of hepatocytes develop necrosis. This is followed by cellular rupture and spillage of intracellular components into the serum, contributing to a massive inflammatory response. Necrosis may occur focally within the liver with relatively preserved hepatic function, or diffuse injury may compromise both synthetic and metabolic function. Acute hepatic necrosis may be identified by a rapid increase in aminotransferases (eg, over days) and is defined by an alanine aminotransferase (ALT) concentration more than twice normal or an ALT to alkaline phosphatase ratio greater than or equal to 5 (**Table 1**).[16] These abnormalities are followed by increases in bilirubin and alkaline phosphatase.[2] This particular injury pattern represents nearly 50% of toxin-induced hepatic injury.[7] It is most commonly seen in severe acetaminophen toxicity, but other less common toxin-induced causes may include acute toxicity from iron or cyclopeptide-containing mushrooms (eg, *Amanita phalloides*), as well as exposure to halogenated hydrocarbons (eg, carbon tetrachloride, halothane), and isoniazid (INH) (**Table 2**).

Cholestasis

Cholestasis occurs when transfer of bile acids cannot be effected from the hepatocyte into the biliary cannaliculus. This may be caused by blockage of the biliary tract (eg, common bile duct cholelithiasis), as a result of genetic insufficiencies (eg, Gilbert

Table 1
Enzymes and their association with common hepatic injury patterns

Hepatic Injury Pattern	AST, ALT	PTT, INR	Bilirubin	Alkaline Phosphatase (AP)	Albumin	Ammonia	Anion Gap Acidosis	Comments
Hepatocellular necrosis								
Focal	>2 × N	N-H	H	N-H	N	N	N	ALT/AP ≥5
Massive	>2 × N	H	H	N-H	N	H	H	
Cholestasis								
Pure	N-H	N	H	>2 × N	N	N	N	
Acute cholestatic hepatitis	H	N	H	>2 × N	N	N	N	
Chronic	H	N	H	>2 × N	N	N	N	
Steatosis								
Microvesicular	H	N	H	N-H	N-L	H	H	Hypoglycemia
Macrovesicular	N-H	N	N	N-H	N	N	N	
Hepatic venoocclusive	N-H	N-H	H	N-H	L-N	N	N	99% have hyperbilirubinemia
Cholelithiasis	H	N	N-H	H	N	N-H	N	
Cirrhosis	H	N-H	N-H	N-H	L	N-H	N	
Chronic alcoholism	N-H	N	N	N	N	N	N	AST/ALT >2

Abbreviations: H, high; L, low; N, normal; PTT, partial thromboplastin time.
Data from Refs. [2,6,9,10,13,16,62,67]

disease, Crigler-Najjar), or secondary to xenobiotic toxicity, such as with anabolic steroids, estrogens (eg, oral contraceptives), cyclosporine, and several antimicrobials (eg, trimethaprim/sulfamethoxazole, tetracycline, macrolides, and rifampin). Both acute and chronic forms exist.

Acute cholestasis is defined by an initial increase in the serum alkaline phosphatase concentration to more than twice the normal concentration (see **Table 1**).[2,16,17] It may be divided into two subtypes: pure cholestasis and cholestatic hepatitis, which are differentiated by the presence of increased aminotransferase concentrations in cholestasis.[16,17]

Chronic cholestasis is most commonly from cardiovascular and central nervous system pharmaceuticals such as atorvastatin, azathioprine, bupropion, carbamazepine, mirtazapine, and tricyclic antidepressants (see **Table 2**).

Steatosis

Hepatic steatosis refers to the abnormal retention of lipids within hepatocytes. Microvesicular and macrovesicular forms may be differentiated by the size of lipid deposits on histology. Steatosis reflects an impairment of the handling or storage of lipids and may be caused by a variety of toxins (see **Table 2**).

Macrovesicular steatosis is more common than microvesicular steatosis and may be caused by the chronic use of alcohol or amiodarone (see **Table 2**). Microvesicular steatosis is characterized by mildly increased serum ALT concentrations in the presence of impaired β-oxidation of fatty acids and mitochondrial dysfunction. This phenomenon is characterized by hypoglycemia, hyperammonemia, hyperlactatemia, and metabolic acidosis (see **Table 1**).[17] Chronic use of valproate, tetracycline, antiretroviral nucleoside analogues (eg, didanosine, zidovudine [AZT]), as well as more rare exposures to margosa oil, hypoglycin (from unripe Jamaican ackee fruit), aflatoxin (*Aspergillus* mycotoxin found in grain), dimethylformamide (an industrial solvent), and cerulide (*Bacillus cereus* food poisoning) present in this fashion.

Chronic hepatitis

Chronic hepatitis may develop after chronic exposure to several xenobiotics, including diclofenac, nitrofurantoin, and methyldopa. This injury should be suspected in the presence of highly increased concentrations (5- to 60-fold) of aminotransferases. Positive antinuclear antibodies and/or smooth muscle antibodies in conjunction with increases in serum concentrations of immunoglobulins suggest an autoimmune etiology.[17] Granulomatous hepatitis may also occur after chronic exposure to many xenobiotics (see **Table 2**) and is characterized by granuloma formation within the hepatic parenchyma.

Hepatic venoocclusive disease

Hepatic venoocclusive disease is rare and may be caused by toxins that induce edema, intimal thickening, and nonthrombotic obstruction of the hepatic veins. Subsequent dilatation of the hepatic sinusoids, a gross appearance of a "nutmeg liver," and hepatic congestion are associated with a mortality rate of 10% to 20%. Toxins that may cause this condition are generally found in plant supplements or teas and contain pyrrolizidine alkaloids. Several examples are comfrey tea (*Symphytum*), *Heliotropium* species, *Senecio* species, and *Crotalaria spectabilis*.

Cirrhosis

Cirrhosis results from progressive fibrosis and scarring of the liver parenchyma with eventual diminution of hepatic function and portal hypertension. Chronic use of alcohol is the most common cause. The chronic ingestion of large amounts of vitamin

Table 2
Agents causing liver injury

Type of Liver Injury	Agents
Acute necrosis	Acetaminophen
	α-Amanitin
	Carbon tetrachloride
	Dantrolene
	Diclofenac
	Halothane
	Iron
	INH (isoniazid)
	Ketoconazole
	Methyldopa
	Minocycline
	Nitrofurantoin
	Pyrazinamide
	Phenytoin
	Tetracycline
	Troglitazone
	Valproic acid
Microvesicular steatosis	Aflatoxin
	Cerulide
	Dimethylformamide
	Fialuridine
	Hypoglycin (ackee fruit)
	Margosa oil
	Nucleoside inhibitors
	Tetracycline
	Transcriptase inhibitors
	Valproic acid
Macrovesicular steatosis	Amiodarone
	Tamoxifen
Cholestasis	ACE inhibitors
	Amoxicillin-clavulate acid
	Anabolic steroids
	Atorvastatin
	Azathioprine
	β-Lactam antibiotics
	Bosentan
	Bupropion
	Carbamazepine
	Chlorpromazine
	Clopidogrel
	Cytabarine
	Erythromycin
	Estrogen
	Floxuridine
	Fosinopril
	Irbersartan
	Mirtazapine
	Phenothiazines
	Phenytoin
	Sulindac
	Sulfonamides
	Terbinafine
	Tricyclic antidepressants
	(continued on next page)

Table 2 *(continued)*	
Type of Liver Injury	**Agents**
Granulomatous	Allopurinol
	Amoxicillin-clavulanate
	Carbamazepine
	Diphenylhydantoin
	Diltiazem
	Interferon α
	INH (isoniazid)
	Phenytoin
	Quinidine
	Sulfonamides
	Verapamil
Fibrosis/cirrhosis	Amiodarone
	Ethanol
	Methotrexate
	Methyldopa
	Perhexilene
	Vitamin A
Chronic/autoimmune hepatitis	α-Methyldopa
	Bentazepam
	Diclofenac
	Ebrotidine
	Fluoxetine
	INH (isoniazid)
	Mesalazine
	Methyldopa
	Minocycline
	Nitrofurantoin
	Paroxetine
	Trazodone
Hepatic venoocclusive	Busulfan
	Cyclophosphamide
	Dacarbazine
	Oral contraceptives
	Pyrrolizidone alkaloids
	Symphytum spp (comfrey)
	Heliotropium spp
	Senecio spp
	Crotalaria spectabilis
	Urethane

Data from Refs.[3,6,17,66]

A (at least 25,000 IU/day for years), as well as chronic use of methyldopa and methotrexate have led to cirrhosis. Methotrexate-induced cirrhosis is dose-dependent.

Acute liver failure

Several of the conditions already mentioned may lead to acute liver failure (ALF), which is defined as the onset of encephalopathy and coagulopathy within a short period (usually 26 weeks) of the onset of symptoms of hepatic toxicity. ALF can be subdivided into hyperacute liver failure (onset <7 days), acute (7–21 days), and subacute (21 days to 26 weeks). Most cases of ALF can be attributed to acetaminophen (39%) and other drug reactions (13%).[18] The diagnostic evaluation and treatment depend on the toxin involved and the severity of toxicity.

When considering pharmaceutical-induced hepatic toxicity, it is helpful to note that when pharmaceuticals are responsible for hepatic injury, patients most commonly (80%) have laboratory abnormalities or symptoms within three months of initiating drug therapy,[10] and within 12 months of drug initiation, with few exceptions.[7]

CLINICAL PRESENTATION

Patients may present to an ED with a range of symptoms. Asymptomatic increased aminotransferase concentrations are a common dilemma in the ED. Conversely, patients less commonly present with acute or chronic hepatic conditions that may be related to a toxin. In these cases, the emergency physician plays a vital role in determining the type of hepatic injury, withdrawing the toxin, and/or initiating treatment.

Symptoms that occur after a drug-induced hepatic insult tend to be nonspecific and may include asthenia, anorexia, nausea, abdominal pain, fever, jaundice, choluria (dark or brown urine due to bile salts), and pruritus.[2,10,18] Toxin-induced hepatic injury should be considered in the setting of these symptoms and laboratory evidence of liver function abnormalities.[2] **Table 1** includes common laboratory abnormalities from toxin-induced hepatic injury that may be used as a starting point for diagnosis.

Mildly increased aminotransferase concentrations without evidence of liver failure (eg, coagulopathy or encephalopathy) are commonly noted in ED evaluations. The pattern of injury may be helpful in determining cause. The AST/ALT ratio is normally less than 1, but a ratio of greater than 2 may indicate alcoholic hepatitis.

Patients may present to the ED with highly increased aminotransferases concentrations or with evidence of liver failure (eg, encephalopathy or coagulopathy) that has developed over two to four days. In these cases, acetaminophen should be considered, as it is the most common cause of ALF in the United States[19,20] and most developed countries, and is the cause of most cases of ALF that develop over days (hyperacute liver failure). Other causes of toxin-induced liver toxicity that should be considered include iron toxicity and ingestion of cyclopeptide-containing mushrooms, as there may be effective antidotes for each. Other causes of toxin-induced ALF are included in **Table 2**.

Other clinical clues may steer the emergency physician to a specific diagnosis. Prominent jaundice and pruritis may suggest cholestasis, subacute symptoms such as nausea, weight loss, and fatigue, may suggest steatosis,[17] and signs of hepatic congestion suggest hepatic venoocclusive disease. Fever, rash, and eosinophilia may suggest chronic hepatitis.[1]

APPROACH TO TOXIN-INDUCED HEPATIC INJURY
Management

The initial approach in the evaluation of a patient who presents to the ED with acute liver injury involves a thorough history and physical examination. A history of recent ingestions, including pharmaceuticals as well as recently consumed foods, herbal products, and supplements should be obtained.[15] Careful assessment should ensure that there is no alternative explanation such as alcohol abuse, risk factors for infectious hepatitis, or recent episodes of either hypoperfusion or heart failure.[3,4,15]

In some patients, nontoxicologic causes of hepatic injury may be evident on history, physical examination, and laboratory evaluation. Common nontoxicologic causes include cholelithiasis, cholecystitis, viral hepatitis, and biliary cirrhosis. These patients may need specific laboratory and imaging evaluations, including abdominal ultrasonography and serologic molecular studies to exclude commonly responsible viruses such as hepatitis B and C, and based on local prevalence or travel history, evaluation for hepatitis A and E.[2,4,10] In patients without obvious nontoxicologic causes, toxins should be considered and a laboratory examination should be initiated including AST, ALT, partial thromboplastin time or internationalized normalized ratio (INR), and acid-base status. If the mental status is altered or there is evidence of acidosis, an ammonia concentration should also be obtained.

In all patients with unexplained increase in aminotransferase concentrations, acetaminophen overuse should be considered because it is a commonly ingested pharmaceutical in overdose, a common coingestant, the most common cause of toxin-related hospital admission, and the most common cause of ALF in the United States.[19,20] If the medical history suggests acetaminophen overuse or it is unobtainable or unreliable, the patient should be immediately treated with N-acetylcysteine (NAC) and a serum acetaminophen concentration should be obtained. NAC may be effective in treating acetaminophen toxicity even when acetaminophen is undetectable in the serum, particularly in cases where liver failure has developed.[21] Because acute ingestion or repeated supratherapeutic ingestion of acetaminophen are common and because there is some evidence that NAC may be effective in treating non–acetaminophen-induced hepatotoxicity in adults,[22–24] it is reasonable to treat highly increased aminotransferase concentrations with NAC until the history or laboratory evaluation either confirms or eliminates acetaminophen as the causative agent.

In the rare patient who presents to the ED with ALF that is toxin-induced, acetaminophen should be strongly considered and NAC should be started unless the history or laboratory evidence rule it out. In one randomized trial, NAC decreased mortality in acetaminophen-induced ALF by almost 50%,[21] and there is limited evidence that NAC may improve outcomes in a subset of patients with non–acetaminophen-induced ALF.[22–24] Patients should be thoroughly evaluated for evidence of infection, coagulopathy, and cerebral edema. Supportive care for the patient with ALF is beyond the scope of this article, but is reviewed elsewhere.[20,25] Hypoglycemia is common in ALF and glucose concentrations should be monitored frequently. Early referral to a regional hepatic transplant center may be prudent.

If cholestasis, chronic hepatitis, or other toxin-induced hepatotoxicity are suspected, then the primary goal of the emergency physician involves discontinuation of the agent responsible.[1,2,7,13] In many cases, clinical improvement may be slow, and sometimes there might be continued deterioration before resolution.[2,10]

In cases of valproate toxicity, hemodialysis is used for severe acidosis or hypotension, and L-carnitine is recommended in the setting of encephalopathy or highly increased ammonia concentrations (see later section on valproate).[1]

If ingestion of cyclopeptide-containing mushrooms is suspected, multidose activated charcoal, penicillin G, silybinin, and NAC may be effective (see later discussion on mushrooms).[26–28]

In cases of cholestasis and toxin-induced hepatitis, corticosteroids are often prescribed but have no proven benefit.[7,10] However, corticosteroids may be beneficial in the setting of hypersensitivity syndromes such as those encountered with carbamazepine or in the setting of drug-induced autoimmune hepatitis.[1,15]

Additional Laboratory Analysis

The laboratory evaluation of a patient with hepatotoxicity may involve exclusion of genetic and metabolic disorders known to cause hepatic injury. Ferritin, iron concentrations, and total iron binding capacity can evaluate hematochromatosis. If autoimmune chronic hepatitis is suspected, serum concentrations of antinuclear and antismooth antibodies may be suggestive.[2,4] α-1-Antitrypsin deficiency can be evaluated with an α-1 antitrypsin concentration and further genotypic studies. Young individuals should be evaluated for Wilson disease by obtaining a ceruloplasmin concentration.[2] Because comorbid conditions such as human immunodeficiency virus and diabetes can lead to hepatic injury and may actually lead to worse outcomes, testing for these may be considered.[6]

Imaging

As part of the workup, individuals may undergo imaging to evaluate for alternative diagnoses, particularly if cholelithiasis or cholecystitis are considered. Abdominal ultrasonography can assist in the evaluation of mechanical biliary obstruction. Cholangiography, magnetic resonance cholangiopancreatography, or hepatobiliary iminodiacetic acid scans may be required.[2–4,13]

Pathology

A biopsy of the liver is not indicated in the ED; however, it may be obtained in the inpatient setting to better define the lesion and determine or suggest drug-induced liver injury, or eliminate alternative diagnoses.[16] Occasionally, biopsy findings may be available to the emergency physician; typical biopsy findings are listed in **Table 3**.

Specialized Care Transfer

In patients with toxin-induced ALF, urgent transfer to a liver transplant center for further evaluation and management should be considered.[1,7]

In the case of acetaminophen-induced ALF, rapid transfer to a transplant center should be considered in certain cases, because death may occur within three to five days of the ingestion and time is needed for patient evaluation and organ matching. There are no set criteria for transplant center transfer. However, patients who meet the King's College criteria have less than a 20% chance of survival; thus, it seems reasonable that a patient who meets, or approaches, any of these criteria should be considered for transfer:[29,30]

pH less than 7.30 or lactate greater than 3 mmol/L after fluid resuscitation
Creatinine greater than 3.3 mg/dL

Table 3
Typical biopsy findings in toxin-induced hepatic injury

Hepatic Injury Pattern	Biopsy Findings
Acute necrosis	Liver cell necrosis with an associated inflammatory cell infiltrate[16]
Cholestasis	Bilirubin deposits in the hepatocytes as well as dilated biliary canaliculi containing biliary pigments[13,16]
Macrovesicular steatosis	Hepatocytes with large lipid droplets within the cell that displace the nucleus of the cell. Mallory bodies (eosinophilic cytoplasmic keratin deposits) may be seen in alcoholic steatosis and lamellated intralysosomal phospholipid inclusion bodies may be evident in amiodarone steatosis
Microvesicular steatosis	Hepatocytes with lipid droplets that do not displace the nucleus
Cirrhosis	Fibrosis with fibrous tissue bands of varying sizes
Fibrosis	Steatosis with associated ballooning of the hepatocytes in the setting of minimal necrosis
Hepatic venoocclusive disease	Congestion and thrombosis of the vasculature with centrizonal necrosis and fibrosis[14]

Prothrombin time greater than 100 seconds (or INR >6.5)
Grade III or IV encephalopathy (somnolence, confusion, disorientation)

Several other criteria have been used to predict severe toxicity or death and may be adequate to use as criteria for transfer to, or discussion with, a transplant center:

Lactate greater than 4.7 mmol/L[29,30]
MELD (Model for End-Stage Liver Disease) score greater than 32[31–33]
SOFA (Sequential Organ Failure Assessment) score greater than 12[31,34]
APACHE II (Acute Physiology And Chronic Health Evaluation) score greater than 12[31,35]

Advanced Modalities

Several modalities attempt to bridge patients with ALF to either transplantation or recovery by supplementing hepatic toxin clearance. These systems may be divided into acellular and bioartificial hepatic support systems. Some have achieved approval for use in drug overdose or hepatic encephalopathy, but not as bridges to transplantation; others are not yet approved beyond trials. There is some evidence of efficacy for these systems.[36] Definitive trials in the setting of toxin-induced ALF, particularly acetaminophen-induced ALF, are needed.[37]

The acellular systems include extracorporeal albumin dialysis (eg, molecular adsorbent recirculation system [MARS] Gambro Lundia AB, Lund, Sweden), sorbent hemoperfusion (eg, Prometheus [Fresenius Medical Care, Bad Homburg, Germany]), and single pass albumin dialysis (SPAD). Currently, MARS is the most commonly used and studied system and has been shown to improve hemodynamics, encephalopathy, and intracranial pressures in patients with ALF,[38–40] while reducing the blood concentration[41] of bilirubin, bile acids, and creatinine. However, it was only found to be effective when used as a bridge to transplant, because it failed to provide survival benefit in those not undergoing transplantation.[37,42] MARS has been used to decrease bile acid concentrations and decrease the clinical manifestations of cholestasis.[43,44]

The Prometheus system is less well studied in toxin-induced ALF. Prometheus yields higher ammonia and bile acid clearance than MARS but has no effect on hemodynamics.[38,45]

SPAD is venovenous hemodialysis with albumin-containing dialysate. SPAD is more available than MARS or Prometheus, which require specialized equipment. SPAD may clear ammonia more effectively than MARS but may not alter hemodynamics or encephalopathy in ALF.[46,47] SPAD is not well studied in toxin-induced hepatic injury.

Bioartificial systems use cell-based bioreactors to conduct extracorporeal perfusion. The patient's blood is placed in contact with either porcine or human hepatocytes through the separation of a semipermeable membrane, which ideally prevents circulatory contamination. Studies of the effectiveness of these systems on ALF have been mixed and concerns for infectious or tumor transmigration have decreased their usefulness.[48,49]

SPECIFIC TOXINS OF INTEREST
Acetaminophen

In the United States, acetaminophen is responsible for almost 50% of cases of ALF, is the most commonly ingested pharmaceutical overdose, and results in more hospital admissions than any other toxin.[1,10,19,20]

Acetaminophen is metabolized to nontoxic metabolites through sulfation and glucuronidation, which account for approximately 95% of all metabolism. The remaining percentage undergoes metabolism by CYP2E1 to N-acetyl-p-benzo-quinoneimine (NAPQI). At therapeutic doses, NAPQI binds to glutathione through interactions with glutathione-S-transferase to a nonreactive metabolite. The liver's glutathione supply and recirculation are ample to bind NAPQI, and no toxicity occurs. With increasing doses of acetaminophen, normal metabolic pathways are saturated (eg, sulfation), and there is a proportionally higher generation of the reactive metabolite. The concentration of NAPQI increases, overwhelms the supply of glutathione, and covalently binds with surrounding proteins, leading to cell damage, necrosis, and inflammation. The use of NAC provides cysteine needed for the generation of glutathione, which prevents its depletion in the setting of acetaminophen overdose.[13,37]

On ingestion of a toxic dose, acetaminophen toxicity clinically presents as an entity with three distinct phases. The first phase corresponds to the immediate time frame following exposure, when the patient may report nausea, anorexia, and vomiting. The second phase is characterized by an improvement in the initial symptoms, although there is an increase of liver enzymes in the serum. AST concentrations increase first, typically between 8 and 24 hours after ingestion (**Fig. 2**). ALT concentrations increase shortly after AST and precedes an increases in INR and creatinine. The final phase involves the rapid development of jaundice, encephalopathy, and coagulopathy (acute liver failure). During the final phase, there may be concomitant development of renal injury.[14]

The toxic dose of acetaminophen is generally accepted as an acute ingestion that is greater than 7.5 g in adults or 150 mg/kg in children[37,50] or a repeated supratherapeutic ingestion of greater than 200 mg/kg/d (or 10 g/day, whichever is less) in a 24-hour period, 150 mg/kg/d (or 6 g/day, whichever is less) in a 48-hour period, or in children less than 6 years old, greater than 100 mg/kg/day over a 3-day period.[51,52]

Management

Appropriate management of acetaminophen toxicity requires separation of patients into acute and chronic ingestion. Acute ingestion is defined as a single ingestion or repeated ingestions in a time period that is less than 8 hours. Repeated supratherapeutic ingestion (chronic ingestion) occurs when the patient takes the acetaminophen over a period that is longer than eight hours.[52]

In acute ingestion when the time of ingestion is known, an acetaminophen concentration should be obtained four hours or later after the ingestion and plotted on the

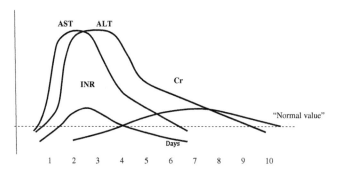

Fig. 2. Typical time course of increase, peak, and decrease of laboratory values in patients with acetaminophen-induced hepatic dysfunction who survive. Peaks are not proportional. Not all laboratory abnormalities occur in all patients and significant individual variation may occur. Cr, creatinine. (*Courtesy of* Robert G. Hendrickson, MD, Portland, OR.)

modified Rumack-Mathew nomogram to assess the risk of hepatotoxicity. An acetaminophen concentration that is higher than the possibly toxic line (treatment line), from 150 μg/mL at four hours to 9 μg/mL at 20 hours, indicates the need for initiation of treatment with NAC. However, this nomogram cannot be used in repeated supratherapeutic ingestions, staggered ingestions, presentations beyond 24 hours, and those with an unknown time of ingestion.[50]

Acetaminophen concentrations that are obtained before four hours should not be interpreted except to exclude the ingestion of acetaminophen (eg, an undetectable concentration). Very high initial concentrations may be below the treatment line at four hours, and very low initial concentrations may exceed the treatment line at four hours. There is no apparent increased risk of hepatotoxicity in waiting until four hours after the ingestion to obtain an acetaminophen concentration.

Initiation of NAC should occur within six to eight hours after acute ingestion if the concentration is above the treatment line, or as soon as possible if a concentration will not be available before the 8-hour mark.

NAC is available for both oral and intravenous regimens. The oral dosing includes an oral loading dose of 140 mg/kg followed by 70 mg/kg orally every 4 hours for a total of 18 doses (72 hours). The intravenous dosing starts with a loading dose of 150 mg/kg over 1 hour, followed by 50 mg/kg over 4 hours, and concluding with 100 mg/kg over the next 16 hours, for a total dosing duration of 21 hours.[50]

In cases of repeated supratherapeutic ingestions, AST and acetaminophen concentrations should be obtained if the patient has ingested more than

200 mg/kg/d (or 10 g/day, whichever is less) in any 24-hour period
150 mg/kg/d (or 6 g/day, whichever is less) in any 48-hour period, or
If <6 years old, greater than 100 mg/kg/d over three or more days

Other useful laboratory data for the management of acetaminophen toxicity include the assessment of aminotransferases, coagulation parameters, with particular attention to the INR and prothrombin time, renal function and electrolytes, all of which reflect the level of hepatic and metabolic compromise (see **Fig. 2**).[50]

Patients with ALF as demonstrated by altered mentation and/or coagulopathy as a result of acetaminophen exposure require intensive care management.[1,37] Transfer to a liver transplant center should be considered in patients who have coagulopathy, acidosis, renal dysfunction, and/or encephalopathy. The King's College criteria referenced previously provide guidelines for transplantation, particularly for patients with little chance of spontaneous recovery (>80%–90% mortality) and transplantation may be the only option for survival.

However, meeting King's College criteria does not ensure meeting transplant requirements; more than 50% of patients who meet the criteria fail to be listed because of a history of coexisting alcohol and/or drug abuse, psychiatric disease, sepsis, hypotension, and cerebral edema. Discussion with a regional transplant center about an individual's potential for transplant is advised. If transplantation does occur, overall survival is nearly 70%; deaths are linked to multiorgan failure, sepsis, and neurologic complications.[37]

If a biopsy is performed, it will reveal extensive centrilobular necrosis without steatosis and some inflammatory cells infiltrating.[37]

Valproic Acid

Valproic acid (valproate), a simple carboxylic acid, is a widely available agent commonly used for seizures. This agent has also been approved for mood stabilization and as a migraine prophylaxis agent. Practitioners are increasingly prescribing it off-label for the management of social phobias and neuropathic pain.[53–55] Its mechanism of action is postulated to involve alterations of central nervous system γ-aminobutyric acid concentration, attenuation of N-methyl-D-aspartate receptor–mediated neuroexcitation, depletion of cellular inositol, and membrane effects via potassium channels.[55,56] Although generally well tolerated, it is known to cause a benign increase in aminotransferase concentrations in up to 20% of patients. The risk of developing liver failure is age dependent, with children younger than two years old having the highest risk (1:550 with valproate use in combination with other drugs, 1:8000 when used as a single agent).[54]

Clinically, two types of hepatic injury are associated with valproic acid. One type leads to an acute and idiosyncratic hepatic failure that involves vesicular steatosis and may progress to necrosis similar to Reye syndrome. This type of injury is more commonly seen in children less than two years of age, as well as those with intellectual disabilities or neurologic disease, viral infections, and metabolic diseases. A second type of injury involves a milder, reversible form of injury associated with increased concentrations of aminotransferase, alkaline phosphatase, and bilirubin, which may develop in up to 44% of patients. This reaction tends to be dose dependent and associated with the initiation of the treatment.[55]

The mechanism for hepatotoxicity is linked to mitochondrial dysfunction as a result of impaired fatty acid metabolism and the depletion of coenzyme A.[55] Coenzyme A deficiency results in impairment of the mitochondrial enzymes responsible for β-oxidation of short-chain, medium-chain, and long-chain fatty acids, shifting metabolism to that of ω-oxidation, which generates the toxic metabolites 2-propyl-4-pentanoic acid, 4-en-valproic acid, and proprionic acid.[53,54] Valproic acid and its metabolites may also directly inhibit the respiratory chain within the mitochondria, leading to intracellular depletion of adenosine triphosphate.[17] The formation of 4-en-valproic acid also inhibits urea production, which leads to accumulation of ammonia.[53]

The clinical presentation of ALF from valproic acid includes lethargy, fatigue, anorexia, nausea, vomiting, jaundice, hemorrhage, and worsening of seizures. Fatalities caused by this hepatic injury tend to occur within three to six months of initiation. Hyperammonemic encephalopathy may start with initiation of valproate or after years of treatment (particularly with physiologic stress). It is characterized by acute onset of cognitive slowing, impaired consciousness, and delirium in the setting of increased concentrations of ammonia.[53]

Management

The most critical action in the management of this agent in the setting of hepatic injury involves cessation of use when the symptoms develop.[54] It is important to obtain valproate as well as ammonia concentrations to further delineate the management. The administration of L-carnitine has been recommended in the management of hepatic injury, particularly with concentrations greater than 450 mg/L.[53,54] Carnitine, a water-soluble amino acid derivative, is widely available in diets rich in red meat and dairy products. The human body is also capable of endogenous synthesis within the liver and the kidneys from dietary amino acids. L-carnitine mitigates valproic acid toxicity by facilitating fatty acid transport into the mitochondria, as well as regulating the ratio of coenzyme A within the mitochondria.[53]

Hemodialysis as a method of extracorporeal elimination may be beneficial in the setting of increased concentrations with severe symptoms, as a result of diminished protein binding in overdose. Criteria for the use of this intervention include concentrations greater than 850 to 1000 mg/L as well as signs of severe compromise such as hemodynamic instability, coma, hyperammonemia, electrolyte abnormalities, or metabolic disturbances.[57]

Mushrooms: Amanita Species

Amatoxins can be found within three fungal families: *Amanita*, *Lepiota*, and *Galerina*. The main toxin leading to morbidity and mortality is α-amanitin. *Amanita phalloides*, commonly called the death cap, is a member of the Amanita family. It contains the highest concentration of α-amanitin and is responsible for most of the fatalities from mushroom ingestions.[26,28] Emergency physicians should not attempt to identify mushrooms by description or Internet photos. Contact the regional poison center to access a local mycologist who may more accurately identify the mushroom. The typical appearance of the most common cyclopeptide-containing mushroom in the United States, *Amanita phalloides*, includes cream-colored gills, a solid stalk with a round base, overlying white volva with a contrasting white universal veil patch and a yellowish-brown cap;[26,58] however, the appearance changes based on the mushroom's age. Other cyclopeptide-containing mushrooms exist in the United States (eg, *Gallerina marginata*), such that nonmycologist identification should be avoided. *Amanita phalloides* grow in oak woodlands, in lawns near oak trees, and at the base of hazelnut trees, particularly in the Pacific Northwest, Pennsylvania, New Jersey, and Ohio. In the United States, two distinct populations occur: a western population ranging from California to British Columbia, and an eastern population found from Maine to Maryland.[58] Most deaths (50–100) occur in western Europe; deaths are less common in the United States, and even fewer are reported in Africa, Asia, Australia, and the Americas.[28]

Amanita phalloides toxicity proceeds from the activity of two distinct toxins. Phallotoxin alters the cellular membrane of the enterocytes.[59] It is responsible for the early gastrointestinal toxicity noted in patients. Although hepatotoxic, it is not absorbed by the intestines and toxicity is limited locally to the gastrointestinal tract.[28] α-Amatinin, a heat-stable toxin, is absorbed and inhibits RNA polymerase II, reducing protein synthesis and causing enterocytes, hepatocytes, and renal tubular cell necrosis.[26,28,58,59] Hepatocyte necrosis leads to the development of hepatic failure with coagulopathy, encephalopathy, renal failure, and death.[26,28] Up to 60% of the toxin is excreted into bile, causing further damage on recycling in the gastrointestinal tract via the enterohepatic circulation.[26] Amatoxin is filtered by the glomerulus and reabsorbed by the renal tubules, resulting in acute tubular necrosis.[28] For an adult, the lethal dose that causes 50% mortality (LD_{50}) is 0.1 mg/kg of body weight, an amount easily contained within one mushroom.[28,58]

Poisoning by *Amanita* is characterized by four distinct stages, which are quite similar to those of acetaminophen toxicity.[28] The initial stage, known as the incubation or lag phase during which time patients are asymptomatic, may range from 6 to 40 hours after ingestion, but is typically less than 24 hours. It is followed by a gastrointestinal phase, which lasts for 12 to 24 hours, characterized by clinical symptoms of nausea, vomiting, abdominal pain, and diarrhea. During this phase, the severe symptoms may lead to dehydration, electrolyte and acid-base disturbances, and hypotension. The convalescent stage, lasting 36 to 48 hours, then follows. During this time, the patient's gastrointestinal symptoms resolve, but hepatic injury evolves as demonstrated by increased aminotransferase concentrations.[28] The final cytotoxic stage heralds ALF. It is characterized by a dramatic increase in aminotransferases, coagulopathy, hepatic encephalopathy, and renal failure.[26,28] The disease may progress to multiorgan failure, disseminated intravascular coagulation, seizures, and coma; death ensues typically within 1 week after ingestion.[28]

Management

Unfortunately, there is no specific antidote available to treat α-amanitin toxicity. However, there are multiple modalities that may be effective, although definitive studies have not been performed. If a patient presents early after ingestion, gastrointestinal decontamination with activated charcoal may be effective in preventing absorption of the toxin. Aggressive supportive care using intravenous hydration should be considered to correct electrolyte and metabolite abnormalities.[28] Multiple-dose activated charcoal aids in reducing absorption of the toxin, particularly due to its enterohepatic circulation.[26,28] Some sources advocate the use of gastroduodenal aspiration through a nasoduodenal tube to aid in the removal of bile, as an attempt to interrupt recirculation of the toxin,[28] although theoretically multidose charcoal serves the same purpose of decreasing the enterohepatic recirculation and is less invasive.

Penicillin G, at doses of 40 million units per day for adults or 10 million units per day for children, has been used as a competitor for binding sites on serum proteins, preventing uptake of α-amantin by the hepatocytes.[26,28] This regimen does have a risk of seizures, and hypernatremia, or hyperkalemia, depending on the penicillin preparation. Ceftazidime in doses of 4.5 g intravenously every 2 hours has also been shown to prevent uptake, and was more effective than penicillin G in some studies.[26]

Silybinum marianum, a falvonolignant that is isolated from milk thistle, inhibits binding of α-amanitin to hepatocytes. It also interferes with the transmembrane transport required for enterohepatic circulation of the toxin. An intravenous formulation, silybinin dihemisuccinate (Legalon SIL), is available in Europe. It is administered as a loading dose of 5 mg/kg over one hour followed by a 20 mg/kg/d infusion for six days.[26,28] Although currently not approved by the US Food and Drug Administration, open phase 2/3 clinical trials are underway for patients diagnosed with amatoxin poisoning by history, signs, and symptoms, as well as increased concentrations of liver enzymes.[27] If the intravenous formulation is unavailable, oral silymarin capsules have also been used at doses of 1.4 to 4.2 g/day.[28]

NAC is another adjuvant used in the treatment of α-amanitin toxicity by providing sulfhydryl groups to aid in the detoxification of reactive metabolites.[26] It is given intravenously as a loading dose of 150 mg/kg over 60 minutes, followed by an infusion of 50 mg/kg over 4 hours, and 100 mg/kg over 16 hours.[28]

A review of all published American and European cases of mushroom hepatotoxicity over 20 years found that penicillin G alone and in combination with other treatments showed little efficacy. Therapies that had support for use included sylibin and NAC.[60]

If patients continue to decompensate despite therapy, liver transplantation may be required. This may be the outcome in 10% to 20% of cases of α-amanitin exposure.[26,28,59] Currently there are two surgical approaches available: orthotopic liver transplantation (OLT) and auxiliary partial orthotopic liver transplantation (APOLT). In OLT, the entire organ is replaced with a graft that requires long-term immunosuppression to prevent rejection. In APOLT, only a partial resection of the native liver occurs and the graft supports the native liver until recovery occurs at which point immunosuppression may be stopped.[28]

Alcohol (Ethanol)

Alcohol toxicity is the third most common cause of morbidity worldwide, and in the United States it is the third leading cause of preventable deaths. The development of hepatic injury in the setting of ethanol ingestion has a spectrum that includes asymptomatic increased aminotransferase concentrations, hepatic steatosis, steatohepatitis, and cirrhosis.[61]

A common conundrum faced by emergency physicians is the asymptomatic patient with a mildly increased aminotransferase concentration. A mild increase is defined as up to 5 times the upper limit of normal. Studies have found this event to occur in up to 4% of the population. Incidental increases in aminotransferase might not solely reflect liver injury. Hyperthyroidism, exercise, diurnal variations, and muscle injury might account for it, and evaluation to exclude these causes should occur. Initial management involves appropriate history gathering focusing on medication, supplements, drug and alcohol use, history of blood transfusions, and symptoms of liver disease. In alcoholics, a ratio of AST/ALT greater than two is characteristic for alcoholic hepatitis, although this ratio should not be used for diagnostic purposes.[62]

Hepatic steatosis involves two distinct entities: macrovesicular steatosis and microvesicular steatosis. Within two weeks of heavy consumption, up to 90% of heavy ethanol consumers can develop macrovesicular steatosis, or large-droplet fat deposition within zone 3 hepatocytes (see **Fig. 1**) without necrosis or inflammation. In severe cases, fatty deposition can occur throughout the liver. In microvesicular steatosis or alcoholic foamy degeneration, small-droplet fat deposition occurs within hepatocytes. Both entities clinically present with asymptomatic hepatomegaly and nonspecific gastrointestinal complaints. Those with microvesicular steatosis tend to have more severe illness and may present with jaundice, acidosis, and increased concentrations of liver aminotransferases. Cessation of ethanol consumption leads to reversal; however, if ethanol use continues, it may progress to steatohepatitis or fibrosis.[61]

In one-third of heavy ethanol drinkers, continued heavy consumption progresses to steatohepatitis.[61] When these patients present, they tend to be ill with fever, anorexia, nausea, vomiting, jaundice, abdominal pain, and weight loss with increased concentrations of aminotransferase.[61,63] If a biopsy is performed, there may be hepatic inflammation and hepatocyte necrosis.[61] There may also be intrahepatic cholestasis, Mallory bodies, and giant mitochondria.[63] Cessation of ethanol consumption can lead to complete regression in up to 10% of patients, although up to 70% develop cirrhosis.[61]

Cirrhosis, the eventual fibrosis of the hepatocytes that occurs as a result of chronic inflammation and necrosis, is the end of the spectrum. In the United States, alcohol-related cirrhosis is responsible for 44% of all deaths caused by liver disease. Clinical decompensation of these patients includes the development of encephalopathy, ascites, or variceal bleeding. If cessation of alcohol consumption occurs, 5-year survival can range from 60% to 90%. Unfortunately, decreased survival (30%–70%) occurs in those with persistent ethanol consumption. The development of cirrhosis also increases the patient's risk of developing hepatocellular carcinoma, further increasing their morbidity and mortality.[61]

Management

The cornerstone of management for all injuries related to ethanol abuse involves cessation of ethanol consumption, which may allow the liver to regenerate. Nutrition, including electrolyte repletion as well as liberal supplementation of multivitamins, folate, and thiamine are important. It may be necessary to supplement caloric intake, because the hepatic derangements present in these patients generate a catabolic state.[63]

Statins

The statin class of drugs act to inhibit the action of 3-hydroxy-3-methylglutaryl coenzyme A, thus aiding in lowering blood cholesterol concentrations.[64] In therapeutic dosing, statins are known to cause mild increases in aminotransferase concentrations.

Asymptomatic mild increases occur in 0% to 3% of patients and it tends to be dose related and likely to occur within the first 12 weeks of treatment.[9,64] However, these increases are no different when compared with placebo. Significant increases leading to ALF are extremely rare.[9]

ALF is rare in these patients, and it is likely to the result of idiosyncratic mechanisms of injury. Data from US transplant recipients from 1990 to 2002 documented only 3 cases of 51,741 with ALF linked to statins. When lovastatin was independently studied, it was found to have the same rate of idiopathic liver failure as that found in the background occurrence of ALF.[9]

When affected, patients tend to present with symptoms consistent with acute hepatitis such as pruritus, jaundice, nausea, abdominal pain, anorexia, and fatigue.[65] Autoimmune hepatitis seems to be the specific liver injury pattern associated with statins. Biopsies have shown minimal to advanced fibrosis, as well as portal inflammation including lymphocytes and sometime eosinophils, with or without cholestasis.[9,65]

Management

As with all toxins leading to hepatic injury, the first step in management should be the cessation of the offending agent. Previous management of these cases has included treatment with prednisone and other immunosuppressants including tacrolimus, azathioprine, or mycophenolate mofetil. Genotypic analysis of the few cases available has revealed positivity of HLA- DR3, DR4 and DR7.[9]

Anabolic Steroids

Anabolic steroids, in particular those with an alkyl group at the 17th carbon, are known to cause hepatotoxicity. Classically, a cholestatic pattern of injury is produced without damage to the hepatic parenchyma. The mechanism of injury is likely dose related. These steroids impair biliary excretion through interference with the sodium-potassium pump, altering permeability, and leading to dysfunction and inability to secrete and transport bile. At therapeutic dosing, most users experience aminotransferase abnormalities. Within 2 to 5 months, a few go on to develop dysfunction leading to jaundice.[14]

Management

The mainstay of management for this condition is cessation of use of the offending agent. Further monitoring should occur to ensure improvement and resolution of dysfunction.[14]

SUMMARY

Toxins such as pharmaceuticals, herbals, foods, and supplements may lead to hepatic damage that presents as nonspecific symptoms in the setting of liver test abnormalities. Most cases of toxin-induced damage are caused by acetaminophen, which is treated with NAC. The most important step in the patient evaluation is gathering an extensive history that includes toxin exposure and excludes common causes of liver dysfunction. Patients with ALF benefit from transfer to a transplant service for further management. The mainstay in management for most exposures is cessation of the offending agent.

REFERENCES

1. Bjornsson E. Review article: drug-induced liver injury in clinical practice. Aliment Pharmacol Ther 2010;32:3–13.

2. Navarro VJ, Senior JR. Drug-related hepatotoxicity. N Engl J Med 2006;354: 731–9.
3. Lucena MI, Garcia-Cortes M, Cueto R, et al. Assessment of drug-induced liver injury in clinical practice. Fundam Clin Pharmacol 2008;22:141–58.
4. Gunawan B, Kaplowitz N. Clinical perspectives on xenobiotic-induced hepato-toxicity. Drug Metab Rev 2004;36:301–12.
5. Estes JD, Stolpman D, Olyaei A, et al. High prevalence of potentially hepatotoxic herbal supplement use in patients with fulminant hepatic failure. Arch Surg 2003;138:852–8.
6. Nathwani RA, Kaplowitz N. Drug hepatotoxicity. Clin Liver Dis 2006;10: 207–17, vii.
7. Fontana RJ. Acute liver failure due to drugs. Semin Liver Dis 2008;28: 175–87.
8. Bronstein AC, Spyker DA, Cantilena LR Jr, et al. 2011 annual report of the American Association of Poison Control Centers' National Poison Data System (NPDS): 29th annual report. Clin Toxicol (Phila) 2012;50:911–1164.
9. Chang CY, Schiano TD. Review article: drug hepatotoxicity. Aliment Pharmacol Ther 2007;25:1135–51.
10. Lozano-Lanagran M, Robles M, Lucena MI, et al. Hepatotoxicity in 2011–advancing resolutely. Rev Esp Enferm Dig 2011;103:472–9.
11. Chalasani N, Bjornsson E. Risk factors for idiosyncratic drug-induced liver injury. Gastroenterology 2010;138:2246–59.
12. Ghany M, Hoofnagle JH. Approach to the Patient with Liver Disease. In: Longo DL, Fauci AS, Kasper DL, et al, editors. Harrison's Principles of Internal Medicine. 18th edition. New York: McGraw-Hill; 2012. Available at: http://www.accessmedicine.com.liboff.ohsu.edu/content.aspx?aID=9132925. Accessed October 27, 2013.
13. Kaplowitz N, Aw TY, Simon FR, et al. Drug-induced hepatotoxicity. Ann Intern Med 1986;104:826–39.
14. Timbrell JA. Drug hepatotoxicity. Br J Clin Pharmacol 1983;15:3–14.
15. Lee WM. Drug-induced hepatotoxicity. N Engl J Med 2003;349:474–85.
16. Larrey D. Drug-induced liver diseases. J Hepatol 2000;32:77–88.
17. Tujios S, Fontana RJ. Mechanisms of drug-induced liver injury: from bedside to bench. Nat Rev Gastroenterol Hepatol 2011;8:202–11.
18. Pathikonda M, Munoz SJ. Acute liver failure. Ann Hepatol 2010;9:7–14.
19. Davern TJ 2nd, James LP, Hinson JA, et al. Measurement of serum acetaminophen-protein adducts in patients with acute liver failure. Gastroenterology 2006;130:687–94.
20. Larson AM, Polson J, Fontana RJ, et al. Acetaminophen-induced acute liver failure: results of a United States multicenter, prospective study. Hepatology 2005; 42:1364–72.
21. Keays R, Harrison PM, Wendon JA, et al. Intravenous acetylcysteine in paracetamol induced fulminant hepatic failure: a prospective controlled trial. BMJ 1991; 303:1026–9.
22. Kortsalioudaki C, Taylor RM, Cheeseman P, et al. Safety and efficacy of N-acetylcysteine in children with non-acetaminophen-induced acute liver failure. Liver Transpl 2008;14:25–30.
23. Lee WM, Hynan LS, Rossaro L, et al. Intravenous N-acetylcysteine improves transplant-free survival in early stage non-acetaminophen acute liver failure. Gastroenterology 2009;137:856–64, 864.e1.

24. Stravitz RT, Kramer AH, Davern T, et al. Intensive care of patients with acute liver failure: recommendations of the U.S. Acute Liver Failure Study Group. Crit Care Med 2007;35:2498–508.
25. Nguyen NT, Vierling JM. Acute liver failure. Curr Opin Organ Transplant 2011;16: 289–96.
26. Chen WC, Kassi M, Saeed U, et al. A rare case of amatoxin poisoning in the state of Texas. Case Rep Gastroenterol 2012;6:350–7.
27. Intravenous milk thistle (Silibinin-Legalon) for hepatic failure induced by amatoxin/ amanita mushroom poisoning. National Library of Medicine. Available at: http:// www.clinicaltrials.gov/ct2/show/NCT00915681?term=nct00915681&rank=1. Accessed October 24, 2013.
28. Santi L, Maggioli C, Mastroroberto M, et al. Acute liver failure caused by *Amanita phalloides* poisoning. Int J Hepatol 2012;2012:487480.
29. Bernal W, Donaldson N, Wyncoll D, et al. Blood lactate as an early predictor of outcome in paracetamol-induced acute liver failure: a cohort study. Lancet 2002;359:558–63.
30. Dabos KJ, Newsome PN, Parkinson JA, et al. A biochemical prognostic model of outcome in paracetamol-induced acute liver injury. Transplantation 2005;80: 1712–7.
31. Cholongitas E, Theocharidou E, Vasianopoulou P, et al. Comparison of the sequential organ failure assessment score with the King's College Hospital criteria and the model for end-stage liver disease score for the prognosis of acetaminophen-induced acute liver failure. Liver Transpl 2012;18:405–12.
32. Llado L, Figueras J, Memba R, et al. Is MELD really the definitive score for liver allocation? Liver Transpl 2002;8:795–8.
33. Schmidt LE, Larsen FS. MELD score as a predictor of liver failure and death in patients with acetaminophen-induced liver injury. Hepatology 2007;45:789–96.
34. Craig DG, Reid TW, Martin KG, et al. The systemic inflammatory response syndrome and sequential organ failure assessment scores are effective triage markers following paracetamol (acetaminophen) overdose. Aliment Pharmacol Ther 2011;34:219–28.
35. Mitchell I, Bihari D, Chang R, et al. Earlier identification of patients at risk from acetaminophen-induced acute liver failure. Crit Care Med 1998;26:279–84.
36. Hassanein TI, Schade RR, Hepburn IS. Acute-on-chronic liver failure: extracorporeal liver assist devices. Curr Opin Crit Care 2011;17:195–203.
37. Chun LJ, Tong MJ, Busuttil RW, et al. Acetaminophen hepatotoxicity and acute liver failure. J Clin Gastroenterol 2009;43:342–9.
38. Laleman W, Wilmer A, Evenepoel P, et al. Effect of the molecular adsorbent recirculating system and Prometheus devices on systemic haemodynamics and vasoactive agents in patients with acute-on-chronic alcoholic liver failure. Crit Care 2006;10:R108.
39. Schmidt LE, Wang LP, Hansen BA, et al. Systemic hemodynamic effects of treatment with the molecular adsorbents recirculating system in patients with hyperacute liver failure: a prospective controlled trial. Liver Transpl 2003;9:290–7.
40. Sen S, Davies NA, Mookerjee RP, et al. Pathophysiological effects of albumin dialysis in acute-on-chronic liver failure: a randomized controlled study. Liver Transpl 2004;10:1109–19.
41. Sorkine P, Ben Abraham R, Szold O, et al. Role of the molecular adsorbent recycling system (MARS) in the treatment of patients with acute exacerbation of chronic liver failure. Crit Care Med 2001;29:1332–6.

42. Khuroo MS, Farahat KL. Molecular adsorbent recirculating system for acute and acute-on-chronic liver failure: a meta-analysis. Liver Transpl 2004;10: 1099–106.
43. Lee KH, Lee MK, Sutedja DS, et al. Outcome from molecular adsorbent recycling system (MARS) liver dialysis following drug-induced liver failure. Liver Int 2005;25:973–7.
44. Stauber RE, Krisper P, Zollner G, et al. Extracorporeal albumin dialysis in a patient with primary sclerosing cholangitis: effect on pruritus and bile acid profile. Int J Artif Organs 2004;27:342–4.
45. Krisper P, Haditsch B, Stauber R, et al. In vivo quantification of liver dialysis: comparison of albumin dialysis and fractionated plasma separation. J Hepatol 2005;43:451–7.
46. Karvellas CJ, Bagshaw SM, McDermid RC, et al. A case-control study of single-pass albumin dialysis for acetaminophen-induced acute liver failure. Blood Purif 2009;28:151–8.
47. Sauer IM, Goetz M, Steffen I, et al. In vitro comparison of the molecular adsorbent recirculation system (MARS) and single-pass albumin dialysis (SPAD). Hepatology 2004;39:1408–14.
48. Detry O, Arkadopoulos N, Ting P, et al. Clinical use of a bioartificial liver in the treatment of acetaminophen-induced fulminant hepatic failure. Am Surg 1999; 65:934–8.
49. Hughes RD, Williams R. Use of bioartificial and artificial liver support devices. Semin Liver Dis 1996;16:435–44.
50. Hodgman MJ, Garrard AR. A review of acetaminophen poisoning. Crit Care Clin 2012;28:499–516.
51. Daly FF, O'Malley GF, Heard K, et al. Prospective evaluation of repeated supratherapeutic acetaminophen (paracetamol) ingestion. Ann Emerg Med 2004;44: 393–8.
52. Dart RC, Erdman AR, Olson KR, et al. Acetaminophen poisoning: an evidence-based consensus guideline for out-of-hospital management. Clin Toxicol (Phila) 2006;44:1–18.
53. Lheureux PE, Hantson P. Carnitine in the treatment of valproic acid-induced toxicity. Clin Toxicol (Phila) 2009;47:101–11.
54. Murray KF, Hadzic N, Wirth S, et al. Drug-related hepatotoxicity and acute liver failure. J Pediatr Gastroenterol Nutr 2008;47:395–405.
55. Silva MF, Aires CC, Luis PB, et al. Valproic acid metabolism and its effects on mitochondrial fatty acid oxidation: a review. J Inherit Metab Dis 2008;31:205–16.
56. Schmid MM, Freudenmann RW, Keller F, et al. Non-fatal and fatal liver failure associated with valproic acid. Pharmacopsychiatry 2013;46:63–8.
57. Thanacoody RH. Extracorporeal elimination in acute valproic acid poisoning. Clin Toxicol (Phila) 2009;47:609–16.
58. Cress CM, Malliah A, Herrine SK. Image of the month. Fulminant hepatic failure caused by Amanita phalloides toxicity. Clin Gastroenterol Hepatol 2011;9:A26.
59. Escudie L, Francoz C, Vinel JP, et al. Amanita phalloides poisoning: reassessment of prognostic factors and indications for emergency liver transplantation. J Hepatol 2007;46:466–73.
60. Enjalbert F, Rapior S, Nouguier-Soule J, et al. Treatment of amatoxin poisoning: 20-year retrospective analysis. J Toxicol Clin Toxicol 2002;40:715–57.
61. Schwartz JM, Reinus JF. Prevalence and natural history of alcoholic liver disease. Clin Liver Dis 2012;16:659–66.

62. Giboney PT. Mildly elevated liver transaminase levels in the asymptomatic patient. Am Fam Physician 2005;71:1105–10.
63. Amini M, Runyon BA. Alcoholic hepatitis 2010: a clinician's guide to diagnosis and therapy. World J Gastroenterol 2010;16:4905–12.
64. Lewis JH. Clinical perspective: statins and the liver–harmful or helpful? Dig Dis Sci 2012;57:1754–63.
65. Russo MW, Scobey M, Bonkovsky HL. Drug-induced liver injury associated with statins. Semin Liver Dis 2009;29:412–22.
66. Kleiner DE. The pathology of drug-induced liver injury. Semin Liver Dis 2009;29: 364–72.
67. Delaney KA. Hepatic Principles. In: Nelson LS, Lewin NA, Howland MA, et al, editors. Goldfrank's Toxicologic Emergencies. 9th editon. New York: McGraw-Hill; 2011. Chapter 26, Table 26-4. p. 376.

Toxin-induced Respiratory Distress

Charles A. McKay Jr, MD[a,b],*

KEYWORDS

- Acute lung injury • Inhalation injury • Simple asphyxiant • Respiratory irritant
- Reactive airways dysfunction syndrome • Impaired oxygen transport
- Water solubility

KEY POINTS

- When an exposure history is unclear or unknown, the presenting symptoms and signs referable to a particular airway component should guide assessment and treatment.
- Useful categories include lack of oxygen delivery from exposure to a simple asphyxiant, airway irritation from a water-soluble irritant, airways irritation from a water-insoluble irritant, direct pulmonary toxicity from a recent or remote event, altered oxygen transport from acquired dyshemoglobinemia, and altered oxygen use by cells because of a mitochondrial toxin.
- Treatment should focus on supportive care and addressing the specific dysfunction identified.

INTRODUCTION

Most poisoning and overdose events involve unintentional or intentional ingestions by the oral route. However, the possibility of inhalation exposure to volatile compounds or suspended particulates is a daily concern for everyone. Most people go through each day without respiratory or systemic complaints, which is as much a tribute to people's pulmonary defensive capabilities as it is to the low ambient concentration of most commonly occurring xenobiotics, allergens, and infectious agents. High-dose exposure, inadequate defenses, and genetic or acquired susceptibility can affect multiple components of the airway from the point of air entry to the level of gas exchange. Examples of these varied maladies include allergic rhinitis, viral pharyngitis, fungal

Funding Sources: None.
Conflict of Interest: None.
[a] Occupational Health Services, Division of Medical Toxicology, Department of Emergency Medicine, Hartford Hospital, 80 Seymour Street, Hartford, CT 06102-5037, USA;
[b] Connecticut Poison Control Center, Division of Medical Toxicology, University of Connecticut Health Center, University of Connecticut School of Medicine, 263 Farmington Avenue, Farmington, CT 06030, USA
* Division of Medical Toxicology, Department of Emergency Medicine, Hartford Hospital, 80 Seymour Street, Hartford, CT 06102-5037.
E-mail address: charles.mckay@hhchealth.org

Emerg Med Clin N Am 32 (2014) 127–147
http://dx.doi.org/10.1016/j.emc.2013.09.003

sinusitis, irritant-induced bronchospasm, chemical or bacterial pneumonitis, alpha-1 antitrypsin deficiency–mediated emphysema, granulomatous diseases such as sarcoidosis or berylliosis, as well as many other occupational pneumoconioses such as silica-mediated pulmonary fibrosis. This article focuses on the variety of chemical compounds that can result in injuries to the airways, resulting in a patient presenting to the emergency department.

PULMONARY ANATOMY AND PHYSIOLOGY AND RESPONSE TO INJURY
Ventilatory Capacity

A basic understanding of respiratory anatomy and physiology is essential in characterizing its response to external insults. Of all biologic systems in the human body, the pulmonary system has the greatest potential surface area of exposure. Under a heavy workload, adult minute ventilation can increase more than 10-fold from an average baseline of 6 L. Roughly equal contributions from increased respiratory rate and recruitment of additional alveolar units contribute to this capacity. The alveoli, estimated at 300 million in the adult, are the sites of gas exchange. One aspect of increased susceptibility to inhalation injury in children is the smaller number of alveolar units (at birth, ~15% of adult capacity), and the requisite higher respiratory rate, resulting in a greater concentration-time exposure at any given pulmonary site.[1] In addition, at all ages, changes in ventilation/perfusion matching with exertion increase the potential for pulmonary and systemic exposure to inhaled compounds.

Gas Exchange

Oxygen delivery and carbon dioxide excretion follow the principles of the gas laws, whereby the total pressure of gas within a system is composed of the partial pressure contributed by each constituent (Dalton's law of partial pressures), and the exchange of those gases at an interface (ie, the alveolar air and the blood of the alveolar capillaries) is proportional to their concentrations (Henry's law). The critical role of a properly functioning gas carrier (hemoglobin) is shown by the Bohr and Haldane effects, which result in increased tissue release of oxygen from, and increased binding of carbon dioxide to, hemoglobin at the tissue level; whereas increasing binding of oxygen and release of carbon dioxide take place at the alveoli, respectively. This efficiently engineered system of gas exchange can be disrupted in several ways, including changes to hemoglobin affinity based on inhaled toxins such as carbon monoxide (CO) and methemoglobin (MetHb) inducers. Other agents can injure the thin gas exchange membrane composed of alveolar epithelial cells and capillary endothelium, increasing diffusion distance by acute lung injury with edema and inflammatory injury, or decreasing the number of functioning alveolar units.

Ventilatory Mechanics

The mechanics of ventilation are not extensively addressed in this article. However, because they can be affected by the toxicity of various compounds, it is important to define a few terms.[2] Air is conducted through the fixed-volume ventilatory dead space of the upper airways and the more dynamic intrathoracic airways. The ventilatory process is depicted in **Fig. 1** as the volumes and capacities present within the lungs. For example, a tidal volume (V_T) of approximately 500 mL for an adult with an average respiratory rate of 12 breaths per minute results in a minute ventilation volume of 6 L. Additional air can be inhaled (inspiratory reserve volume [IRV]) and actively exhaled beyond the passive recoil of the chest wall (expiratory reserve volume [ERV]) to make up the total lung capacity (TLC; total lung volume of a single maximal

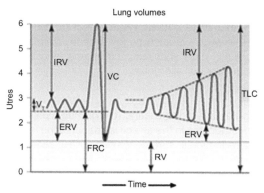

Fig. 1. Lung volumes and capacities. ERV, expiratory reserve volume; FRC, functional residual capacity; IRV, inspiratory reserve volume; RV, residual volume; TLC, total lung capacity; VC, vital capacity. (*From* Jennett S. Churchill Livingstone's dictionary of sport and exercise science and medicine. Philadelphia: Churchill Livingstone/Elsevier; 2008; with permission.)

breath), which is approximately 5 to 6 L in healthy adults. The functional residual capacity (FRC) comprises that amount of air within the lungs that is not readily exchanged with each breath, plus an amount that is unable to be exhaled, termed the (absolute) residual volume (RV). Various pathologic processes within the lungs can significantly impair ventilation. As examples, fibrosis following pulmonary inflammation reduces ventilatory capacity by restricting lung expansion; pulmonary function tests show a proportional reduction in the rate of airflow, both early in forced exhalation (forced expiratory volume in 1 second [FEV_1]) and over the course of the exhalation (forced vital capacity [FVC]). Other agents, such as respiratory irritants, can cause bronchoconstriction or air trapping, which lead to changes in effective pulmonary volumes, as well as impairing the ability to exhale, effectively increasing the RV. This process is shown on pulmonary function testing as a markedly low FEV_1, a prolonged slow rate of exhalation during the middle portion of exhalation (forced expiratory flow, 25%–75% [$FEV_{25\%-75\%}$]), and a mildly to moderately reduced FVC. The hallmark of reversible versus nonreversible obstructive lung disease is the improvement in the FEV_1/FVC ratio with bronchodilators or treatment of an underlying condition or exposure. In the absence of formal pulmonary function tests, a peak expiratory flow rate (PEFR) is often substituted for monitoring the progression of an obstructive process or its response to therapy. Although this test is effort dependent, this feature can be used to advantage when monitoring processes that may also affect ventilatory muscle function, such as exposure to paralytic agents affecting acetylcholine transmission.

Cellular Airway Components

Although designation of the airways as either those of air conduction or gas exchange allows adequate representation of the mechanics of ventilation and gas exchange mechanisms, it is inadequate to encompass the diversity of cell types present within the airways and their response to injury. The airways can be considered to consist of all mucosal and cell barrier systems from the nares to the alveoli. If the conducting airways are considered as those from the nares to the alveolar ducts, the degree of diversity present in this continuum is obvious.

Mucosal surfaces

The mucosal surfaces of the nares and oral pharynx are susceptible to irritation by water-soluble compounds. The production of mucus in the upper airways and epithelium lining the terminal bronchioles and smaller conducting airways can mitigate injury by retrograde transport of irritants via an intact mucociliary transport mechanism. However, these airways can also become obstructed by the mucin output of goblet cells, direct cellular injury with resulting edema, and by bronchoconstriction mediated by extrinsic irritants or allergens.

Alveolar epithelium

In contrast with the potentially complicating role of mucin production, the release of surfactin by type II pneumocytes in the alveoli is critical to the maintenance of patency and gas exchange via reduction in surface tension. These cells only occupy a fraction of the alveolar surface (5%), but are more numerous than the thinned squamous type I pneumocytes that form the airway side of the gas exchange membrane. The type I pneumocytes also serve as a barrier to fluid accumulation via their intercellular tight junction complexes. Once this barrier has been overwhelmed, pulmonary edema ensues. Transudative pleural effusions or pulmonary edema caused by congestive heart failure or chronic liver failure are primarily mediated by intravascular pressure, with oncotic pressure as an important covariant. For poisoned patients, direct pulmonary injury or the impact of mitochondrial poisoning altering the energy-dependent process of maintaining tight junctions are often the cause of acute lung injury. Oncotic pressure is not usually a major concern. Even therapies that significantly alter oncotic pressure, such as high-dose lipid emulsion rescue following lipid-soluble medication overdose, have not been shown to result in pulmonary toxicity as was once feared.[3] In addition, multiple other causes may play a role in causing acute lung injury in critically ill poisoned patients, including aspiration of gastric contents, ingestion of agents causing cardiovascular collapse, and pulmonary toxicity from continuous high-flow oxygen therapy.

Interstitial airway components

The supporting connective tissue of the pulmonary unit is not static; it can contribute significantly to the initial and chronic response to toxic exposures. Although reversible bronchoconstriction to acute airways irritants is a familiar component of reactive airways disease, whether labeled as asthma or reactive airway dysfunction syndrome (RADS) in the wake of exposure to several irritants, structural remodeling of the airways with both muscular and fibrous proliferation are also important contributors to disease, and impediments to effective treatment with bronchodilators alone. Following chronic exposures or manifesting as chronic sequelae of acute exposures, macrophage-initiated or macrophage-mediated inflammatory response plays a major role in exposures such as asbestos, beryllium, hexavalent chromium, and cigarette smoke. Whether circulating monocytes or airway-resident macrophages serve as the source for pulmonary macrophages in steady state or in response to injury is debated[4]; the importance of their role in mitigating or exacerbating injury is not. In addition, understanding of the roles for other airway components and pathways, such as the neural responsiveness of autonomic innervation of the lungs, is still evolving.[5,6] A range of neurally mediated pulmonary responses are commonly seen in poisoned patients, including the primary respiratory alkalosis characteristic of the stimulation of the medullary respiratory center by salicylates, or the respiratory acidosis characteristic of opioid-mediated respiratory depression. These aspects affecting pulmonary toxicity are not addressed further in this article.

As can be seen from the previous descriptions, the interacting or competing influences that dictate normal pulmonary function are prone to alteration by a variety of potential toxins and toxicants. Using the sites or mechanism of injury shown in **Table 1,**

Table 1
General categories of pulmonary toxicants and injury. The acronym AIR-OUT can be used as a memory aide

Injury Type or Mechanism	Examples	Comments
Asphyxiants, simple	Nitrogen, noble gases, methane, carbon dioxide	Oxygen displacement leading to hypoxia and CNS symptoms; recover on removal from source
Irritants, water-soluble	Ammonia, MIC, chlorine, chloramines, sulfur dioxide	Prominent upper respiratory symptoms; generally good warning properties
Irritants, water-insoluble	Oxides of nitrogen, phosgene	Predominantly delayed-onset, lower respiratory symptoms; poor warning properties
RBC Dyshemoglobinemias	Carbon monoxide, MetHb inducers	Impaired oxygen tissue delivery; treat with high-flow oxygen (and methylene blue for MetHb)
Organ/cellular asphyxiants	Mitochondrial toxicity from cyanide, salicylates, phosphine	Impaired tissue oxygen use; secondary pulmonary toxicity
Unique mechanisms	Hydrocarbons, paraquat, asbestos, silica, beryllium	Particular features of uptake or inflammatory response generate characteristic clinical or radiographic features
Usual combinations of agents	Smoke Smog Metal fume fever	All categories of toxins Predominantly respiratory irritants, but concern with particulates Metal oxides induce cytokine-mediated pulmonary inflammation (flu-like illness)
Thermal/physical	Heat, caustics	Direct thermal or caustic injury, the latter usually restricted to upper airway
Transfer of systemic toxins	Multiple	Systemic delivery of toxins/toxicants via pulmonary route without specific pulmonary injury

Abbreviations: CNS, central nervous system; MetHb, methemoglobin; MIC, methyl isocyanate; RBC, red blood cell.

groups of compounds or inciting agents that can affect health via pulmonary injury can be categorized.

AGENTS CAUSING PULMONARY INJURY
Simple Asphyxiants

Several agents can alter oxygen delivery by simple displacement. These agents, for the most part nonmetabolically active, follow Dalton's law of partial pressures. The presence of other gases in sufficient concentration (eg, the inert noble gases helium, neon, argon, krypton, and xenon, some of which are used in industrial reactor vessels or mixtures used to treat asthma exacerbations; methane in sewer mains; carbon dioxide off-gassing of dry ice) leads to lower oxygen tensions and hypoxia based on decreased availability of oxygen to diffuse through the alveoli, causing central nervous system and cardiac impairment.[7–9]

Carbon dioxide

Carbon dioxide (CO_2), although able to cause asphyxia, can have a varied presentation, determined by concentration and exposure rate. Carbon dioxide causes a centrally mediated respiratory stimulation,[10] and also acts as a central nervous system depressant in high doses. Although this latter effect is most often seen in patients with chronic obstructive pulmonary disease whose respiratory response to CO_2 has been blunted, it is operative in fatalities attributed to enclosed-space exposure to dry ice. Large-scale experiences with CO_2-induced hypoxia and death are seen following the displacement of CO_2 dissolved from limestone at depth in volcanic lakes, releasing clouds of CO_2 in violent discharges. Being heavier than air, the CO_2 settles in the surrounding communities and causes immediate death to those overcome by it. The most recent large-scale event of this kind occurred around Lake Nyos in Cameroon, Africa, in 1986, resulting in the immediate death of more than 1700 people and thousands of livestock up to 12 miles away.[11] A similar geologic situation currently exists in the Rift Valley of Rwanda and the Democratic Republic of Congo, where the larger Lake Kivu is situated with a surrounding population of 2 million people. Attempts at degassing lakes in Cameroon are slowly decreasing the dissolved CO_2.[12] Treatment of individuals overcome by CO_2 and other simple asphyxiants is straightforward:

- Remove from the exposure
- Apply oxygen and provide adequate ventilation
- Supportive measures to restore hemodynamic competence, if necessary

Rescuers should take care not to enter an oxygen-deficient environment without adequate supplied oxygen to ensure that they do not become secondary victims.

Respiratory Irritants

Respiratory irritants differ from simple asphyxiants in that the chemical interaction of the agent and the water at the mucosal surface of the airways and/or other cellular components result in direct tissue injury via the generation of acids, alkali, or other reactive compounds. Although toxicity depends on dose, pH, and volatility, the most important characteristic of these agents in their gaseous state is their water solubility. Water solubility dictates warning properties, the area and possibly extent of tissue involvement, and the nature of treatment.

Water-soluble irritants

Water-soluble irritants cause upper airway irritation and injury manifested initially as a sense of mucous membrane burning, sneezing, runny nose, watery eyes, and cough. These symptoms are sufficiently uncomfortable to cause the victim to flee continued exposure unless trapped, thus limiting total inhaled dose (agent concentration multiplied by time of exposure and minute ventilation). Exposure to ammonia or chlorine gas, the latter of which is generated when bleach (sodium hypochlorite) and acid toilet bowl cleaners are mixed, are common examples of the noxious nature of these water-soluble gases. In cases in which escape is not possible, or if there are particularly high (eg, industrial) concentrations, continued exposure results in ongoing injury with the potential for upper airway obstruction and additional lower airway findings of bronchospasm with wheezing, dyspnea, and pulmonary edema. In the setting of severe exposure, pulmonary fibrosis may complicate recovery. Numerous railway and industrial accidents show the potential scale of releases from pressurized tank cars transporting or storing these agents and the resultant impact on patients requiring acute care (**Table 2**).

Table 2
Examples of large-scale releases of respiratory irritants[a]

Agent[b]	Event	Release	Killed/Injured[c]	Water Solubility	Vapor Density	Vapor Pressure (mm Hg)[d]	Warning Properties	Location of Airway Symptoms
Anhydrous ammonia	Minot, ND (2002)	555,320 L (initial)	1/333 (11,600 shelter in place)	High	0.6	6000	Adequate; acrid odor	Upper
Chlorine	Graniteville, SC (2005)	34,826 L	9/554 (5400 evacuated)	Intermediate	2.5	4500	Adequate; irritating odor	Upper and lower
Hydrofluoric acid	Texas City, TX (1987)	13,608 kg	0/>1000 (4000 evacuated)	High	0.7	783	Adequate; irritating odor	Upper, aystemic
Methyl isocyanate	Bhopal, India (1984)	39,916 kg	~3800/170,000	High	1.4	348	Inadequate; pungent odor	Upper and lower
Phosgene	Lake Charles, LA (1984)	17 kg	1/40	Low	3.5	1215	Inadequate; odor of fresh-cut hay	Lower
Phosphorous trichloride	Somerville, MA (1980)	49,210 L	0/817 (23,000 evacuated)	High (exothermic)	4.75	150	Adequate; pungent odor	Upper

[a] At standard temperature and pressure: 20°C to 25°C (68–77°F) and 1 atm absolute (760 mm Hg).
[b] Concentrated forms under pressure.
[c] As per number of people seeking care.
[d] Approximate.
Data from Refs.[66–72]

RADS as a consequence of irritant exposure

Some water-soluble irritants are associated with the occurrence of RADS, in which subsequent exposure to small concentrations of the same agent or other potential respiratory irritants results in an asthmalike condition with bronchospasm, bronchoconstriction, and decreased airflow. This respiratory sensitization should not be confused with typical allergic phenomena, because it occurs following exposure to small molecules or elements, and is not associated with immunoglobulin E–mediated histamine release. Diagnosis of this syndrome requires:

- Absence of prior chronic respiratory illness or competing pulmonary diagnosis
- Documented significant exposure to suspect chemical irritant
- Onset of initial symptoms (cough, dyspnea, wheezing) within 24 hours and persistence for longer than 3 months
- Demonstration of airway obstruction/bronchial hyper-responsiveness by pulmonary function testing

As noted earlier, the criteria for this diagnosis require that preexisting asthma be ruled out as far as possible and that the nature of the inciting event be adequately characterized.[13] A methacholine challenge test may be useful in diagnosis for questionable cases.[14]

The largest industrial accident to date is an example of both the acute and chronic impact of a water-soluble irritant exposure. Shortly after midnight, December 3, 1984, a cloud of methyl isocyanate (MIC) was generated when water was introduced into a tank of MIC. This resulted in up to 5000 deaths and an estimated 100,000 to 200,000 symptomatic individuals in Bhopal, India. Many of these people still have chronic eye and respiratory dysfunction.[15]

Treatment following exposure to water-soluble respiratory irritants includes:

- Removal from exposure
- Decontamination of exposed skin and mucous membranes (with particular attention to the eyes)
- Administration of oxygen (humidified to decrease laryngeal irritation)
- Administration of nebulized bronchodilators, if indicated by clinical symptoms
- Consideration of inhaled and/or systemic corticosteroids for severe reactive airways symptoms

Some case reports describe use of nebulized sodium bicarbonate (generally as a 3.75% solution; eg, sodium bicarbonate 44 mEq/50 mL diluted 1 to 1 with saline, and placed in a nebulizer) in addition to inhaled bronchodilators, perhaps to decrease the impact of hydrochloric acid generated in the airway. Although neutralization therapy is not generally recommended in the management of caustic injury, there have not been reports of adverse effects of this therapy.[16,17]

Water-insoluble irritants

Compared with water-soluble irritants, water-insoluble irritants have poor warning properties following exposure. These agents slowly hydrolyze in water or react with other cellular components, causing damage that tends to be more prominent distally in the pulmonary tree, because of the more insidious nature of tissue injury. This lower airway injury is characterized by delayed onset (hours to days) of pulmonary edema and pulmonary fibrosis on healing, with significant scarring. Features of both obstructive and restrictive airways disease may be present.

Oxides of nitrogen Oxides of nitrogen (NO_x) are a low-water-solubility pulmonary irritant component of smog. Nitrogen dioxide is also generated by ice resurfacing machines in enclosed arenas,[18,19] and in the process of grain fermentation in the setting of trapped moisture. In the latter case, this condition is called silo-filler's disease, and is characterized by the insidious progression of dyspnea on exertion, leading to shortness of breath at rest and pulmonary fibrosis or bronchiolitis obliterans in farmworkers.[20]

Phosgene Phosgene is another example of a poorly water-soluble respiratory irritant. It is a chemical intermediate in many industrial processes including manufacture of pesticides and polycarbonate plastics. It is also potentially released as a combustion product when any chlorine-containing hydrocarbon is burned. The warning properties of phosgene are noted to include an odor like new-mown hay or green corn. However, this odor is not a good warning property because the slow hydrolysis to form hydrochloric acid or the covalent binding to amine constituents within cells results in the delayed onset of tissue injury and pulmonary edema at concentrations below its odor threshold. The ensuing inflammatory process can result in pulmonary fibrosis.

In general, patients presenting after exposure to water-insoluble respiratory irritants have discontinued exposure, but they may have ongoing episodic exposure based on their workplace or avocation. Treatment following exposure to water-insoluble respiratory irritants includes:

- Administration of oxygen
- Administration of nebulized bronchodilators, if indicated by clinical symptoms
- Early administration of inhaled and/or systemic corticosteroids to modify inflammatory healing
- Sufficient observation to ensure that acute progressive pulmonary injury (which may require advanced oxygenation and ventilation strategies) does not occur
- Referral for formal pulmonary function testing
- Evaluation of potential exposure settings to prevent ongoing exposure, and identification of other potentially affected individuals

Warning Properties of Irritant Gases

The differences in warning properties between the water-soluble and water-insoluble gases can be demonstrated by the difference in the typical concentrations of ammonia and phosgene needed for odor detection or perceptible airway irritation versus the concentrations required for injury or danger to human health.[21] The odor threshold and irritant properties of ammonia can be appreciated as low as 5 to 50 parts per million (ppm), whereas phosgene's odor (described as that of fresh-cut hay or green corn) is approximately 0.5 to 1.5 ppm. Although this 3-fold to 100-fold difference suggests that phosgene has better warning properties, the truth is the reverse. The Acute Emergency Guideline Level (AEGLs) 3 exposure limit (major or life-threatening impact with 30 minutes' exposure) for phosgene is 1.5 ppm, whereas the ammonia AEGL 3 concentration in air is 1600 ppm, indicating that phosgene is more than 1000 times as toxic as ammonia. Thus, the warning properties for ammonia are protective, resulting in upper airway and other mucous membrane discomfort well before tissue injury, whereas phosgene's low water solubility can result in severe delayed-onset lower pulmonary injury if there is a perceptible odor or mild irritation present acutely.

DIRECT AIRWAY INJURY
Ingested Caustic Agents

There are several compounds that can be separated out artificially from the respiratory irritants as caustics and that, by the nature of their degree of alkalinity or acidity, cause immediate and direct injury to epithelial surfaces that they contact. Although the caustics are predominately considered to cause esophageal and other gastrointestinal injury following ingestion, direct injury to the glottis area may occur as well, particularly in children or in adults with suicidal ingestions of large volumes. Upper airway symptoms are generally obvious shortly after ingestion.[22] Treatment should focus on assessment and control of the airway should there be concern for airway obstruction secondary to edema. Nebulized epinephrine has been used in some cases,[23] but should not be considered definitive treatment.

Thermal Airway Injury

Another common localized direct injury is that caused by superheated gases making direct contact with the respiratory epithelium. This injury can be a component of smoke inhalation during fire exposure (discussed later), but there is generally poor correlation between severity of respiratory symptoms and signs (cough, carbonaceous sputum), bronchoscopic grade of mucosal injury, and survival. However, the presence of pulmonary injury from smoke inhalation does contribute to a poor outcome and presumably increases the risk of infectious complications of pneumonia.[24] Localized upper airway injuries from inhalation of freebase cocaine vapors include palatal and uvular edema, hypopharyngeal edema, and localized necrosis.[25]

Hydrocarbon Aspiration

Hydrocarbon aspiration is another common cause of direct airway injury, resulting in the rapid onset of choking, coughing, dyspnea, and hypoxia. The greatest concern is for those hydrocarbons with low viscosity and high vapor pressure, notably kerosene derivatives and mineral seal oil. Acute lung injury occurs secondary to necrosis of pulmonary epithelium, initiation of an inflammatory cascade, and loss of pulmonary surfactant.[26] Patients may require supplemental oxygenation, intubation, positive end-expiratory pressure, and occasionally extracorporeal membrane oxygenation, or other heroic measures.[27]

UNIQUE PULMONARY TOXINS AND TOXICANTS

Although many of the agents already listed produce significant airway injury based on their interaction with specific airway components or processes, there are numerous agents that interact with airway components in a unique fashion, highlighting toxin-mediator relationships. A few of these agents are described here.

Paraquat

Paraquat is a diquaternary amine aromatic nonselective herbicide. Although severely restricted for use in the United States, it is one of the most common herbicides in use around the world. Unintentional or intentional ingestion and mucosal exposure can result in frequently fatal pulmonary toxicity. Although paraquat can induce oxygen radical formation in all tissues, a structural homology results in its active uptake by pneumocytes from the circulation. The high concentration of polyamine transporters on the luminal side of the type I and type II pneumocytes and club (formerly Clara) cells result in as much as a 10-fold concentration of paraquat in the pneumocytes.[28,29] With prolonged exposure and slower clearance, the lung thus becomes the target organ for paraquat. Should patients survive the initial caustic ingestion, progressive pulmonary fibrosis with death occurring up to a month later can be expected. Attempts to mitigate this course focus on avoiding supplemental oxygen administration, even for moderate hypoxia. Early interventions, such as activated charcoal administration or hemodialysis, are ineffective if delayed even 3 hours after ingestion. A recent Cochrane Review provided some support for the use of corticosteroids and cyclophosphamide in an attempt to modulate the inflammatory response following paraquat ingestion.[30]

Asbestos

The mineral fibers of asbestos consist of silicates (Si_xO_y) bound to other elements, predominantly iron and magnesium. The needlelike amphiboles, with the base structure of Si_8O_{22}, consist of tremolite, crocidolite, amosite, actinolite, and anthophyllite, which have traditionally been considered the primary cause of asbestosis and asbestos-related malignancies (adenocarcinoma and mesothelioma) because their short fiber length could be engulfed by alveolar macrophages, but not broken down (frustrated endocytosis), initiating an inflammatory cascade and progressive fibrosis over a period of years. The International Agency for Research on Cancer (IARC) and other organizations recently concluded that there is sufficient evidence of carcinogenicity by the longer, thinner serpentine fibers of chrysotile asbestos, which has the base structure $Mg_3(Si_2O_5)(OH)_4$.[31] This type is the predominant form of asbestos used in the United States and the only form of asbestos mined today. These fibers have had multiple industrial uses as insulators, with extensive mining occurring over the last 100 years. Current levels of industrial exposure are a fraction of what they were 50 years ago, but the delayed impact of restrictive lung disease characteristic of asbestosis (pleural plaques and interstitial fibrosis most prominent in the lower lung fields) and malignancy will continue for decades to come. An uncertain source of ongoing exposure comes from vermiculite insulation that is contaminated with tremolite asbestos mined from Libby, Montana. Operations ceased in 1990, but widespread use of this product in household insulation and soil treatments have raised concern for exposure far distant from the severely affected mining community.[32]

Silica

Crystalline silica is a nonsubstituted silicon dioxide (SiO_2) mineral compound. Even though it shares a structural relationship with asbestos and can sometimes be found in the same ore, silica's toxicity differs in important ways. Inhaled silica dust results in the same ineffective alveolar macrophage interaction that is seen with asbestos, but the clinical features, progression, and nature of associated diseases are different. With large-scale silica inhalation, as might be seen in sandblasting or mining, a proliferation of type II pneumocytes can occur, with alveolar proteinosis from excessive surfactant production. This condition is known as acute silicosis. More commonly, chronic inhalation of small amounts of silica, as reflected in the National Institute for Occupational Health and Safety Recommended Exposure Limit (NIOSH REL) for silica particles of only 0.05 mg/m^3, results in predominantly upper lung zone deposition of silica dust that leads to the formation of 1-mm 10-mm inflammatory nodules and resulting local tissue damage. Migration of silica to regional lymph nodes results in egg-shell rims of calcification in hilar lymph nodes. Although associations with pulmonary malignancy have been described with silicosis, studies have been inconsistent, likely secondary to inadequate control of such confounders as tobacco smoking. At times, pulmonary nodules are noted to coalesce and increase in size. This process predisposes to rapid growth of the resulting inflammatory nodules, with central necrosis and cavitation. This disease is also associated with an increased risk of tuberculosis. Restrictive lung disease can occur, although features of obstructive lung disease may also be present. Because this condition can progress even with removal from ongoing exposure, proper respiratory protection or engineering controls (such as wet drilling) should be in place whenever silica-containing rock or manufactured products are likely to be encountered. Some forms of crystalline silica, such as quartz, are less prone to initiate the silica-related inflammatory cascade and fibrosis.[33]

The difference in pulmonary response to asbestos (with lower lung zone fibrosis and pleural plaques, and causation of mesothelioma) and crystalline silica (with a prominence of type II pneumocyte response, upper zone inflammatory nodules, and lymph node calcification) despite similar inabilities of the alveolar macrophages to successfully manage these mineral fibers highlights the importance of as yet undefined pulmonary cellular interactions.

Beryllium

Beryllium, one of the hard metal elements, is an example of a workplace inhalation exposure in which the nature of the pulmonary response highlights the developing understanding of toxicity and tolerable exposure limits. Acute beryllium disease, a chemical pneumonitis induced by exposure to beryllium from grinding (often occurring in airplane turbine blade manufacturing or metallurgy) is a disease that is now uncommon because of increased workplace controls on dust and fume exposure. As the regulatory limits for beryllium exposure became more stringent, the potential for this type of exposure decreased. However, with the disappearance of this acute illness, it became clear that safe exposures still put workers at risk of a more chronic inflammatory response characterized by the development of pulmonary granulomas and hilar adenopathy that were similar in distribution and histologic appearance to those of sarcoidosis.[34,35] Basic science and epidemiologic studies have shown that this condition, berylliosis or chronic beryllium disease (CBD), is not strictly a dose-response process, but is a delayed cellular hypersensitivity reaction (type IV allergic response) determined by a person's genetic susceptibility.[36] Identification of individuals with sensitization to beryllium (positive response on a beryllium lymphocyte proliferation test [BeLPT]) can be by either blood or lavage fluid obtained during bronchoscopy, although only the latter is considered diagnostic of disease. BeLPT can also serve to identify the likelihood of the diagnosis in patients with unclear exposure histories. The use of a biomonitoring tool to identify exposure, rather than to monitor the consequences of a known exposure, raises the possibility of false-positive ascertainment, and positive findings in this population should be confirmed.[37] Many people with positive BeLPT do not go on to develop CBD, particularly if further exposure is prevented by a change in job or workplace practices. Beryllium is slowly cleared once inhaled and absorbed or incorporated into granulomas.

Symptoms of CBD include exertional dyspnea. Initial diagnostic studies such as chest radiograph show interstitial lung disease with some predominance of upper lung zone findings. Pulmonary function tests (PFTs) may only show a reduced diffusion capacity for CO indicating the interstitial inflammatory nature of this cytokine-mediated lymphocyte and macrophage response. With progression over decades, both restrictive and obstructive PFT abnormalities can develop. Treatment is directed at limiting any ongoing exposure. Systemic corticosteroids, particularly if instituted early in the course of the disease, offer an improved prognosis.

Usual Combinations

There are some inhaled mixtures that are commonly encountered or have sufficient public health impact to mention specifically.

Fire smoke

Smoke inhalation presents a particular challenge, because multiple chemical compounds in addition to heated gases and particulate material cause damage throughout the respiratory system.[38] The requirement for fluid resuscitation can be complicated by the presentation of acute lung injury following exposure to acrolein and other caustic compounds.[39] Cyanide is generated from almost all modern structure fires and there is a rough correlation between degree of CO and cyanide exposure.[40] As a practical matter, fire victims presenting with hypotension, metabolic acidosis, and/or a worsening cardiovascular state despite intubation and oxygenation should be considered to have a component of cyanide toxicity. Treatment with hydroxocobalamin and/or sodium thiosulfate is appropriate in the management of these critically ill patients.

Smog

Air pollution has generally improved throughout the country with decrements in all of the 6 commonly monitored criterion air pollutants (SO_x, NO_x, CO, ground-level ozone, lead, and particulates).[41] However, poor air quality days in the United States and worldwide are still associated with statistical increases in presentations of acute respiratory exacerbations of asthma and increased cardiovascular mortality attributable to acute coronary syndromes.[42,43] An additional concern has been raised that improvements in air quality because of removal of larger particulates (particles less than 10 μm in diameter) has resulted in a predominance of smaller particulates (eg, fine and ultrafine particulates, particles less than 2.5 μm in diameter) that carry other pulmonary toxins deeper into the airways, resulting in an increase in asthma exacerbations.

Metal fume fever

This cytokine-mediated flulike illness is classically associated with inhalation of zinc oxide fumes during welding or metal smelting operations, although it has been described with several other metal fumes. Increases of interleukin-6 correlated with temperature increases in one study designed to test the adequacy of the workplace threshold limit value–time-weighted average of 5 mg/m³ for 8 hours.[44] Obtaining a good environmental/occupational exposure history is essential to making the correct diagnosis and avoiding inappropriate antibiotic treatment; as well as preventing ongoing exposure. One characteristic of this syndrome is lessening of symptoms with ongoing exposure, with recrudescent symptoms after a period of time away from exposure. This work-week tachyphylaxis underlies one of the common terms applied to this syndrome: Monday morning fever.[45]

Pulmonary Carcinogens

Tobacco smoking is the most common cause for a variety of lung cancers (including small cell carcinoma, squamous carcinoma, and some types of adenocarcinoma), accounting for perhaps 90% of all lung cancer diagnoses in the United States.[46] Several other inhaled agents have also been shown to contribute to the risk of lung cancer. Household exposure to radon is considered the second leading cause of lung cancer;[47] concomitant tobacco smoke exposure increases this risk. Other pulmonary carcinogens include:

- Second-hand tobacco smoke
- Asbestos
- Arsenic
- Cadmium
- Hexavalent chromium (Cr^{6+})
- Nickel

Note that some of these agents are more likely to be ingested than inhaled (eg, arsenic). It is likely that all putative carcinogens affect pulmonary health in a multifactorial way, with initial inflammation and inflammatory cascades overwhelming local reducing capacity, proliferation of alveolar macrophages and release of proto-oncogenes, epigenetic alterations in methylation and other reparative processes, as well as impaired clearance of additional irritants.[48–52]

TOXINS INHIBITING OXYGEN TRANSPORT

Oxygen transport by red cells depends on the configuration of the 4 binding sites for oxygen in each hemoglobin tetramer. This feature is used to advantage by endogenous 2,3-bisphosphoglyceric acid, which binds to deoxyhemoglobin, reducing affinity for oxygen by remaining binding sites, thus increasing oxygen delivery to cells (so-called rightward shift of the oxyhemoglobin dissociation curve). There are several exogenous compounds that bind to hemoglobin, preventing oxygen binding, and/or increasing the affinity of remaining binding sites for oxygen (resulting in a leftward shift of the oxyhemoglobin dissociation curve), which can have a deleterious impact on oxygen transport to tissues (**Fig. 2**).

MetHb Inducers

Methemoglobinemia is a state of oxidized hemoglobin in which the hemoglobin iron is in the ferric state (Fe^{3+}) and is unable to bind to or transport oxygen. This conformational change results in other nonferric oxygen-binding sites having an increased affinity for oxygen, and decreased release to tissues.[53] There are numerous agents that can cause methemoglobinemia, including:

- Benzocaine
- Dapsone
- Nitrites (or high nitrate concentrations in water or food)
- Aromatic amines (including aniline dyes)
- Chlorates

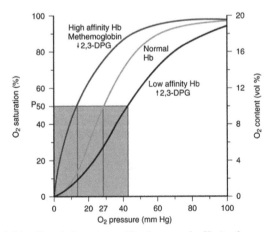

Fig. 2. Oxyhemoglobin dissociation curve. The increased affinity for oxygen occurs with a leftward shift (lower partial pressure of oxygen = decreased release to tissues), as is also seen with increasing carboxyhemoglobin and methemoglobin concentrations. (*From* Nagel RL. Methemoglobinemias and unstable hemoglobins. In: Goldman L, Ausiello DA, editors. Cecil Medicine. 23rd edition. Philadelphia: Saunders Elsevier; 2007; with permission.)

The change in conformation results in a shift in light absorbance by hemoglobin, imparting a blue-gray discoloration to mucous membranes and other highly vascularized tissues. This cyanosis is largely nonresponsive to oxygen, but is readily reversed by reduction of MetHb. In the acute setting of exposure to MetHb inducers, methylene blue has been used for this purpose with good success. However, this treatment depends on an intact hexose monophosphate shunt, which is missing in patients with glucose 6-phosphodehydrogenase deficiency. In those patients, administration of methylene blue can increase oxidation of hemoglobin and cause hemolysis.

Pulse oximetry in MetHb

Routine pulse oximetry can be misleading in methemoglobinemia because the bluish discoloration of the blood is read by the pulse oximeter's 2 monitoring wavelengths as being similar to deoxyhemoglobin. The pulse oximeter typically plateaus in the 80% to 85% saturation range, in the presence of marked cyanosis.[54] This misinformation is useful, in that typical cyanosis caused by hypoxia is expected to yield a lower reading. Note that immediately following administration of methylene blue, the pulse oximeter reading may decrease, potentially causing concern among providers; however, this rapidly resolves, because the intense blue dye is distributed, metabolized to leukomethylene blue, and excreted. Newer point-of-care monitoring devices, such as the pulse CO-Oximeter (Masimo Corporation, Irvine, CA) use 8 to 12 monitoring wavelengths, and may more accurately approximate MetHb and carboxyhemoglobin (COHb) concentrations.[55]

CO

CO is produced as a combustion product whenever a carbon-based fuel is burned. It is therefore a frequently encountered inhaled poison in settings of inadequate ventilation of car exhaust or malfunctioning oil-fired or gas-fired heating systems, and with inappropriate use of gas-powered tools or generators. CO is also produced by hepatic metabolism of inhaled methylene chloride, which is used as a paint stripper. CO induces a leftward shift of the oxyhemoglobin dissociation curve, impairing tissue oxygen delivery and use. CO also binds to ferrous (Fe^{2+}) iron in myoglobin and mitochondria as some of the multiple mechanisms for CO toxicity, primarily affecting the central nervous system and heart. Because CO binds approximately 220 times as tightly to hemoglobin as does oxygen, and this effect is more pronounced at low oxygen tensions,[56] delivery of 100% oxygen by a tight-fitting mask with reservoir or by tracheal intubation is considered the standard of care when CO exposure is suspected or diagnosed. Increased oxygen delivery was also the theoretic rational for administration of hyperbaric oxygen (HBO). On a practical basis, initiation of HBO therapy is rarely rapid enough to significantly affect the clearance of COHb; although HBO has several other theoretic or proven effects on cell function, its role in the treatment of CO poisoning is far from settled.[57]

Pulse oximetry in COHb

Routine pulse oximetry is useless in the setting of CO poisoning. The conformational change of COHb makes the blood appear pink, simulating oxyhemoglobin. Even with high COHb values, the pulse oximeter's two monitoring wavelengths yield values near 95% apparent saturation.[58] In contrast with MetHb, in which the discrepancy in pulse oximetry and clinical appearance can be diagnostically useful, the false readings with increased COHb are misleading.[59] Again, newer devices may circumvent these limitations, and pulse CO oximetry has been used to screen for CO poisoning.[60]

INHIBITION OF OXYGEN USE BY TISSUES (MITOCHONDRIAL POISONS)

This important mechanism for systemic toxicity does not generally cause direct pulmonary injury, although the sequela of impaired mitochondrial oxygen use can present with cardiovascular collapse and pulmonary edema. Refer an article by Wiener elsewhere in this issue, for a brief review of toxins may interfere with oxygen utilization, including mitochondrial toxins.

SYSTEMIC DELIVERY OF TOXINS BY RESPIRATORY ROUTE

Inhalation is a common delivery route for systemic toxins, requiring only that the agent be adequately volatile to be inhaled in sufficient concentrations or duration for systemic effect. Some agents, such as heroin, cocaine, tobacco, and marijuana, have well-described pulmonary effects,[61,62] whereas other agents tend to cause few direct acute or chronic pulmonary effects compared with their systemic toxicity. Because of the intimate anatomic association of olfactory sensors and the airway, those agents that are both irritating and associated with an odor tend to be readily discernible and prolonged voluntary exposure is not expected. This feature has been exploited for agents such as natural gas and fumigants by the addition of mercaptans or lachrymators as warning agents, respectively. The association of an odor with the presence of chemicals can also lead to misattribution of symptoms, as occurred with the gasoline additive, methyl tert-butyl ether.[63] This odor association is likely a major component to such poorly defined symptom complexes as multiple chemical sensitivity syndrome.[64,65] Systemic toxicity of many other agents delivered by inhalation are described elsewhere in this issue.

SUMMARY: ASSESSMENT OF PATIENTS PRESENTING WITH RESPIRATORY SYSTEM COMPLAINTS OR SIGNS

Diagnosis and management of an exposure to a respiratory system toxin is straightforward in the setting of a history of exposure to a known compound with complaints referable to a particular airway component. In such situations, treatment should be focused on the symptomatic region as guided by knowledge of the causative agent. For example, someone choking and coughing after mixing cleaning agents has been exposed to a water-soluble respiratory irritant (likely chlorine or chloramine gas) and should receive humidified oxygen with bronchodilators if the pulmonary examination identifies wheezes or the cough persists on removal from exposure. However, knowing that a water-soluble agent is involved, an assessment should be done to make sure there is no ocular injury.

When history of recent exposure is unclear or the identity of an agent is unknown, the presenting symptoms and signs referable to a particular airway component should still guide assessment and treatment. Using the categories described in this article, an assessment should be made to define the problem. Is the problem:

- Lack of oxygen delivery from exposure to a simple asphyxiant?
  - This would be supported by rapid onset of breathlessness or syncope with rapid recovery (if removed from site).
- Irritated airways from exposure to a water-soluble irritant?
  - This would be supported by the presence of acute onset of tearing, eye burning, nasal and throat irritation, with or without coughing, stridor, or wheezing.

- Irritated airways from exposure to a water-insoluble irritant?
  - This would be supported by a history of subacute or chronic symptoms of chest tightness, decreased exercise tolerance, or wheezes; and a finding of rales or rhonchi, with abnormal pulmonary function tests on follow-up.
- Altered oxygen transport because of an acquired dyshemoglobinemia?
  - The presence of cyanosis unresponsive to supplemental oxygen with a pulse oximetry reading of a mid-80% saturation level is consistent with methemoglobinemia, or less commonly, sulfhemoglobinemia.
  - The absence of cyanosis, but the presence of prominent central nervous system (CNS) effects is consistent with CO.
- Altered oxygen use by cells because of exposure to a mitochondrial toxin?
  - As described elsewhere in this issue, the rapid onset of metabolic acidosis with cardiac and CNS symptoms, particularly in the presence of similar measured oxygen saturations of mixed venous and arterial specimens, suggests cyanide or other mitochondrial toxins.
- Direct pulmonary toxicity from a recent event?
  - This should be evaluated in the presence of acute lung injury with hypoxia or pulmonary edema.
- Direct pulmonary toxicity from remote, chronic exposure or as a sequela to a remote event?
  - This should be evaluated in the presence of imaging evidence of scarring, diffuse nodules, or cavities.

Once an assessment or tentative diagnosis is considered, treatment should focus on supportive care and addressing the particular dysfunction. Diagnostic testing should be tailored to rule in the condition(s) under consideration. Additional history regarding potential workplace exposures, personal protective equipment use and compliance, hobbies, identification of others with similar symptoms, prior exposures, hospitalizations, and history of chronic medical problems such as asthma, atopy, chronic obstructive pulmonary disease, and smoking status assist in the diagnostic process. Should there be concern about multiple victims or workplace safety issues, additional resources are available through the regional poison control centers (accessible via 1-800-222-1222). The poison specialists and clinical toxicologists have a list of outpatient clinics managed by medical toxicologists or occupational medicine physicians. As a component of evaluation in these outpatient settings, additional recommendations or involvement of state departments of labor can be initiated to assist employees and employers in evaluating and improving workplace safety.

REFERENCES

1. Burri PH. Structural aspects of postnatal lung development – alveolar formation and growth. Biol Neonate 2006;89:313–22.
2. CDC. NIOSH Spirometry training guide [electronic resource]. 2003. Available at: http://www.cdc.gov/niosh/docs/2004-154c/pdfs/2004-154c-ch1.pdf. Accessed August 29, 2013.
3. Weinberg GL. Lipid emulsion infusion: resuscitation for local anesthetic and other drug overdose. Anesthesiology 2012;117:180–7.
4. Hashimoto D, Chow A, Noizat C, et al. Tissue-resident macrophages self-maintain locally throughout adult life with minimal contribution from circulating monocytes. Immunity 2013;38:792–804.
5. Kummer W. Pulmonary vascular innervation and its role in responses to hypoxia. Proc Am Thorac Soc 2011;8:471–6.

6. Brooks SM, Bernstein IL. Irritant-induced airway disorders. Immunol Allergy Clin North Am 2011;31:747–68.
7. Musshoff F, Hagemier L, Kirschbaum K, et al. Two cases of suicide by asphyxiation due to helium and argon. Forensic Sci Int 2012;223:e27–30.
8. Dunford JV, Lucas J, Vent N, et al. Asphyxiation due to dry ice in a walk-in freezer. J Emerg Med 2009;36:353–6.
9. Gill JR, Ely SF, Hua Z. Environmental gas displacement: three accidental deaths in the workplace. Am J Forensic Med Pathol 2002;23:26–30.
10. Dahan A, Teppema LJ. Influence of anesthesia and analgesia on the control of breathing. Br J Anaesth 2003;91:40–9.
11. Baxter PF, Kapila M, Mfonfu D. Lake Nyos disaster, Cameroon, 1986: the medical effects of large scale emission of carbon dioxide? BMJ 1989;298:1437–41.
12. Kling GW, Evans WC, Tanyileke G, et al. Degassing Lakes Nyos and Monoun: defusing certain disaster. Proc Natl Acad Sci U S A 2005;102: 14185–90.
13. Bardana EJ Jr. Reactive airways dysfunction syndrome (RADS): guidelines for diagnosis and treatment and insight into likely prognosis. Ann Allergy Asthma Immunol 1999;83:583–6.
14. Crapo RO, Casaburi R, Coates AL, et al. Guidelines for methacholine and exercise challenge testing-1999. This official statement of the American Thoracic Society was adopted by the ATS Board of Directors July 1999. Am J Respir Crit Care Med 2000;161:309–29.
15. Dhara VR, Dhara R. The Union Carbide disaster in Bhopal: a review of health effects. Arch Environ Health 2002;57:391–404.
16. Bosse G. Nebulized sodium bicarbonate in the treatment of chlorine gas inhalation. J Toxicol Clin Toxicol 1994;32:233–41.
17. Cevik Y, Onay M, Akmaz I, et al. Mass casualties from acute inhalation of chlorine gas. Southampt Med J 2009;102:1209–13.
18. Soparkar G, Mayers I, Edouard L, et al. Toxic effects from nitrogen dioxide in ice-skating arenas. Can Med Assoc J 1993;148:1181–2.
19. Pelham TW, Holt LE, Moss MA. Exposure to carbon monoxide and nitrogen dioxide in enclosed ice arenas. Occup Environ Med 2002;59:224–33.
20. Iowa Department of Public Health, Division of Environmental Health. Silo Filler's Disease. 2012. Available at: http://www.idph.state.ia.us/idph_universalhelp/MainContent.aspx?glossaryInd=0&TOCId=%7B7DFAF174-77E8-4F50-97BD-4E2FC3345E4E%7D. Accessed August 29, 2013.
21. Environmental Protection Agency. Acute exposure guideline levels (AEGLs) [web page]. 2012. Available at: http://www.epa.gov/oppt/aegl. Accessed August 29, 2013.
22. Turner A, Robinson P. Respiratory and gastrointestinal complications of caustic ingestion in children. Emerg Med J 2005;22:359–61.
23. Ziegler D. Caustic-induced upper airway obstruction responsive to nebulized adrenaline. Pediatrics 2001;1074:807.
24. Dries DJ, Endorf FW. Inhalation injury: epidemiology, pathology, treatment strategies. Scand J Trauma Resusc Emerg Med 2013;21:31.
25. Meleca RJ, Burgio DL, Carr RM, et al. Mucosal injuries of the upper aerodigestive tract after smoking crack or freebase cocaine. Laryngoscope 1997;107: 620–5.
26. Sertogullarindan B, Bora A, Sayir F, et al. Hydrocarbon pneumonitis; clinical and radiologic variability. J Clin Analyt Med 2012;1–3. Available at: www.jcam.com.tr/files/KATD-869.pdf. Accessed October 11, 2013.

27. Mastropietro CW, Valentine K. Early administration of intratracheal surfactant (calfactant) after hydrocarbon aspiration. Pediatrics 2011;127:e1600–4.
28. Gawarammana IB, Buckley NA. Medical management of paraquat ingestion. Br J Clin Pharmacol 2011;72:745–57.
29. Dinis-Oliveira RJ, Duarte JA, Sánchez-Navarro A, et al. Paraquat poisonings: mechanism of lung toxicity, clinical features, and treatment. Crit Rev Toxicol 2008;38:13–71.
30. Li LR, Sydenham E, Chaudhary B, et al. Glucocorticoid with cyclophosphamide for paraquat-induced lung fibrosis. Cochrane Database Syst Rev 2012;(7):CD008084. http://dx.doi.org/10.1002/14651858.CD008084.pub3.
31. International Agency for Research on Cancer, World Health Organization (IARC) Working Group on the Evaluation of Carcinogenic Risks to Humans. Asbestos (chrysotile, amosite, crocidolite, tremolite, actinolite, and anthophyllite). IARC Monographs 2012;100:219–309. Available at: http://monographs.iarc.fr/ENG/Monographs/vol100C/mono100C-11.pdf. Accessed August 29, 2013.
32. ATSDR. Asbestos. Libby, Montana. Agency for Toxic Substances and Disease Registry. 2009. Available at: http://www.atsdr.cdc.gov/asbestos/sites/libby_montana/. Accessed August 29, 2013.
33. Greenberg MI, Waksman J, Curtis J. Silicosis: a review. Dis Mon 2007;53:394–416.
34. Madl AK, Unice K, Brown JL, et al. Exposure-response analysis for beryllium sensitization and chronic beryllium disease among workers in a beryllium metal machining plant. J Occup Environ Hyg 2007;4:448–66.
35. OSHA. Preventing adverse health effects from exposure to beryllium on the job. US Department of Labor Occupational Safety and Health Administration, Directorate of Science, Technology and Medicine, Office of Science and Technology Assessment. 2010. Available at: https://www.osha.gov/dts/hib/hib_data/hib19990902.html. Accessed August 29, 2013.
36. Van Dyke MV, Martyny JW, Mroz MM, et al. Risk of chronic beryllium disease by HLA-DPB1 E69 genotype and beryllium exposure in nuclear workers. Am J Respir Crit Care Med 2011;183:1680–8.
37. Stange AW, Furman FJ, Hilmas DE. The beryllium lymphocyte proliferation test: relevant issues in beryllium health surveillance. Am J Ind Med 2004;46:453–62.
38. Alarie Y. Toxicity of fire smoke. Crit Rev Toxicol 2002;32:259–89.
39. Enkhbaatar P, Traber DL. Pathophysiology of acute lung injury in combined burn and smoke inhalation injury. Clin Sci 2004;107:137–43.
40. Grabowska T, Skowronek R, Nowicka J, et al. Prevalence of hydrogen cyanide and carboxyhaemoglobin in victims of smoke inhalation during enclosed-space fires: a combined toxicologic risk. Clin Toxicol 2012;50:759–63.
41. EPA. Air and radiation. Air trends. United States Environmental Protection Agency; 2012. Available at: http://www.epa.gov/airtrends. Accessed August 29, 2013.
42. Samoli E, Nastos PT, Paliatsos AG, et al. Acute effects of air pollution on pediatric asthma exacerbation: evidence of association and effect modification. Environ Res 2011;111:418–24.
43. Raaschou-Nielsen O, Andersen ZJ, Jensen SS, et al. Traffic air pollution and mortality from cardiovascular disease and all causes: a Danish cohort study. Environ Health 2012;11:60.
44. Fine JM, Gordon T, Chen LC, et al. Metal fume fever: characterization of clinical and plasma IL-6 responses in controlled human exposures to zinc oxide fume at and below the threshold limit value. J Occup Environ Med 1997;39:722–6.

45. Wong A, Greene S, Robinson J. Metal fume fever: a case review of calls made to the Victorian Poisons Information Centre. Aust Fam Physician 2012;41:141–4.

46. Hashimoto T, Tokucchi Y, Hayashi M, et al. Different subtypes of human lung adenocarcinoma caused by different etiological factors: evidence from p53 mutational spectra. Am J Pathol 2000;157:2133–41.

47. Lubin JH, Tomasek L, Edling C, et al. Estimating lung cancer mortality from residential radon using data for low exposures in miners. Radiat Res 1997;147: 126–34.

48. Fong KM, Sekido Y, Gazdar AF, et al. Lung cancer 9: molecular biology of lung cancer: clinical implications. Thorax 2003;58:892–900.

49. Hubaux R, Becker-Santos DD, Enfield KS, et al. Molecular features in arsenic-induced lung tumors. Mol Cancer 2013;12:20.

50. Urbano AM, Ferreira LM, Alpoim MC. Molecular and cellular mechanisms of hexavalent chromium-induced lung cancer: an updated perspective. Curr Drug Metab 2012;13:284–305.

51. Wild P, Bourgkard E, Paris C. Lung cancer and exposure to metals: the epidemiological evidence. Methods Mol Biol 2009;472:139–67.

52. Zhao J, Shi X, Castranova V, et al. Occupational toxicology of nickel and nickel compounds. J Environ Pathol Toxicol Oncol 2009;28:177–208.

53. Ash-Bernal R, Wise R, Wright SM. Acquired methemoglobinemia: a retrospective series of 138 cases at 2 teaching hospitals. Medicine (Baltimore) 2004; 83:265–73.

54. Barker SJ, Tremper KK, Hyatt J. Effects of methemoglobinemia on pulse oximetry and mixed venous oximetry. Anesthesiology 1989;70:112–7.

55. Feiner JR, Bickler PE. Improved accuracy of methemoglobin detection by pulse CO-oximetry during hypoxia. Anesth Analg 2010;111:1160–7.

56. Westphal M, Weber TP, Meyer J, et al. Affinity of carbon monoxide to hemoglobin increases at low oxygen fractions. Biochem Biophys Res Commun 2002; 295:975–7.

57. Buckley NA, Juurlink DN, Isbister G, et al. Hyperbaric oxygen for carbon monoxide poisoning. Cochrane Database Syst Rev 2011;(13):CD002041. http://dx. doi.org/10.1002/14651858.CD00201.pub3.

58. Barker SJ, Curry J, Redford D, et al. Measurement of carboxyhemoglobin and methemoglobin by pulse oximetry: a human volunteer study. Anesthesiology 2006;105:892–7.

59. Buckley RG, Aks SE, Eshom JL, et al. The pulse oximetry gap in carbon monoxide intoxication. Ann Emerg Med 1994;24:252–5.

60. Chee KJ, Nilson D, Partridge R, et al. Finding needles in a haystack: a case series of carbon monoxide poisoning detected using new technology in the emergency department. Clin Toxicol 2008;46:461–9.

61. Fligiel SE, Roth MD, Kleerup EC, et al. Tracheobronchial histopathology in habitual smokers of cocaine, marijuana, and/or tobacco. Chest 1997;112:319–26.

62. Tashkin DP. Airway effects of marijuana, cocaine, and other inhaled illicit agents. Curr Opin Pulm Med 2001;7:43–61.

63. Fiedler N, Kelly-McNeil K, Mohr S, et al. Controlled human exposure to methyl tertiary butyl ether in gasoline: symptoms, psychophysiologic and neurobehavioral responses of self-reported sensitive persons. Environ Health Perspect 2000;108:753–63.

64. Lehrer PM. Psychophysiological hypotheses regarding multiple chemical sensitivity syndrome. Environ Health Perspect 1997;105(Suppl 2):479–83.

65. Leikin JB, Mycyk MB, Bryant S, et al. Characteristics of patients with no underlying toxicologic syndrome evaluated in a toxicology clinic. J Toxicol Clin Toxicol 2004;42:643–8.

66. Methyl isocyanate. EPA air toxics Web site. Environmental Protection Agency. Available at: http://www.epa.gov/ttnatw01/hlthef/methylis.html. Accessed August 29, 2013.

67. National Transportation Safety Board. Derailment of Canadian Pacific railway freight train 292-16 and subsequent release of anhydrous ammonia near Minot, North Dakota. Railroad accident report NTSB/RAR-04/01. Washington, DC: National Transportation Safety Board; 2002. Available at: http://www.ntsb.gov/doclib/reports/2004/RAR0401.pdf. Accessed August 29, 2013.

68. National Transportation Safety Board. Collision of Norfolk Southern freight train 192 with standing Norfolk Southern local train P22 with subsequent hazardous materials release: Graniteville, South Carolina January 6, 2005. Railroad accident report NTSB/RAR-05/04. Washington, DC: National Transportation Safety Board; 2005. Available at: https://www.ntsb.gov/doclib/reports/2005/RAR0504.pdf. Accessed August 29, 2013.

69. National Transportation Safety Board. Phosphorous trichloride release in Boston and Maine Yard 8 during switching operations Somerville, Massachusetts April 3, 1980. Washington, DC: National Transportation Safety Board; 1981. Available at: http://babel.hathitrust.org/cgi/pt?id=ien.35556021345897;view=1up;seq=25. Accessed August 29, 2013.

70. National Transportation Safety Board. Safety recommendations 1-81-1 and -2 re. Collision of Boston and Maine Corporation (BM) Boston switcher with standing draft of cars, Somerville, Massachusetts April 3, 1980. Washington, DC: National Transportation Safety Board; 1981. Available at: http://www.ntsb.gov/doclib/recletters/1981/I81_1_2.pdf. Accessed August 29, 2013.

71. Woodward J, Woodward HZ. Analysis of hydrogen fluoride release at Texas City. Process Saf Progr 2004;17:213–8.

72. Occupational Safety & Health Administration (OSHA). Accident: 14259261 – inhalation of phosgene gas. Report ID: 0625700 – event date: 09/10/1984. Washington, DC: US Department of Labor, Occupational Safety & Health Administration. Available at: https://www.osha.gov/pls/imis/accidentsearch.accident_detail?id=14259261. Accessed August 29, 2013.

Toxicologic Acid-Base Disorders

Sage W. Wiener, MD[a,b,c,]*

KEYWORDS

- Acid-base • Acidemia • Alkalemia • Anion gap • Delta gap • Osmol gap • Toxicity

KEY POINTS

- Draw a blood gas with lactate and a chemistry panel in patients presenting after poisoning of unknown etiology.
- The toxicologic differential diagnosis of respiratory alkalosis, respiratory acidosis, metabolic alkalosis, and nonanion gap metabolic acidosis is fairly narrow.
- When approaching the patient with an anion gap metabolic acidosis, check for lactate first and ketones second, as these account for the vast majority of patients with anion gap metabolic acidosis.
- Patients with alcoholic ketoacidosis rapidly improve with fluids, dextrose, and thiamine.
- The osmol gap can sometimes be an important clue, but a normal osmol gap never excludes toxic alcohol poisoning.

INTRODUCTION

Interpretation of a patient's acid-base status can be critical to the evaluation of the poisoned patient. Many toxins will lead to a characteristic acid-base changes, and a blood gas analysis helps to establish a differential diagnosis that can be instrumental in narrowing down the potential cause of toxicity.

BASIC ACID-BASE PHYSIOLOGY

Human respiration is regulated by the brainstem to attempt to maintain a constant partial pressure of carbon dioxide (P_{CO_2}) of approximately 40 mm Hg. Carbonic anhydrase converts carbon dioxide and water to carbonic acid, with a concentration of carbonic acid linearly related to the P_{CO_2}. Carbonic acid can dissociate to

Disclosures: Nothing to disclose.
[a] Department of Emergency Medicine, SUNY Downstate Medical Center, 450 Clarkson Avenue, Box 1228, Brooklyn, NY 11203, USA; [b] Department of Emergency Medicine, Kings County Hospital Center, 451 Clarkson Avenue, Brooklyn, NY 11203, USA; [c] New York City Department of Health and Mental Hygiene, New York City Poison Control Center, 455 First Avenue, New York, NY 10016, USA
* Department of Emergency Medicine, SUNY Downstate Medical Center, 450 Clarkson Avenue, Box 1228, Brooklyn, NY 11203.
E-mail address: sagewiener-em@yahoo.com

Emerg Med Clin N Am 32 (2014) 149–165
http://dx.doi.org/10.1016/j.emc.2013.09.011

bicarbonate and hydrogen ion (a proton). This equilibrium is the primary buffering system of the body, and it is governed by the Henderson-Hasselbalch equation (**Fig. 1**). Acidemia (pH <7.35) results from either excess carbon dioxide (acid) or a paucity of bicarbonate (base). Alkalemia (pH >7.45) results from either a low P_{CO_2} or an excess of bicarbonate.

INTERPRETATION OF THE ARTERIAL BLOOD GAS
Identifying the Primary Acid Base Disorder

Interpretation of the arterial blood gas (ABG) starts with an assessment of the pH for acidemia or alkalemia. Most typically, a blood gas will have been drawn because of a suspicion of metabolic acidosis due to a low bicarbonate on a serum chemistry analysis. When this occurs, the pH can be used to distinguish metabolic acidosis from respiratory alkalosis as the primary process. If the serum bicarbonate is low and the pH is low, the primary process is a metabolic acidosis. If the pH is high, then the primary process must be a respiratory alkalosis. When the serum bicarbonate is high, a low pH indicates a respiratory acidosis, whereas a high pH indicates a metabolic alkalosis.

Determining Whether a Respiratory Disorder is Chronic or Acute

If there is a respiratory acidosis or alkalosis, the next step is to determine whether the process is acute or chronic. In an acute respiratory acidosis or alkalosis, for every 10 mm Hg change from 40 mm Hg in the P_{CO_2}, the pH should change from 7.40 by 0.08. If the process is chronic, the pH should change by approximately 0.03 for every 10 mm Hg change in the P_{CO_2}.

Determining Whether Compensation is Appropriate

If the primary process is a metabolic acidosis or alkalosis, it must next be determined whether respiratory compensation is appropriate. For a metabolic acidosis, this can be calculated using Winter's formula. The expected P_{CO_2} when compensation is appropriate should be approximately 1.5 times the serum bicarbonate concentration plus 8.

$$\text{Predicted } P_{CO_2} = (1.5 \times [\text{observed } HCO_3^-]) + 8 \pm 2$$

$$CO_2 + H_2O \xrightleftharpoons{\text{carbonic anhydrase}} H_2CO_3$$

$$H_2CO_3 \rightleftharpoons HCO_3^- + H^+$$

$$[H_2CO_3] = P_{CO_2} \times 0.03$$

$$pH = \log 6.1 \times \frac{\overset{\text{Base}}{[HCO_3^-]}}{\underset{\text{Acid}}{[H_2CO_3]}}$$

Fig. 1. Relationship among carbon dioxide, carbonic acid, and bicarbonate. Carbon dioxide and water are converted to carbonic acid by carbonic anhydrase. Carbonic acid is in equilibrium with bicarbonate, a relationship governed by the Henderson-Hasselbalch equation. The concentration of carbonic acid is a linear function of the partial pressure of carbon dioxide.

For a metabolic alkalosis, the appropriate compensation can be estimated using the formula:

Predicted P_{CO_2} = 15 + (observed HCO_3^-)

If the P_{CO_2} does not fall within the predicted range, there is a second acid-base disorder, respiratory acidosis or respiratory alkalosis depending on whether the P_{CO_2} is above or below the predicted P_{CO_2}, respectively. This generally indicates a problem with ventilation, and must be addressed immediately.

Determining Whether a Metabolic Acidosis is Associated with an Anion Gap

If a metabolic acidosis is present, the next step is to calculate the anion gap. The anion gap is the difference between the serum sodium concentration (the primary cation in the body) and the sum of the chloride and bicarbonate concentrations (the primary anions in the body).

Anion gap = $(Na^+) - ([Cl^-] + [HCO_3^-])$

Normally, the difference is 8 to 12 because there are more unmeasured anions (eg, phosphates, sulfates, albumin, organic acids) than unmeasured cations (magnesium, potassium). When there is an excess of an organic acid, the anion gap rises because the sum of all anions and the sum of all cations must always be equal, and the amount of unmeasured anions rises. When there is a metabolic acidosis, distinguishing between acidosis with an elevated anion gap from acidosis with a normal anion gap is critical, because they suggest different underlying etiologies. The anion gap may be elevated by toxins that produce deficiencies in calcium, potassium, or magnesium. Conversely, it may lowered by cationic toxins such as lithium, or halides other than chlorine such as bromine or iodine.

Distinguishing a Mixed Acid-Base Disorder from an Isolated Anion Gap Acidosis

When a metabolic acidosis with an elevated anion gap is present, the next step is to calculate the *delta gap*. The delta gap allows the distinction between a pure anion gap metabolic acidosis and a mixed acid base disorder with both anion gap and non–anion gap acidosis. The delta gap is calculated as follows:

delta gap = delta anion gap – delta bicarbonate

The delta anion gap is the rise in the anion gap from 12, whereas the delta bicarbonate is the fall in bicarbonate from 24. For a pure anion gap metabolic acidosis, the delta gap should approximate zero. If the delta gap is significantly positive, there is a metabolic alkalosis in addition to the anion gap metabolic acidosis. If the delta gap is significantly negative, there is a concomitant non−anion gap metabolic acidosis.[1]

The Stewart Strong Ion Difference

The Stewart strong ion theory is another approach to acid-base problems that takes into account all of the major ions that are normally in the plasma, and separates them into dependent and independent variables. The independent variables are P_{CO_2}, the total weak nonvolatile acids, such as phosphate and proteins (A_{TOT}) and the strong ion difference (SID). The SID is defined as follows:

(SID) = $(Na^+) + (K^+) + (Ca^{2+}) + (Mg^{2+}) - (Cl^-) - $ (Other Strong Anions)

In a sense, this is similar in concept to the anion gap, in that it is based on the law of electroneutrality, which is that the sum of all anions must equal the sum of all cations in the body. The strong ion theory is useful because it explains some concepts, such as dilutional acidosis and contraction alkalosis, which are more difficult to explain using a standard approach to acid-base problems, and because it includes the effects of changes in other buffers, such as albumin and phosphate, all in one master equation.[2,3] However, it is more complicated to calculate and proportionately more affected by small errors in measurement, and thus less commonly used in the clinical setting. Additionally, although it is mathematically correct, it does not correspond to actual physiology, in that the body regulates pH and bicarbonate, not strong ion difference.[2,4,5]

RESPIRATORY ALKALOSIS

The most common reason for respiratory alkalosis is compensation for a metabolic acidosis, but compensatory respiratory alkalosis cannot be the primary disorder, because compensation does not overcorrect (does not change the pH past 7.40). The major toxicologic causes of respiratory alkalosis include salicylate toxicity and hyperventilation compensating for impaired oxygenation from pulmonary toxins.

Salicylates

Salicylates are complex metabolic toxins that cause a characteristic acid-base pattern that changes somewhat depending on how far along the course of illness the patient presents. Early in poisoning, patients will have a respiratory alkalosis. This is because of direct stimulation of the medulla, where salicylates increase respiratory rate and tidal volume.[6] This stage may be missed in younger children, because of the lack the ventilatory reserve that adults are able to mobilize.[7] As toxicity progresses, patients may display double, or even triple, acid-base disorders as they develop metabolic alkalosis from vomiting and metabolic acidosis through multiple mechanisms (see later in this article).

Hyperventilation due to Impaired Oxygenation

Patients with impaired gas exchange compensate by increasing their ventilation, becoming tachypneic and hyperpneic. Several toxins may cause impaired gas exchange by causing pulmonary edema or pulmonary fibrosis, or interstitial lung disease (**Table 1**). Some of these patients may also have a concomitant metabolic acidosis due to lactate from anaerobic metabolism if oxygenation is severely impaired.

RESPIRATORY ACIDOSIS

Respiratory acidosis is a marker of hypoventilation. Hopefully, by the time a blood gas result demonstrates respiratory acidosis, the hypoventilation will have already been recognized based on the physical examination, and addressed. However, it is important to be aware that hypoventilation may occur even with a normal respiratory rate if the tidal volume is decreased. When this occurs, not only is there a resulting diminished minute ventilation, proportionally more dead space ventilation occurs, and this poor gas exchange leads to CO_2 accumulation and respiratory acidosis. The major toxicologic causes of primary respiratory acidosis are opioid intoxication and sedative-hypnotic intoxication.

Table 1
Some toxins and toxicants that cause respiratory alkalosis by inducing tachypnea due to impaired gas exchange[a]

Toxicologic Causes of Respiratory Alkalosis	
Pulmonary Edema	Pulmonary Fibrosis
Calcium channel antagonists	Amiodarone
Deferoxamine	Bleomycin
Glyphosate	Busulfan
Meprobamate, ethchlorvynol	Cyclophosphamide
Nonsteroidal anti-inflammatory drugs	Environmental (bird and animal droppings)
Opioids	Methotrexate
Phenobarbital	Nitrofurantoin
Pulmonary irritant inhalants	Occupational (silica, asbestos, coal, beryllium, grain)
Salicylates	Propranolol
Scorpion envenomation	Sulfasalazine

[a] Selected data elements contained in reference.[8]

Opioids

Opioids lead to hypoventilation through mu-opioid receptor–mediated blockade of specialized respiratory neurons in the brainstem.[9] These lead to tolerance of hypercapnea, suppressing the normal drive for respiration. In fact, hypoventilation is the best predictor of response to naloxone (an opioid antagonist) in the prehospital setting.[10] Other signs may provide clues to opioid intoxication, including miosis, hypoactive bowel sounds, "track marks" on the forearms, or drug paraphernalia found on the scene, but the absence of these signs do not exclude opioid intoxication as the cause of hypoventilation. A history of opioid abuse or chronic pain may also suggest the diagnosis. In patients with chronic pain with opioid overdose, it is important to perform a careful skin examination to exclude adherent opioid analgesic patches. If found, these should be immediately removed from the skin to prevent further absorption.

Most cases of opioid intoxication are readily reversed by the opioid antagonist naloxone. However, if a patient has a respiratory acidosis due to an opioid, the patient should be ventilated by bag valve mask before administering the antidote. Abrupt reversal of opioid effect in a patient who is still hypercapneic may precipitate acute lung injury (ALI),[11] although ALI may also result from opioid overdose alone. Rapid reversal of opioid effect on the brainstem in a patient who is still hypercapneic leads to release of catecholamines that increase the permeability of the vascular bed in the lungs. If the patient is ventilated before administration of naloxone, the Pco_2 will be normalized once the opioid effect on the brain is reversed, so the catecholamine surge should not occur.

Sedatives/Hypnotics

Sedatives/hypnotics classically cause coma with normal vital signs. However, some sedative/hypnotic agents may be associated with hypoventilation and respiratory acidosis, particularly barbiturates, GHB (gamma-hydroxybutyrate) and its congeners, and propofol. Additionally, combinations of sedative hypnotics (eg, ethanol and benzodiazepines) can cause respiratory depression. Although a competitive antagonist for benzodiazepines exists (flumazenil), it should not be used in patients who may be benzodiazepine tolerant or dependent, because it may induce seizures and life-threatening withdrawal.[12] There is no reversal agent for other sedative/hypnotics. If hypoventilation and respiratory acidosis occur, they can be treated with intubation and mechanical ventilation.

METABOLIC ALKALOSIS

The underlying mechanisms for metabolic alkalosis can be separated into five basic categories:

- Compensation for respiratory acidosis (never a primary process)
- Addition of bicarbonate
- Loss of chloride
- Appropriate mineralocorticoid excess
- Inappropriate mineralocorticoid excess (renin, aldosterone-producing tumors, renal artery stenosis, Bartter syndrome)

The urine chloride can help distinguish between causes of metabolic alkalosis (**Table 2**).

Vomiting

Vomiting is a common adverse effect of many toxins. When vomiting is severe, metabolic alkalosis may occur due to the loss of hydrochloric acid in emesis. Additionally, patients with severe vomiting can become volume depleted and develop a contraction alkalosis (from appropriate mineralocorticoid excess). Although recent data suggest that the chloride loss may be the underlying factor causing acidosis, not the volume depletion (see contraction alkalosis/chloride depletion acidosis later in this article),[3] there is not yet universal consensus on this point.[5]

Increased Bicarbonate Intake

Patients who ingest too much bicarbonate (antacid abuse/milk-alkali syndrome) may develop metabolic alkalosis directly due to absorption of the bicarbonate. This most commonly occurs in people who take excessive antacids for symptoms of dyspepsia. Milk-alkali syndrome, a triad of metabolic alkalosis, hypercalcemia, and renal insufficiency results from excess calcium and alkali intake.[13] Calcium carbonate taken as an antacid (with or without milk intake) is the most common cause, although it may also occur in people taking calcium carbonate as a calcium

Table 2 Distinguishing causes of metabolic alkalosis by urinary chloride	
Differential Diagnosis of Metabolic Alkalosis by Urinary Chloride	
[Urine Cl⁻] <25 mEq/L	**[Urine Cl⁻] >45 mEq/L**
Vomiting or nasogastric suction[a]	Mineralocorticoid excess[a]
Diuretics (late)[a]	Diuretics (early)[a]
Posthypercapnea	Alkali load (bicarbonate overdose)[a]
Cystic fibrosis	Severe hypokalemia (<2.0 mEq/L)[a]
Low chloride intake	—
Refeeding	—

[a] Toxicologic or potentially toxicologic causes.

supplement or as a phosphate binder in chronic renal insufficiency. In one series, milk-alkali syndrome was responsible for 12% of patients presenting with hypercalcemia.[14]

Licorice Abuse

Ingestion of natural licorice can lead to acidosis among other effects due to the *glycyrrhizin* in natural licorice (not the candy typically sold as "licorice" in the United States). Glycyrrhizin and related compounds are inhibitors of 11-beta-hydroxysteroid dehydrogenase in the kidney. This enzyme normally inactivates cortisol, which has significant mineralocorticoid activity, by converting it to cortisone, which does not. When this enzyme is inhibited, cortisol in the kidney leads to excess sodium retention and excess potassium and hydrogen ion excretion.[15] Inhibition of the enzyme is reversible, and discontinuing exposure will resolve the problem.

Contraction Alkalosis/Chloride Depletion Alkalosis

Patients with volume depletion characteristically develop what has traditionally been termed "contraction alkalosis." If patients lose water without losing bicarbonate (typically due to diuretics), the concentration of bicarbonate rises. Because the P_{CO_2} is regulated by ventilation to remain constant, alkalosis results.[16] Additionally, volume depletion stimulates the renin-angiotensin-aldosterone system, which leads to increased sodium and bicarbonate reabsorption in the proximal tubule and increased proton and potassium secretion in the distal tubule.

A newer understanding of the process suggests that the underlying problem is not volume depletion (contraction), but chloride depletion, and it has been suggested that the condition be renamed "chloride depletion alkalosis." A chloride/bicarbonate exchanger called pendrin has been identified as being key to the process. In both a rat model and in healthy human volunteers with acidosis induced by furosemide and dietary chloride restriction, repletion of chloride corrects the acidosis even when volume depletion and sodium depletion persist.[3]

METABOLIC ACIDOSIS

There are five common mechanisms by which a metabolic acidosis is generated:

- Compensation for a respiratory alkalosis (never a primary process)
- Addition of acid (eg, HCl)
- Increase in the generation of H^+ from endogenous (eg, lactate, ketones) or exogenous acids (eg, salicylate, ethylene glycol, methanol)
- Inability of the kidneys to excrete the hydrogen from dietary protein intake (types 1 and 4 renal tubular acidosis [RTA])
- The loss of bicarbonate due to wasting through the kidney (type 2 RTA) or the gastrointestinal tract (diarrhea)

As described previously, calculating the anion gap is the first step to distinguishing between causes of metabolic acidosis.

Non–Anion Gap Metabolic Acidosis

There are a limited number of mechanisms whereby a non–anion gap metabolic acidosis is generated (**Table 3**). These include the following:

- RTA-inducing toxins (**Table 4**)
- Diarrhea-inducing toxins (**Table 5**)
- Ingestion of an absorbable acid

Table 3
Distinguishing underlying mechanisms of non–anion gap acidosis based on serum potassium concentration, urine pH, and urine ammonia

			Hyperchloremic (Non–Anion Gap) Metabolic Acidosis		
			Proximal Acidification	Distal Acidification	
Disease	Renal Defect	Plasma [K^+]	HCO_3^- Reabsorption	Urine pH	Urine NH_3
Recovery DKA	None	↓	normal or ↑	<5.5	↑
Diarrhea	None	↓	normal or ↑	≤5.5	↑
Proximal RTA (Type 2)	↓ proximal acidification	↓	↓	<5.5	normal or ↑
Classic distal RTA (Type 1)	↓ distal acidification	↓	normal or ↑	>5.5	↓
Generalized distal RTA (Type 4)	↓ aldosterone action	↑	normal or ↑	<5.5	↓
Renal failure	↓ ammonia production	normal or ↑	normal or ↑	<5.5	↓

Abbreviations: ↑, increased; ↓, decreased; DKA, diabetic ketoacidosis; RTA, renal tubular acidosis.

- Carbonic anhydrase inhibition
- Toluene, ethylene glycol
- Dilutional acidosis

Toxins that Cause RTA

There are three types of RTA: type 1 (defect of distal tubule bicarbonate absorption), type 2 (defect of proximal tubule bicarbonate absorption), and type 4 (hyporeninemic hypoaldosteroneism). Any of the three may be caused by toxins. Examples are provided in **Table 4**. Metabolic acidosis due to RTA, unlike anion gap acidosis, should be treated with bicarbonate, because the underlying problem is loss of bicarbonate.

Toxins that Cause Diarrhea

Toxins may cause diarrhea through several mechanisms (see **Table 5**). Osmotic agents, like most laxatives, draw fluid into the gastrointestinal (GI) tract by introducing

Table 4
Selected toxins causing renal tubular acidosis

Distal (Type 1)	Proximal (Type 2)	Hypoaldosterone (Type 4)
Amphotericin B	Cadmium	Angiotensin-converting enzyme inhibitors
Ifosfamide	Antiretroviral therapy	Angiotensin receptor antagonists
Lithium carbonate	Ifosfamide	Eplerenone
Toluene	Lead	Nonsteroidal anti-inflammatory drugs
Zoledronate	—	Pentamidine
—	—	Spironolactone
—	—	Trimethoprim

Table 5	
Examples of various mechanisms of toxin-mediated diarrhea	
Mechanism	**Examples**
Malabsorption	Cholestyramine, olestra, tetrahydrolipstatin, alpha-glucosidase inhibitors
Motility	Erythromycin, metoclopramide
Mucosal necrosis	Colchicine, methotrexate, antineoplastics
Osmotic	Sorbitol, magnesium citrate, lactose, mannitol, sodium polystyrene sulfonate, polyethylene glycol (some formulations)
Secretory	Stimulant laxatives

molecules that cannot be absorbed into the lumen. Secretory diarrhea occurs from toxins that irritate the GI mucosa. Other toxins interfere with absorption in the gut. Motility agents may cause diarrhea by speeding transit through the GI tract. Finally, some chemotherapeutic drugs cause necrosis of the GI mucosa. Severe diarrhea may also cause a contraction alkalosis.

Ingestion of an Absorbable Acid

Unlike ingestion of alkalis, ingestion of some strong acids leads to systemic absorption of those acids. For example, when sulfuric acid is absorbed, the sulfate becomes an unmeasured anion, leading to an elevated anion gap. However, when hydrochloric acid is absorbed, the excess chloride is accounted for in the measured anions, so an anion gap elevation does not occur. This is generally not clinically occult, because hydrochloric acid has significant caustic effects; signs and symptoms of the caustic effect are often present.

Carbonic Anhydrase Inhibition

Carbonic anhydrase inhibitors (acetazolamide, topiramate) can induce non–anion gap metabolic acidosis, particularly in patients with impaired renal function.[17,18] The underlying mechanism is increased renal bicarbonate loss due to inability to absorb protons with bicarbonate in the kidney.[19] The protons are instead absorbed with chloride, leading to a hyperchloremic acidosis.

Non–anion Gap Metabolic Acidosis from Toluene and Ethylene Glycol

Although non-gap acidosis from toluene has been attributed to distal RTA in the past, this has recently been called into question. The acidosis may in fact be due to toluene's metabolism to hippuric acid. Although hippurate is an unmeasured anion, and could cause anion gap acidosis, it is postulated that the presence or absence of an anion gap elevation is dependent on the kidney's ability to excrete that anion.[20] Similarly, patients have been identified that develop non-gap acidosis after ethylene glycol poisoning, presumably for similar reasons.[21]

Dilutional Acidosis

It seems counterintuitive that the addition of a neutral solution such as saline could acidify the blood. The reason this occurs is that respiration is regulated to maintain a constant Pco_2. When saline is administered, the bicarbonate buffer gets diluted while the Pco_2 remains constant, thus the pH drops.[2] This is conceptually the exact opposite of what happens in contraction alkalosis.

Anion Gap Metabolic Acidosis

Basic approach to anion gap acidosis

Most medical students are familiar with the mnemonic "MUDPILES" or its extension "CAT-MUDPILES" for the differential diagnosis of metabolic acidosis with an elevated anion gap. This stands for the following:

- C = cyanide
- A = alcoholic ketoacidosis
- T = toluene
- M = methanol, metformin
- U = uremia
- D = DKA (diabetic ketoacidosis)
- P = phenformin, paraldehyde
- I = iron, INH (isoniazid), ibuprofen
- L = lactate
- E = ethylene glycol
- S = salicylates, SKA (starvation ketoacidosis)

Although this is an easy way to remember most of the common causes of anion gap elevation, it is not exhaustive, nor does it provide a rational approach to the evaluation of the patient with an anion gap acidosis. For example, numerous mitochondrial poisons, vasoactive agents, systemic toxins (aluminum phosphide) and nonsteroidal anti-inflammatory drugs are excluded from this list. It is highly inefficient to take a "shotgun" approach to anion gap metabolic acidosis, sending tests to rule out all of the "CAT-MUDPILES" causes when the acid-base disorder is recognized. In most centers, tests for methanol and ethylene glycol are not done on-site, so results may take several days. If toxic alcohols are suspected, treatment should not be delayed for these results, and an alcohol dehydrogenase (ADH) inhibitor, ethanol or fomepizole, should be administered. This is potentially expensive, unnecessary, and can lead to other complications, particularly if ethanol is used as the ADH inhibitor.

A more rational approach to the patient with an elevated anion gap is to rule out the most common causes before considering more rare causes (**Fig. 2**). The vast majority of patients with anion gap acidosis have an elevated lactate as the cause. Thus, when sending a sample for blood gas analysis, it is critical to also request a lactate concentration. Ketoacidosis is also common, so serum and/or urine should be analyzed for ketones. Uremia is also a common cause of anion gap acidosis, but it is typically apparent whether a patient is uremic by the time it is determined that there is an anion gap elevation. It is also rare for the metabolic acidosis to occur from uremia unless the serum creatinine approaches 5 to 6 mg/dL. Once these common causes have been evaluated, the diagnosis of toxic alcohols may be pursued, unless the diagnosis is suspected based on the history or other clues.

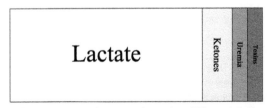

Fig. 2. Metabolic acidosis. A rational approach to the differential diagnosis of metabolic acidosis with an elevated anion gap focuses on what causes are most common.

LACTATE

Metabolic acidosis with an elevated lactate is typically classified as Type A (associated with underlying tissue hypoxemia or hypoperfusion) or Type B (associated with inborn errors of metabolism, toxins, or underlying diseases). However, this is generally less useful from a toxicologic perspective, as some toxins lead to lactate excess because of underlying tissue hypoxemia or hypoperfusion. Toxins such as iron can cause both a Type A and Type B lactic acidosis. It is more useful to consider which of two basic mechanisms is the underlying cause of an elevated lactate: excess production of lactate or inability to clear lactate. Most toxin-associated lactic acidosis is due to excess production of lactate. Production of excess lactate is generally due to one of the several underlying mechanisms (**Table 6**):

- Seizure-inducing toxins: seizures cause excess motor activity, causing a basic imbalance between oxygen supply and demand, particularly in generalized seizures, during which ventilation may be impaired. In this situation, skeletal muscle tissue turns to anaerobic metabolism for energy, generating lactate (**Fig. 3**).
- Toxins causing oxygen demand to exceed oxygen supply: lactate is a nonspecific marker of severe illness and hypovolemia in many disease states, from sepsis to trauma. Some toxins can also cause lactate elevation by causing hypovolemia and/or mismatch of oxygen supply and demand. This is characteristic of iron toxicity (the "I" in MUDPILES). Lactate is also a marker of poor prognosis after acetaminophen poisoning, likely for similar reasons.[22] Another example is the lactate elevation that may occur after beta-agonist poisoning.[23,24]
- Tissue ischemia due to vasoconstriction and local hypoperfusion: toxins that cause vasoconstriction, primarily alpha-adrenergic agonists and ergot derivatives, lead to local tissue hypoperfusion and resultant anaerobic metabolism in that tissue, producing lactate (see **Fig. 3**).
- Interference with oxygen utilization: toxins may interfere with oxygen utilization either by directly interfering with the electron transport chain and oxidative phosphorylation (eg, carbon monoxide, cyanide, or hydrogen sulfide binding to

Table 6
Various mechanisms of generating metabolic acidosis with an elevated serum lactate concentration

Mechanism of Lactic Acidosis		Examples
Seizures[a]		INH, bupropion, camphor, theophylline
Oxygen demand exceeds supply		Iron, acetaminophen, beta-agonists
Interference with oxygen utilization	Oxidative phosphorylation inhibitors	Carbon monoxide, cyanide, hydrogen sulfide, rotenone
	Mitochondrial toxins	Nucleoside reverse transcriptase inhibitors, non-nucleoside reverse transcriptase inhibitors, propofol
Local ischemia		Cocaine, ergots, amphetamines, cathinones
Metabolism to lactate		Propylene glycol
Inability to clear lactate		Metformin/phenformin, ethanol

Abbreviation: INH, isoniazid.
[a] Seizures are themselves an example in which oxygen demand exceeds oxygen supply, but because toxins that cause acidosis by this mechanism have a clinically apparent manifestation, they are listed as a separate category.

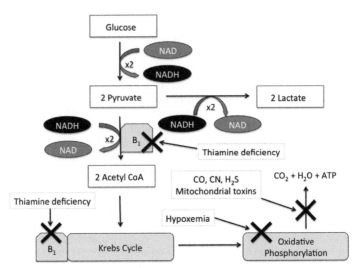

Fig. 3. Effects of hypoxemia, thiamine deficiency, and mitochondrial toxins on glucose metabolism. Ultimately, by blocking different stages of metabolism after glycolysis, all of these mechanisms prevent aerobic metabolism. When pyruvate cannot enter into the Krebs cycle by conversion to acetyl CoA, the only way to maintain glycolysis is to convert pyruvate to lactate, regenerating oxidized NAD.

cytochrome aa3 oxidase) or by poisoning mitochondria. These include nucleoside reverse transcriptase inhibitors and non-nucleoside reverse transcriptase inhibitors which interfere with mitochondrial DNA chlordecone and amphotericin induced changes in mitochondrial permeability, and mitochondrial uncoupling agents such as dinitrophenol and pentachlorophenol). In either case, when oxidative phosphorylation cannot proceed, NADH must be cleared by converting pyruvate to lactate to permit continued glycolysis (see **Fig. 3**). There is some evidence that metformin-associated lactic acidosis may also involve inhibition of oxidative phosphorylation.[25]

- Direct metabolism of a toxin to lactate: propylene glycol, a diol, is metabolized successively by ADH and aldehyde dehydrogenase to lactate. Patients who ingest propylene glycol can have markedly elevated serum lactate concentrations to values that would in most circumstances be incompatible with life. These values are well tolerated in propylene glycol cases because the excess lactate is not reflective of underlying pathology.

Some toxin-associated lactic acidosis is due to an inability to clear lactate. Extensive metabolism of ethanol leads to a reduced redox state of the body (excess NADH relative to NAD). This shifts the lactate/pyruvate equilibrium toward lactate, preventing its metabolism (**Fig. 4**). Metformin-associated lactic acidosis may involve inhibition of pyruvate dehydrogenase, preventing pyruvate metabolism to acetyl CoA and further metabolism.[26] This also shifts the pyruvate/lactate equilibrium toward lactate.

One non-physiological reason for an elevated lactate is ethylene glycol poisoning. Ethylene glycol may interfere with some lactate assays, yielding a high false-positive lactate reading, typically on blood gas analyzers. To help decipher true elevations from spurious values, both serum and blood gas sample lactates can be obtained to determine if a "lactate gap" (a difference between the two samples) exists.

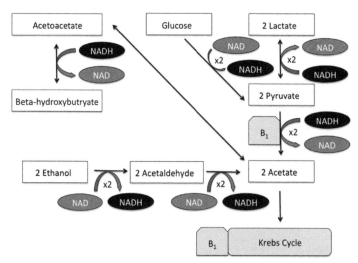

Fig. 4. Relationship between pyruvate and lactate, acetoacetate and beta-hydroxybutyrate, and ethanol and acetate. When NADH is abundant, the equilibrium between pyruvate and lactate shifts to favor lactate and the equilibrium between acetoacetate and beta-hydroxybutyrate shifts to favor beta-hydroxybutyrate. States that lead to abundance of NADH include glucose metabolism when aerobic metabolism is not possible (due to relative hypoxemia, inhibition of the Krebs cycle or oxidative phosphorylation by toxins, or absence of thiamine preventing conversion of pyruvate to acetyl CoA), and extensive metabolism of ethanol. The shift from pyruvate to lactate in chronic drinkers also makes pyruvate unavailable as a starting point for gluconeogenesis.

KETONES

From a toxicologic perspective, the main causes of ketosis are isopropanol or acetone intoxication and alcoholic ketoacidosis (AKA). Salicylates and valproate poisoning may also be associated with ketosis. However, of these, only AKA and salicylates cause a metabolic acidosis. When isopropanol is metabolized by alcohol dehydrogenase, the end product is acetone. Acetone is a ketone, but not an acid, so it is not associated with acidemia. Further, because it is a ketone, not an aldehyde, it cannot be further metabolized to an acid by aldehyde dehydrogenase. This is why acute and isolated isopropanol ingestions may present with "ketosis without acidosis."

Alcoholic ketoacidosis typically occurs in chronic drinkers during a period of abstinence after a binge. Chronic drinkers have depleted glycogen stores, and usually have depleted thiamine as well. This scenario leads to fatty acid breakdown, and generation of acetyl CoA. The absence of thiamine inhibits the Krebs cycle (as it is a cofactor for alpha-ketoglutarate dehydrogenase), so the excess acetyl CoA is converted to acetoacetate (**Fig. 5**). Because of the excess NADH from ethanol metabolism, the equilibrium between acetoacetate and beta-hydroxybutyrate shifts toward mostly beta-hydroxybutyrate (see **Fig. 4**); thus, there may be only trace serum ketones even when there is extensive acidosis (because beta-hydroxybutyrate is a carboxylic acid and not a ketone).[27]

It is common for patients with a history of alcoholism to present with anion gap acidosis of unclear etiology, and trace ketones. Although toxic alcohols may be considered in the differential diagnosis in this setting, it is reasonable to attempt treatment of AKA first. If thiamine, dextrose, and fluids are administered, the anion gap

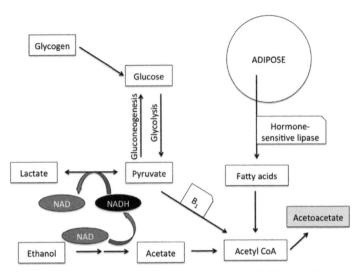

Fig. 5. Starvation, thiamine deficiency, and ethanol metabolism lead to ketoacidosis. Glycogen reserves are quickly exhausted, and glucose intake is low. Existing pyruvate is converted to lactate because of excess NADH from ethanol metabolism, and becomes relatively unavailable for gluconeogenesis. Low glucose impairs insulin release, and hormone-sensitive lipase is activated, liberating fatty acids from fat. These fatty acids are broken down to acetyl CoA in the liver. Absence of thiamine inhibits the Krebs cycle, and the excess acetyl CoA is converted to acetoacetate.

generally improves rapidly if due to AKA, which is not expected in toxic alcohol poisoning without specific antidotal therapy or concurrent ingestion of ethanol.

SALICYLATES

In addition to the respiratory alkalosis (previously discussed in this article), salicylates characteristically cause an anion gap metabolic acidosis. Although early in poisoning it may not yet be present, eventually an acidosis is generated through several mechanisms:

- Lactate from anaerobic metabolism due to lack of oxidative phosphorylation[28]
- Ketones due to inhibition of dehydrogenases in the Krebs cycle, leading to accumulation of acetyl CoA[29]
- Salicylic acid
- Proton shifts due to uncoupling of oxidative phosphorylation
- Sulfuric and phosphorous-containing acids due to effects of salicylate on renal function

In fact, salicylate can cause even more complex acid-base disorders. Patients with severe toxicity may have respiratory alkalosis, anion gap metabolic acidosis by the mechanisms noted previously, and hypochloremic metabolic alkalosis/contraction alkalosis from vomiting and/or osmotic diuresis.

TOXIC ALCOHOLS

Toxic alcohols are "toxic" because they have toxic metabolites. Methanol, ethylene glycol, and other "toxic" alcohols (eg, diethylene glycol, benzyl alcohol) cause metabolic acidosis because they are converted to carboxylic acids through successive metabolism by ADH and aldehyde dehydrogenase. These acids are unmeasured anions and thus cause an elevated anion gap. The formate metabolite of methanol is particularly toxic to the retina, and may cause blindness. The glycolate metabolite of ethylene glycol is responsible for metabolic acidosis, whereas the oxalate metabolite is responsible for nephrotoxicity. Blindness or renal failure may be clues to diagnosis in a patient who presents late after ingestion. As discussed previously, when evaluating a patient with an anion acidosis of unclear etiology, it is important to rule out the more common causes before pursuing toxic alcohols, unless the history or symptoms strongly suggest this etiology. When toxic alcohols are suspected, toxic alcohol concentrations should be obtained also. However, in most hospitals, these are "send-out" tests, and take several days for results to be available. Thus, in the absence of a clear history, decisions about therapy must be made based on collateral information, such as a serum ethanol concentration and serum osmolality, both of which should be obtained during the initial laboratory evaluation.

- Serum ethanol: ethanol is the preferred substrate for ADH, and if present, will prevent metabolism of other alcohols. Thus, if there is significant serum ethanol, an anion gap acidosis cannot have been due to a toxic alcohol, because the ethanol present would have precluded metabolism to the carboxylic acid metabolite that would generate an acidosis. The exception to this is if the patient ingested a toxic alcohol several hours before ingesting ethanol, but this scenario is exceedingly uncommon.
- Osm gap: The osm gap is the difference between the measured osmolality (commonly measured by freezing point depression), and the calculated osmolarity. It is unitless because of the unit differences in osmolality and osmolarity, although they are similar at low solute concentrations. The calculated osmolarity has traditionally been calculated using the formula:

$$Osm_{calc} = 2 \times (Na^+) + (glucose)/18 + BUN/2.8 + (ETOH)/4.6,$$

although a recent study found that it may be more accurate to use 4.25 as the denominator for ethanol.[30] The osm gap is useful to calculate, as long as one considers potential pitfalls. A normal osm gap ranges from −14 to 10.[31] Because of this, a "normal" osm gap cannot completely exclude toxic alcohol poisoning, because a potentially consequential concentration of methanol or ethylene glycol may still be present with an osm gap in this range (if an individual's osm gap had changed from −14 to +10, for example). In addition, as the alcohol is metabolized, the osm gap decreases as the anion gap increases. If toxic alcohols are only being considered in the differential diagnosis because of an elevated anion gap, it may be too late to find an osm gap that may initially have been present. In contrast, a mildly elevated osm gap does not necessarily mean that a patient is poisoned by a toxic alcohol. Patients with either alcoholic ketoacidosis or lactic acidosis may have osm gap elevations significantly above the normal range.[32,33] However, a markedly elevated osm gap (40–60 osms) is almost always a toxic alcohol.

SUMMARY

Understanding the interpretation of a patient's acid-base status can be invaluable in caring for poisoned patients. Obtaining a few critical tests, including serum chemistry, blood gas with lactate, urine or serum ketones, and occasionally serum osmolality, serum ethanol concentration, or urine electrolytes, pH and ammonia can markedly narrow the differential diagnosis and guide therapy. The acid-base status is closely tied to the underlying pathophysiology of many toxicologic processes, so understanding the acid-base status also means better understanding the disease.

ACKNOWLEDGMENTS

Special thanks to Dr Richard Sinert for his help with several of the tables in this article.

REFERENCES

1. Wrenn K. The delta (delta) gap: an approach to mixed acid-base disorders. Ann Emerg Med 1990;11:1310–3.
2. Doberer D, Funk GC, Kirchner K, et al. A critique of Stewart's approach: the chemical mechanism of dilutional acidosis. Intensive Care Med 2009;35:2173–80.
3. Luke RG, Galla JH. It is chloride depletion alkalosis, not contraction alkalosis. J Am Soc Nephrol 2012;23:204–7.
4. Doberer D, Funk GC. Reply to Gatz and Ring. Intensive Care Med 2009;35:2185–6.
5. Worthley LI. Strong ion difference: a new paradigm or new clothes for the acid-base emperor. Crit Care Resusc 1999;1:211–4.
6. Tenney SM, Miller RM. The respiratory and circulatory action of salicylate. Am J Med 1955;19:498–508.
7. Gaudreault P, Temple AR, Lovejoy FH Jr. The relative severity of acute versus chronic salicylate poisoning in children: a clinical comparison. Pediatrics 1982;70:566–9.
8. Mullen WH. Toxin-related noncardiogenic pulmonary edema. PCCSU article, American College of Chest Physicians. Available at: http://69.36.35.38/accp/pccsu/toxin-related-noncardiogenic-pulmonary-edema?page=0,3. Accessed July 27, 2013.
9. Takeda S, Eriksson LI, Yamamoto Y, et al. Opioid action on respiratory neuron activity of the isolated respiratory network in newborn rats. Anesthesiology 2001;95:740–9.
10. Hoffman JR, Schriger DL, Luo JS. The empiric use of naloxone in patients with altered mental status: a reappraisal. Ann Emerg Med 1991;20:246–52.
11. Elman I, D'Ambra MN, Krause S, et al. Ultrarapid opioid detoxification: effects on cardiopulmonary physiology, stress hormones, and clinical outcomes. Drug Alcohol Depend 2001;61:163–72.
12. Spivey WH. Flumazenil and seizures: analysis of 43 cases. Clin Ther 1992;14:292–305.
13. Orwoll ES. The milk-alkali syndrome: current concepts. Ann Intern Med 1982;97:242–8.
14. Beall DP, Scofield RH. Milk-alkali syndrome associated with calcium carbonate consumption. Medicine (Baltimore) 1995;74:89–96.
15. Isbrucker RA, Burdock GA. Risk and safety assessment on the consumption of licorice root (*Glycyrrhiza* sp.), its extract and powder as a food ingredient, with emphasis on the pharmacology and toxicology of glycyrrhizin. Regul Toxicol Pharmacol 2006;46:167–92.
16. Garella S, Chang BS, Kahn SI. Dilution acidosis and contraction alkalosis: review of a concept. Kidney Int 1975;8:279–83.
17. Lastnick G. Metabolic acidosis secondary to acetazolamide therapy—a possible hazardous side effect after prolonged use of acetazolamide in geriatric patients. A case report. Ariz Med 1975;32:19–21.

18. Maisey DN, Brown RD. Acetazolamide and symptomatic metabolic acidosis in mild renal failure. Br Med J 1981;283:1527–8.
19. Leaf DE, Goldfarb DS. Mechanisms of action of acetazolamide in the prophylaxis and treatment of acute mountain sickness. J Appl Physiol 2007;102:1313–22.
20. Carlisle EJ, Donnelly SM, Vasuvatkul S, et al. Glue-sniffing and distal renal tubular acidosis: sticking to the facts. J Am Soc Nephrol 1991;1:1019–27.
21. Soghoian S, Sinert R, Wiener SW, et al. Ethylene glycol toxicity presenting with non-anion gap metabolic acidosis. Basic Clin Pharmacol Toxicol 2009;104:22–6.
22. Bernal W, Donaldson N, Wyncoll D, et al. Blood lactate as an early predictor of outcome in paracetamol-induced acute liver failure: a cohort study. Lancet 2002;359:558–63.
23. Claret PG, Bobbia X, Boutin C, et al. Lactic acidosis as a complication of β-adrenergic aerosols. Am J Emerg Med 2012;30:1319.
24. Hoffman RS, Kirrane BM, Marcus SM. A descriptive study of an outbreak of clenbuterol-containing heroin. Ann Emerg Med 2008;52:548–53.
25. Protti A, Russo R, Tagliabue P, et al. Oxygen consumption is depressed in patients with lactic acidosis due to biguanide intoxication. Crit Care 2010;14:R22.
26. Radziuk J, Zhang Z, Wiernsperger N, et al. Effects of metformin on lactate uptake and gluconeogenesis in the perfused rat liver. Diabetes 1997;46:1406–13.
27. Fulop M, Hoberman HD. Alcoholic ketoacidosis. Diabetes 1975;24:785–90.
28. Krebs HG, Woods HG, Alberti KG. Hyperlactaetemia and lactic acidosis. Essays Med Biochem 1975;1:81–103.
29. Kaplan E, Kennedy J, David J. Effects of salicylate and other benzoates on oxidative enzymes of the tricarboxylic acid cycle in rat tissue homogenates. Arch Biochem Biophys 1954;51:47–61.
30. Carstairs SD, Suchard JR, Smith T, et al. Contribution of serum ethanol concentration to the osmol gap: a prospective volunteer study. Clin Toxicol (Phila) 2013;51(5):398–401.
31. Hoffman RS, Smilkstein MJ, Howland MA, et al. Osmol gaps revisited: normal values and limitations. J Toxicol Clin Toxicol 1993;31:81–93.
32. Almaghams AM, Yeung CK. Osmolal gap in alcoholic ketoacidosis. Clin Nephrol 1997;48:52.
33. Schelling JR, Howard RL, Winter SD, et al. Increased osmolal gap in alcoholic ketoacidosis and lactic acidosis. Ann Intern Med 1990;113:580–2.

An Approach to Chemotherapy-Associated Toxicity

Zhanna Livshits, MD[a],*, Rama B. Rao, MD[a], Silas W. Smith, MD[b]

KEYWORDS

- Adverse effects • Chemotherapy • Cancer • Extravasation • Toxicity

KEY POINTS

- Chemotherapy-induced adverse effects are common and may mimic common disease processes.
- Evaluation of infectious causes of symptoms is important in immunocompromised patients.
- Emergency medicine management of oral and parenteral chemotherapeutic toxicity entails excellent supportive care.
- Intrathecal medication errors may require emergent cerebrospinal fluid drainage.
- Extravasation of vesicants may require emergent administration of specific antidotes.

INTRODUCTION

Cancer is the leading cause of death worldwide and the second leading cause of death in the United States.[1] Approximately 13.7 million Americans with a cancer history were alive in January 1, 2012.[2] Given anticipated increases in cancer incidence and prevalence, the emergency medicine physician is likely to encounter patients receiving chemotherapeutic agents. The breadth of chemotherapeutic agents is vast, and adverse effects are, unfortunately, common. Given disease complexity, most patients receive multidrug regimens. Distinguishing disease pathology from the adverse chemotherapeutic effects remains challenging. Cessation of exposure is often necessary to manage severe toxicity.

Disclosure: The authors have no financial relationships to disclose.
[a] Weill Cornell Medical College, New York Presbyterian Hospital, 525 East 68th Street, New York, NY 10065, USA; [b] Department of Emergency Medicine, New York City Poison Control Center, Bellevue Hospital Center, NYU School of Medicine, 462 First Avenue, Room A-345A, New York, NY 10016, USA
* Corresponding author.
E-mail address: zhl9006@med.cornell.edu

Emerg Med Clin N Am 32 (2014) 167–203
http://dx.doi.org/10.1016/j.emc.2013.09.002
0733-8627/14/$ – see front matter © 2014 Elsevier Inc. All rights reserved.

CHEMOTHERAPEUTIC AGENT CLASSIFICATION

Table 1 lists common chemotherapeutic agents, their mechanisms of action, and commonly used antidotes.[3]

Given the rapid advances in cancer research and the evolving complexity of treatment regimens, it is challenging to provide a comprehensive treatment list for each malignancy. In the absence of definitive patient information, **Table 2** provides several

Table 1
Chemotherapeutic drugs

Class	Agents	Mechanism of Action	Antidotes
Alkylating agents	Busulfan Dacarbazine Nitrogen mustards 　Chlorambucil 　Cyclophosphamide 　Ifosfamide 　Mechlorethamine 　Melphalan Nitrosoureas 　Carmustine 　Lomustine 　Semustine[c] 　Streptozotocin Platinoids 　Cisplatin 　Carboplatin 　Iproplatin 　Oxaliplatin Procarbazine Temozolomide	DNA alkylation; formation of DNA crosslinks and adducts; inhibition of DNA synthesis	Mesna[a] 　Cyclophosphamide and ifosfamide-induced hemorrhagic cystitis Methylene blue[b] 　Ifosfamide-induced encephalopathy Thiosulfate[b] 　Nitrogen mustard skin extravasation Amifostine[a] 　Prevention of cisplatin-induced nephrotoxicity
Antimetabolites	Methotrexate Purine analogues 　Fludarabine 　Mercaptopurine 　Pentostatin 　Thioguanine Pyrimidine analogues 　Capecitabine 　Cytarabine 　5-Fluorouracil (5-FU) 　Gemcitabine	Methotrexate 　Inhibition of dihydrofolate reductase; inhibition of purine synthesis Purine/pyrimidine analogues 　Inhibition of DNA synthesis	Leucovorin[a] and levoleucovorin[a] 　Methotrexate toxicity/overdose Glucarpidase[a] 　Methotrexate toxicity/overdose Uridine triacetate (PN401)[b,d] 　5-Fluorouracil overdose
Antimitotics	Taxanes 　Docetaxel 　Paclitaxel Vinca alkaloids 　Vinblastine 　Vincristine 　Vindesine 　　(unavailable in United States) 　Vinorelbine	Taxanes 　Microtubule stabilization; disruption of microtubule polymerization/depolymerization Vinca alkaloids 　Inhibition of microtubule polymerization; microtubule destabilization	—

(continued on next page)

Table 1
(continued)

Class	Agents	Mechanism of Action	Antidotes

Antibiotics	Anthracyclines
	  Daunorubicin
	  Doxorubicin
	  Epirubicin
	  Idarubicin
	Dactinomycin
	Mitomycin C
	Mitoxantrone
	Bleomycin
	Plicamycin
	  (mithramycin)
		Anthracyclines
		  DNA intercalation;
		  free radical
		  formation
		Dactinomycin
		  DNA binding; RNA
		  synthesis inhibition
		Mitomycin C
		  DNA synthesis
		  inhibition
		Mitoxantrone
		  DNA intercalation;
		  topoisomerase II
		  inhibition
		Bleomycin
		  Inhibition of DNA
		  and RNA synthesis
		Plicamycin
		  Inhibition of RNA
		  transcription
			Dexrazoxane[a]
			  Anthracycline-
			  associated cardiac
			  toxicity and
			  extravasation

Monoclonal antibodies	L-asparaginase
	Alemtuzumab (CD52)
	Apolizumab
	Bevacizumab (VEGFR)
	Cetuximab (EGFR)
	Gemtuzumab (CD33)
	Ibritumomab (CD20)
	Panitumumab (EGFR)
	Rituximab (CD20)
	Tositumomab (CD20)
	Trastuzumab (HER2)
		Monoclonal
		  antibodies specific
		  for cell surface
		  markers
			—

Protein kinase inhibitors	Dasatinib (BCR/ABL, Src) Erlotinib (EGFR) Gefitinib (EGFR-TK) Imatinib Lapatinib (EGFR, HER2) Sorafenib Sunitinib	Protein kinase inhibition	—
Selective estrogen receptor modulators	Tamoxifen	Estrogen receptor antagonism	—

Topoisomerase inhibitors	Camptothecins
	  Irinotecan
	  Topotecan
	Epipodophyllotoxins
	  Etoposide
	  Teniposide
		Camptothecins
		  Topoisomerase I
		  inhibition
		Epipodophyllotoxin
		  Topoisomerase II
		  inhibition
			—

Abbreviations: CD20, B-lymphocyte antigen CD20; CD33, Siglec-3; CD52, cluster of differentiation 52; EGFR, epidermal growth factor receptor; EGFR-TK, epidermal growth factor receptor tirosine kinase; HER2, human epidermal growth factor receptor 2; Src, rous sarcoma oncogene cellular homolog; VEGFR, vascular endothelial growth factor receptor.

[a] Approved by the Food and Drug Administration for this indication.
[b] Not approved by the Food and Drug Administration for this indication.
[c] Withdrawn from marketing.
[d] Food and Drug Administration orphan drug designation.

Table 2
Selected adult chemotherapeutic regimens

Malignancy	Chemotherapeutic Drugs and Regimens
Acute lymphoblastic leukemia	Anthracycline, imatinib, ± L-asparaginase, mercaptopurine, prednisone, teniposide, vincristine
Acute myeloid leukemia	Cytarabine, daunorubicin, gemtuzumab, idarubicin, mercaptopurine, ± thioguanine
Bladder	CMV: cisplatin, methotrexate, vinblastine Intravesical: doxorubicin, mitomycin C, thiotepa MVAC: cisplatin, doxorubicin, methotrexate, vinblastine Systemic: docetaxel, gemcitabine, ifosfamide, paclitaxel
Brain	Carmustine, semustine, temozolomide
Breast	AC: cyclophosphamide, doxorubicin AC-T: cyclophosphamide, doxorubicin, taxane CAF: cyclophosphamide, doxorubicin, 5-FU CMF: cyclophosphamide, 5-FU, methotrexate FEC: cyclophosphamide, epirubicin, 5-FU Other agents: capecitabine, carboplatin, cisplatin, gemcitabine, mitomycin C, mitoxantrone, paclitaxel, vinblastine, vincristine, vinorelbine Receptor-specific therapy: lapatinib, tamoxifen, trastuzumab TAC: cyclophosphamide, docetaxel, doxorubicin TC: cyclophosphamide, docetaxel
Cervical	Cisplatin, 5-FU, gemcitabine, ifosfamide, irinotecan, paclitaxel, topotecan, vinorelbine
Chronic lymphocytic leukemia	CHOP: cyclophosphamide, doxorubicin, prednisone, vincristine CVP: cyclophosphamide, prednisone, vincristine Cyclophosphamide, fludarabine, pentostatin, rituximab
Chronic myelogenous leukemia	Busulfan, cytarabine, imatinib/dasatinib (Philadelphia-chromosome +), vincristine
Colorectal	Cetuximab, 5-FU, irinotecan, oxaliplatin, panitumumab
Endometrial	Cisplatin, doxorubicin, paclitaxel
Esophageal	Carboplatin, cisplatin, etoposide, 5-FU, paclitaxel, vinblastine
Gallbladder	Cisplatin, docetaxel, gemcitabine
Gastric	Capecitabine, cisplatin, docetaxel, epirubicin, 5-FU, mitomycin C, oxaliplatin
Hepatocellular	Sorafenib
Laryngeal	Cisplatin, 5-FU
Lung (non–small cell)	Bevacizumab, carboplatin, cetuximab, cisplatin, docetaxel, erlotinib, etoposide, gefitinib, gemcitabine, irinotecan, paclitaxel, vinorelbine
Lung (small cell)	Cyclophosphamide, doxorubicin, etoposide, gemcitabine, ifosfamide, irinotecan, paclitaxel, platinoids (carboplatin, cisplatin, oxaliplatin), topotecan, vincristine, vinorelbine
Lymphoma (Hodgkin)	ABVD: bleomycin, dacarbazine, doxorubicin, vinblastine BEACOPP: bleomycin, cyclophosphamide, doxorubicin, etoposide, prednisone, procarbazine, vincristine MOPP: mechlorethamine, prednisone, procarbazine, vincristine

(continued on next page)

Table 2 *(continued)*	
Malignancy	**Chemotherapeutic Drugs and Regimens**
Lymphoma (non-Hodgkin)	C-MOPP: cyclophosphamide, doxorubicin, prednisone, procarbazine, vincristine Chlorambucil, cyclophosphamide, fludarabine, ibritumomab, rituximab, tositumomab CHOP: cyclophosphamide, doxorubicin, prednisone, vincristine CVP: cyclophosphamide, prednisone, vincristine FND: dexamethasone, fludarabine, mitoxantrone R-CHOP: CHOP, rituximab
Lymphoma (CNS)	Carmustine, cyclophosphamide, cytarabine, doxorubicin, methotrexate, methylprednisolone/dexamethasone, procarbazine, teniposide, vincristine
Malignant mesothelioma	Carboplatin, cisplatin, cyclophosphamide, doxorubicin, epirubicin, ifosfamide, mitomycin C
Melanoma	Carmustine, dacarbazine, lomustine, temozolomide
Polycythemia vera	Busulfan, chlorambucil
Ovarian epithelial	Cyclophosphamide, doxorubicin, gemcitabine, paclitaxel, platinoids (carboplatin, cisplatin, oxaliplatin)
Ovarian germ cell tumors	BEP: bleomycin, cisplatin, etoposide PVB: bleomycin, cisplatin, vinblastine VAC: cyclophosphamide, dactinomycin, vincristine
Pancreatic	Capecitabine, cisplatin, erlotinib, 5-FU, gemcitabine, mitomycin C, oxaliplatin
Penile	Bleomycin, cisplatin, 5-FU, methotrexate, vincristine
Renal cell	Bevacizumab, sorafenib, sunitinib
Testicular (seminoma)	BEP: bleomycin, etoposide, cisplatin EP: etoposide, cisplatin
Testicular (nonseminomas)	BEP: bleomycin, cisplatin, etoposide EP: cisplatin, etoposide PVB: cisplatin, bleomycin, vinblastine VAB VI: bleomycine, cisplatin, cyclophosphamide, dactinomycin, vinblastine VIP: cisplatin, etoposide, ifosfamide VPV: cisplatin, etoposide, vinblastine
Vaginal	Bleomycin, cisplatin, 5-FU, mitomycin C, vincristine
Vulvar	Bleomycin, cisplatin, 5-FU, mitomycin C

Abbreviations: CNS, central nervous system; 5-FU, 5-fluorouracil.
Some chemotherapeutic regimens in this table may be used off-label.

common chemotherapeutic regimens.[4] These regimens are continually evolving, and their application may vary.

CHEMOTHERAPEUTIC EMERGENCIES
Neurologic Emergencies

Chemotherapeutic agents cause both central and peripheral neurotoxicity. The diagnosis of central neurotoxicity is challenging because it may clinically mimic cancer burden or central nervous system (CNS) infection. Toxicity manifests as encephalopathy with or without seizures, cerebellar syndrome, posterior and multifocal leukocencephalopathies, psychosis, and cranial nerve (CN) palsies. A change in mental status may be due to nonconvulsive status epilepticus and is seen with ifosfamide and cisplatin.[22,23] Encephalopathy occurs most commonly with ifosfamide and typically resolves several days following cessation of therapy. Vincristine is a potent neurotoxin and leads to a variety of neurologic symptoms from encephalopathy and focal CN palsies to peripheral neuropathy. Other neurologic complications may be due to the route of drug administration. The intrathecal (IT) section provides additional information.

Peripheral neuropathy is often a debilitating condition with limited treatment options and potential for irreversible damage. Peripheral neuropathies are typically sensorimotor and most frequently associated with axonal degeneration. Vincristine, paclitaxel, cisplatin, and oxaliplatin are frequently implicated in development of peripheral neuropathy. **Table 3** summarizes commonly encountered neurotoxic effects of respective chemotherapeutic agents.[16]

Clinical evaluation

Altered mental status, hallucinations, psychosis, seizures, and coma may be clinical signs of encephalopathy. A persistent change in mental status may reflect nonconvulsive status epilepticus. CN palsies and hemiparesis may be evident on physical examination. Acute cerebellar syndrome with ataxia may be marked with gait instability and vertigo with clinically abnormal cerebellar examination and gait. Reversible posterior leukoencephalopathy syndrome is characterized by headache, altered mental status, seizures, and visual loss. Progressive multifocal neuro-encephalopathy manifests with altered mental status, changes in vision and speech, motor weakness and paralysis, and cognitive deterioration.

Peripheral neuropathy is often a clinical diagnosis. Symptoms of small-fiber neuropathy include burning pain and loss of pain and temperature sensation. Large-fiber neuropathy may present with muscle weakness and loss of proprioception and reflexes.

Diagnostic evaluation

The following laboratory studies and diagnostics may be helpful in the assessment of patients with chemotherapy-induced neurotoxicity:

- Finger stick glucose in patients with altered mental status to evaluate for hypoglycemia
- Serum electrolytes
- Complete blood count (CBC): evaluation of neutropenia, leukocytosis
- Prothrombin time (PT)/international normalized ratio (INR), partial thromboplastin time (PTT): if considering performing lumbar puncture (LP)
- Computed tomography (CT) brain without contrast: initial diagnostic tool to exclude hemorrhage and brain mass as causes of neurologic symptoms
- LP: consider as a part of infectious workup in immunocompromised patients with altered mental status
- Electroencephalogram: evaluation of nonconvulsive status epilepticus in persistently altered patients
- Magnetic resonance imaging (MRI): a sensitive modality for evaluation of leukoencephalopathy, nonemergent
- Electromyography and nerve conduction studies: nonemergent

Management

The management of chemotherapy-induced neurologic toxicity remains supportive following the exclusion of infectious causes. Methylene blue has been used in the

Table 3
Chemotherapeutic neurotoxins

Toxicity	Drug
Acute cerebellar syndrome with ataxia	Cytarabine 5-FU
Cerebrovascular accident, transient ischemic attack	Bevacizumab[5] Cisplatin Erlotinib[6]
CNS hemorrhage	L-asparaginase[7] Bevacizumab[5]
Cranial nerve palsy	Ifosfamide[8] Paclitaxel[9] Vincristine[10]
Encephalopathy	Cisplatin Fludarabine 5-FU Ifosfamide[8] Methotrexate[11] Pentostatin Vincristine[10]
Hemiparesis	Methotrexate[11]
Occipital encephalopathy	Cisplatin Cytarabine Fludarabine
Parkinson-like syndrome	L-asparaginase[7]
Peripheral mixed sensorimotor neuropathy	Fludarabine Vincristine[10] Vinorelbine[12] Taxanes
Peripheral sensory neuropathy[9,13]	Carboplatin[14] Cisplatin[15] Oxaliplatin Paclitaxel
Peripheral neuropathy with autonomic instability[9]	Cisplatin Paclitaxel Vincristine[10]
Progressive multifocal neuro-encephalopathy	Capecitabine Fludarabine Rituximab[17]
Reversible posterior leukoencephalopathy syndrome	Bevacizumab[5] Cisplatin Cytarabine Gemcitabine[18] Sorafenib Sunitinib[19]
Sagittal sinus thrombosis	L-asparaginase[7]
Seizures	Busulfan[20] Chlorambucil Encephalopathy agents Procarbazine Temozolomide Vinblastine[21]

Abbreviations: CNS, central nervous system; 5-FU, 5-fluorouracil.

management of ifosfamide-induced encephalopathy but is not recommended as a part of emergency department management.

Antidote considerations: Methylene blue

Methylene blue currently does not have approval by the Food and Drug Administration (FDA) for use in ifosfamide-induced encephalopathy and, at this time, cannot be recommended as a part of the emergency department management of ifosfamide-induced encephalopathy. Methylene blue modulates ifosfamide neurotoxicity via different mechanisms.[24,25] It inhibits monoamine oxidase (MAO), preventing generation of the neurotoxic chloroacetaldehyde metabolite. It promotes oxidation of NADH to NAD^+ and, thus, stimulates ifosfamide metabolism and hepatic gluconeogenesis. Methylene blue modulates electron transfer flavoproteins in the mitochondria, restoring oxidative phosphorylation and efficient energy utilization. Methylene blue 1% solution is administered intravenously with an initial dose of 50 mg in adults and a variable daily schedule.[24] Although some studies have demonstrated a decrease in the duration of symptoms, others failed to show a benefit. A transient decrease in numerical oxygen saturation value via pulse oximeter may be seen because of the blue discoloration of the methylene blue. Hemolysis may be seen in neonates or patients with G6PD deficiency.

Intrathecal (IT) Emergencies

Patients may present to the emergency department because of errors in IT medication administration associated with chemotherapy. The term *intrathecal* refers to the space enclosing the cerebrospinal fluid (CSF). Medications may be intentionally placed into the CSF for therapeutic or diagnostic purposes. Examples include IT administration of baclofen via an indwelling catheter or direct administration of antibiotics or chemotherapeutic agents via lumbar puncture. Errors involving the IT space are potentially life threatening because this area can affect the nervous system directly. The routes of IT access are listed in **Boxes 1** and **2**. Scenarios may include administration of the wrong agent or wrong route, dosage errors caused by miscalculation, or, in some cases, errors relating to pumps.

Wrong agent or wrong route

Agents that are therapeutic when administered intravenously may produce acute toxicity or present altered toxicity profiles when delivered IT. Typically, agents that are ionic or hyperosmolar injure the CNS, often in a neuroanatomical distribution. For example, there are several high osmolar radiocontrast agents intended for intravenous (IV) use only. High osmolar radiocontrast agents administered IT via LP may precipitate a progression of symptoms termed *ascending tonic clonic syndrome*, reflecting contrast effects as it moves cephalad. If high osmolar contrast is administered into the ventricles of the brain via an Ommaya reservoir, or during an operative

---

Box 1
Routes of IT access

Lumbar Puncture

Indwelling device

  Spinal catheter

  Ommaya reservoir

Surgical exposure in operating room

Box 2
Management of IT emergencies
If possible, elevate head
Consider CSF drainage[a]
Consult the Poison Control Center (1-800-POISONS)
Consult neurosurgery
ᵃ Institute life-saving measures (intubation and paralysis) as needed.

procedure requiring neuroimaging, the clinical presentation may skip the ascending neurologic signs and symptoms seen with lumbar administration (see radiocontrast agents later).[55] Agents such as methotrexate (MTX) may produce a chemical arachnoiditis, even when administered IT with therapeutic intent.

The timing of toxicity onset may depend on the dose and nature of the agent administered. For example, vincristine is intended for IV administration only. It is commonly administered in a chemotherapeutic regimen that also includes IT MTX. Multiple reports document syringe confusion when the treatments are scheduled concurrently. Vincristine toxicity in the CNS may take hours to days to present, often in a neuroanatomical fashion, and may begin with paresthesias and paralysis, ultimately progressing to coma and death.[56] Inadvertent IT vincristine is almost universally fatal despite a benign patient appearance immediately after administration. Another example is local anesthetics intended for the epidural space with inadvertent penetration of the dura. CNS toxicity may manifest as numbness, weakness, or seizures. Patients receiving such treatments in outpatient facilities may present to the emergency department requiring emergent interventions.

Intrathecal dosage errors and pumps
Dosage miscalculations of medications can result in CNS toxicity in a manner that is sometimes paradoxic to the effects noted in IV overdose. An example is IT morphine toxicity. Morphine administered IV has a predictable dose-dependent effect of sedation, miosis, and respiratory depression. An IT overdose of morphine may cause neuroexcitation,[57] which may happen during refilling errors of subcutaneous pumps that deliver IT morphine through a surgically placed tunneled IT catheter. The pump contains a reservoir with an access port for refilling. Medication is pumped in small increments via the catheter into the IT space. The pump also has a second access port contiguous with the catheter and the IT space. Refilling the pump reservoir requires a template and proper training, because access sites are palpated rather than directly visualized. If the wrong port is identified, several weeks of IT morphine may enter the CSF as a bolus and cause profound hypertension and seizures.[57]

Sometimes external pumps are used to administer medication IT. An example is baclofen. If the pump empties, malfunctions, or there is a loss of continuity, there may be an abrupt cessation of medication, which may result in withdrawal. Patients administered baclofen by this route for the treatment of spasticity have sometimes suffered life-threatening autonomic instability and seizures with pump malfunction.[58–60]

Most common intrathecal scenarios
The Emergency Medicine practitioner may encounter patients from a radiology suite who were given the wrong IT contrast agent for neuroimaging. Confusion in drug administration is complicated by the multiple names and numbers of contrast agents

that do not reflect the osmolarity of the agent. Unfortunately, many radiocontrast dyes that are benign when given IV are hyperosmolar and/or ionic agents and potentially fatal when given IT. This ascending tonic clonic syndrome consists of paresthesias, weakness, and a severe form of myoclonus and muscle spasm that results in rhabdomyolysis, hyperthermia, and contractions severe enough to fracture bones.[55,61]

Management of intrathecal emergencies

There may be IT administration of agents for which there is no prior experience. The presumption should be that the agent is potentially fatal, and timely removal of the CSF is warranted. There is no predictable model for knowing how much medication can be removed after IT drug administration because each drug has unique properties affecting CSF movement. IT drugs administered simultaneously may have different percentages of drug recovery when the CSF is subsequently drained. The only common factor is that the sooner the CSF removal, the more likely the toxic effect is blunted. This point is especially true for an agent such as vincristine in which time to drainage affects survivability. The only documented survivors of erroneous IT vincristine administration had immediate recognition of the error before withdrawal of the lumbar needle and prompt CSF drainage. Even in these cases, the neurologic injuries were devastating.[56,61] For EM physicians attending to patients with a wrong drug error for CSF, a lumbar needle or catheter, if not already in place, should be accessed. CSF can be drained passively in 10 mL to 20 mL aliquots with interval instillation of *preservative-free* isotonic fluid equivalent to the aliquot removed. This procedure can be performed repeatedly while other providers investigate if there is any experience with the exposure in the literature.

On very rare occasions, a neurosurgeon will perform a washout with the placement of an IT catheter either in the ventricles or along the spine for infusion of preservative-free isotonic fluid. This catheter is paired with another more distal IT catheter for CSF drainage. This method has been used for life-threatening chemotherapeutic errors.[56]

In general, antidotes commonly used for IV or oral overdoses should be *avoided* IT because such antidotes may be dangerous or even fatal in the CSF. A single exception is carboxypeptidase G_2, which can cleave MTX in cases of inadvertent IT MTX overdose. Although carboxypeptidase G_2 is FDA approved for IV use only, experience with IT dosing has been well tolerated and efficacious in the setting of IT MTX overdose.[62] Note that, however, MTX's other antidote, leucovorin, is *contraindicated* by the IT route.

Cardiovascular Emergencies

Anthracyclines, especially doxorubicin, cause cardiac toxicity in the acute, subacute, and chronic setting. The generation of hydroxyl radicals leading to DNA disruption and myocyte death is thought to underlie cardiotoxicity.[63] Dysrhythmias, ischemic electrocardiographic (ECG) changes, congestive heart failure (CHF), left ventricular dysfunction, pericarditis, myocarditis, and sudden death have been reported within 24 hours of administration. Subacute toxicity is seen within a few weeks, clinically appears as myocarditis with diastolic dysfunction, and is associated with 60% mortality.[64,65] Chronic toxicity clinically manifests as CHF, left ventricular dysfunction, and dilated cardiomyopathy, with symptoms as early as one month to 10 to 30 years following anthracycline therapy.[63,65–67] A cumulative dose is the most important risk factor for chronic toxicity.[63,65,66] Mitoxantrone may be associated with dose-dependent cardiac effects similar to anthracyclines. Trastuzumab, an HER2-targeted monoclonal antibody, also carries significant CHF risk. In contrast to anthracyclines, cardiac dysfunction is typically reversible.[63,66] High-dose cyclophosphamide and 5-fluorouracil (5-FU) may also cause significant cardiac toxicity manifested by dysrhythmias, CHF, and hemorrhagic pericarditis.[63,65] **Table 4** contains a comprehensive list of chemotherapeutic cardiac toxins and their respective clinical effects.[63–67]

Clinical evaluation

The evaluation of chemotherapy-induced cardiac toxicity is fraught with challenges. A physician should maintain a broad differential diagnosis and exclude common causes of cardiac symptoms. CHF resulting from left ventricular dysfunction manifests with symptoms of shortness of breath, orthopnea, and signs of pulmonary edema on auscultation. Hypoxia and severe respiratory distress may be seen clinically with significant pulmonary edema. Cardiac ischemia and pericarditis typically present with chest pain or referred cardiac pain. Pericarditis symptoms often improve with sitting forward and worsen with the supine position. Pericardial effusion may be asymptomatic or may lead to significant hemodynamic compromise caused by cardiac tamponade. Thromboembolic complications may affect any vascular system and result in strokes, myocardial infarction, pulmonary embolism, and vascular compromise of extremities. The clinical evaluation of myocarditis may be challenging. Symptoms are often vague, with the presence or absence of chest pain, generalized weakness, signs of hemodynamic instability, and pulmonary edema with advanced disease. Dysrhythmia may manifest as syncope, transient lightheadedness, weakness or frank cardiac arrest from a nonperfused rhythm. Capillary leak syndrome, described following gemcitabine administration, may clinically appear similarly to CHF with peripheral and pulmonary edema.

Diagnostic evaluation

The following laboratory studies and diagnostics are recommended for the assessment of patients with chemotherapy-induced cardiac toxicity:

- ECG
- Cardiac monitor
- Chest radiograph (CXR)
- Brain natriuretic peptide
- Cardiac troponin
- Liver function testing (LFTs): hypoalbuminemia may be seen with capillary leak syndrome
- Serum electrolytes to exclude correctable causes of dysrhythmia
- Bedside cardiac ultrasound: evaluation of pericardial effusion or tamponade

Management

Patients who develop anthracycline-associated cardiotoxicity should avoid further anthracycline exposure. The emergency department management of cardiovascular toxicity (ischemia, CHF, dysrhythmia, pericarditis, tamponade, and thromboembolic events) is similar to the management from cardiogenic and vascular causes. Capillary leak syndrome may be managed with volume repletion if hypotension is present, vasopressor therapy, albumin repletion, diuresis, and steroids.[78] Patients with advanced CHF may require inotropic support. Patients receiving anthracycline chemotherapy may also receive dexrazoxane. This decision is made by the oncology team and is typically not a part of emergent management.

Antidotal considerations: Dexrazoxane

Dexrazoxane inhibits doxorubicin-induced generation of hydroxyl radicals.[66] The coadministration of dexrazoxane in patients receiving doxorubicin chemotherapy demonstrated statistically lower incidence of anthracycline-associated CHF and left

Table 4
Chemotherapeutic cardiovascular toxins

Toxicity	Drug
Capillary leak syndrome: increase in endothelial permeability	Gemcitabine[78]
Cardiac ischemia	Bevacizumab[5] Capecitabine Cisplatin Dasatinib[39] Docetaxel Erlotinib[6] Fludarabine 5-FU Paclitaxel Rituximab Sorafenib[68] Vinblastine Vincristine
CHF and left ventricular dysfunction	Anthracyclines (daunorubicin, doxorubicin, epirubicin, idarubicin)[28,41,43,45] Cisplatin Cyclophosphamide (high dose)[71,72] Cytarabine Dasatinib[39] Docetaxel Ifosfamide Imatinib[30] Lapatinib[74] Mitomycin C[70] Mitoxantrone[69] Paclitaxel Pentostatin Sorafenib Sunitinib[19] Trastuzumab[73]
Dysrhythmia	Capecitabine Cisplatin Cyclophosphamide (high dose) Daunorubicin Docetaxel Doxorubicin Epirubicin Fludarabine 5-FU Idarubicin Ifosfamide Mitoxantrone Paclitaxel[75] Pentostatin Rituximab
Hypertension	Bevacizumab[5] Cisplatin Etoposide[47] Sorafenib[68] Sunitinib[19] Vinblastine Vincristine Vinorelbine

(continued on next page)

Table 4 (continued)	
Toxicity	**Drug**
Hypotension	Carmustine (rate related)
	Etoposide[47]
	Fludarabine
	MTX[11]
	Paclitaxel
	Procarbazine[42]
Myocardial necrosis	Cyclophosphamide[71]
Myocarditis	Cyclophosphamide[71]
Pericardial fibrosis	Bleomycin
Pericarditis and pericardial effusion	Bleomycin
	Busulfan
	Cyclophosphamide[71]
	Cytarabine
	Dasatinib
	Imatinib[30]
	MTX[11]
	Pentostatin
QT prolongation	Dasatinib[39]
	Lapatinib[74]
	Sorafenib[68]
	Sunitinib[19]
Sudden cardiac death	Cetuximab[76]
Thromboembolic complications	Bevacizumab[5]
	Cisplatin[63]
	Erlotinib
	Gemicitabine[18]
	Irinotecan
	L-asparaginase[7]
	MTX[11]
	Sunitinib[19]
	Tamoxifen[77]

Abbreviations: CHF, congestive heart failure; MTX, methotrexate.

ventricular dysfunction.[79–81] According to the American Society of Clinical Oncology, dexrazoxane may be recommended in patients who received more than 300 mg/m^2 doxorubicin and may benefit from continued doxorubicin therapy.[82,83]

Hematopoietic Emergencies

Most chemotherapeutic agents are associated with transient bone marrow suppression. **Box 3** contains a comprehensive list of agents that lead to significant myelosuppression. A decrease in the bone marrow cell lines may have the potential for serious complications as well as early cessation of chemotherapy. **Box 3** outlines agents most commonly associated with myelosuppression.

Neutropenia is one of the most significant dose-limiting complications of chemotherapy, especially seen with docetaxel and paclitaxel. Granulocytopenia is a dose-limiting reaction of vinorelbine administration. Leukopenia is frequently seen with MTX, mitomycin C, mitoxantrone, dacarbazine, trastuzumab, and dose-dependent cyclophosphamide therapy. Hemolytic anemia has been described following procarbazine and fludarabine therapy.

Box 3
Agents most commonly associated with bone marrow suppression

Alemtuzumab[26]	Gemtuzumab
Busulfan[20]	Ibritumomab[27]
Capecitabine[29]	Idarubicin[28]
Carboplatin[14]	Ifosfamide[8]
Carmustine[31]	Imatinib[30]
Chlorambucil	Irinotecan[32]
Cisplatin[15]	Lomustine[33]
Cytarabine[34]	Mechlorethamine
Dacarbazine[36]	Melphalan[35]
Dactinomycin[38]	Mercaptopurine[37]
Dasatinib[39]	Methotrexate[11]
Daunorubicin[41]	Oxaliplatin
Docetaxel	Paclitaxel
Doxorubicin[43]	Pentostatin[40]
Epirubicin[45]	Procarbazine[42]
Etoposide[47]	Rituximab
Fludarabine[49]	Streptozotocin[44]
5-fluorouracil[51]	Temozolomide[46]
Gemcitabine[53]	Teniposide[48]
	Thioguanine[50]
	Topotecan[52]
	Tositumomab[54]
	Vinblastine[21]
	Vinorelbine

Thrombocytopenia is noted with bone marrow suppression and thrombotic angiopathy. Thrombotic thrombocytopenic purpura (TTP) and hemolytic uremic syndrome (HUS) are manifestations of thrombotic angiopathy. TTP is a pentad of microangiopathic hemolytic anemia (MAHA), thrombocytopenia, fever, neurologic abnormalities, and renal injury. HUS shares features of MAHA and thrombocytopenia without neurologic abnormalities. Mitomycin C and gemcitabine are the most commonly implicated agents in HUS.[53,70] The following chemotherapeutic agents are also associated with thrombotic angiopathy: daunorubicin, bleomycin, carboplatin, cisplatin, tamoxifen, as well as targeted therapy with alemtuzumab, bevacizumab, erlotinib, sunitinib, and imatinib.[6,84–86] Alemtuzumab therapy has been associated with severe hemolytic anemia. Coagulopathy and subsequent bleeding is described with L-asparaginase therapy because of depression of clotting factors.[7] Bleeding has also been noted with dasatinib therapy due to both thrombocytopenia and platelet dysfunction.[39]

Clinical manifestations

Clinical manifestations of bone marrow suppression may be challenging to distinguish from those of cancer burden. Neutropenia and leukopenia may lead to local or disseminated infection given severe immunocompromised state. Anemia typically manifests with a variety of symptoms depending on the degree and the organ affected. Clinical symptoms include generalized weakness, exercise intolerance, shortness of breath, and pallor. Severe anemia and subsequent lack of oxygen delivery may result in end-organ ischemia. Thrombocytopenia may be asymptomatic or may manifest with petechiae, ecchymosis, purpura, and may result in life-threatening bleeding. Thrombotic microangiopathy presents as a constellation of symptoms, including hemolysis, thrombocytopenia, and impaired neurologic or renal function. Symptoms of hemolytic anemia vary depending on severity of hemolysis and include generalized weakness, pallor, abdominal pain, and altered mental status. TTP is associated with hemolysis and signs of thrombocytopenia. Other symptoms such as nausea, vomiting, abdominal pain, malaise, joint pain, and myalgia have been described. HUS is often seen in children and is associated with petechiae and purpura of the lower extremities and renal compromise.

Diagnostic evaluation

The following laboratory studies and diagnostics may be helpful in the assessment of patients with chemotherapy-induced hematologic toxicity:

- CBC with differential and platelets
- Peripheral blood smear: evaluate for presence of schistocytes seen with hemolysis, disseminated intravascular coagulation
- PT/INR, PTT fibrinogen
- LFTs: elevated indirect bilirubin with hemolysis
- Lactate dehydrogenase (LDH): elevated during hemolysis
- Serum haptoglobin: decreased during hemolysis
- Direct Coombs assay: exclusion of immunologic cause of hemolysis

Management

The management of neutropenia and leukopenia is supportive. Recombinant hematopoietic growth factors, such as granulocyte colony-stimulating factor or granulocyte-macrophage colony-stimulating factor (GM-CSF), may be used to stimulate the production of bone marrow cell lineages.[87,88] The treatment of anemia and thrombocytopenia is supportive. Symptomatic patients may require transfusion of blood products. Coagulopathy is treated with factor repletion. The management of thrombotic microangiopathy depends on the severity of hemolysis and thrombocytopenia. Platelet transfusion may be necessary for patients with severe thrombocytopenia or major bleeding. Consultation with a hematology specialist is recommended in cases of severe hemolysis and a potential need for plasma exchange.[85] Febrile neutropenic patients should have rapid assessment for a source of infection and empiric antibiotic coverage to prevent overwhelming sepsis.

Ophthalmologic Emergencies

Chemotherapy-induced ocular toxicity may range from self-resolving conjunctivitis to loss of vision. **Table 5** lists common chemotherapeutic ocular toxins and their respective toxicity.[89,90]

Clinical evaluation

Symptoms may range from blurry vision to ocular pain and loss of vision. Patients with ocular complaints necessitate a thorough eye examination that entails the documentation of visual acuity, slit lamp examination, and fluorescein staining. Ocular pressure determination is important if there is clinical concern for glaucoma.

Diagnostic evaluation

Although MRI may be useful in the evaluation of the optic nerve, it is often beyond the scope of an emergency department evaluation.

Management

The management is typically supportive. Ophthalmology follow-up is important for patients with chemotherapy-induced ocular toxicity.

Table 5	
Chemotherapeutic ocular toxins	
Toxicity	**Drug**
Conjunctivitis	Busulfan
	Cetuximab
	Cyclophosphamide
	Cytarabine
	Doxorubicin
	5-FU
	Ifosfamide
	Imatinib
	MTX[11]
Corneal perforation	Erlotinib[6]
Corneal ulceration	Erlotinib[6]
Cortical blindness	Carboplatin
	Cisplatin[15]
	Etoposide
	Vincristine
Glaucoma	Carmustine
Keratitis	Busulfan
	Chlorambucil
	Cyclophosphamide
	Cytarabine
	5-FU
Keratoconjunctivitis sicca	Busulfan
	Cyclophosphamide
Ocular CN palsy	Vincristine
Optic atrophy	Lomustine
	Vincristine
Optic neuritis	Carboplatin
	Carmustine
	Cisplatin[15]
	Etoposide
	Oxaliplatin
	Paclitaxel
Optic neuropathy	Cytarabine
	5-FU
	MTX (IT)
	Paclitaxel
	Vincristine
Papilledema	Chlorambucil
	Cisplatin[15]
	Procarbazine[42]
Retinal hemorrhage	Carmustine
	Chlorambucil
	Procarbazine[42]

Otolaryngologic Emergencies

Ototoxicity is a recognized complication of cisplatin and carboplatin chemotherapy.[14,15,91,92] Both agents are associated with sensorineural bilateral high-frequency hearing loss and eventually low-frequency hearing loss with cumulative dose.[93] Ototoxicity is consequential in both adults and children and may affect language development in children. CN VIII dysfunction may occur following vincristine chemotherapy. Jaw osteonecrosis has been reported with sunitinib therapy.[19]

Clinical evaluation
Changes in hearing are seen in patients with ototoxicity. Patients with CN VIII dysfunction may have vertigo. Jaw osteonecrosis typically presents with pain at the affected site.

Diagnostic evaluation
Patients with clinical signs of ototoxicity, such as tinnitus, decreased hearing, and impaired balance, should be referred for audiologic testing. CT imaging may be necessary for the diagnosis of jaw osteonecrosis.

Management
Although there are several trials evaluating the role of antioxidants for otoprotection during chemotherapy, the treatment of hearing loss remains supportive. Therapy for jaw osteonecrosis may require multidisciplinary involvement.

Pulmonary Emergencies

Chemotherapy-induced pulmonary toxicity may be challenging to diagnose given its rare occurrence (<10%) and propensity to mimic infection or metastatic lung disease. It may present a diagnostic challenge with a normal appearance of CXR for days despite the presence of clinical symptoms. Bleomycin is the most well-studied chemotherapeutic pulmonary toxin.[94,95] Chemotherapy-induced pulmonary toxicity may manifest as a hypersensitivity reaction, interstitial pneumonitis, noncardiogenic pulmonary edema, pleural effusions, nodular changes, and bronchiolitis obliterans and organizing pneumonitis (BOOP), and progressive pulmonary fibrosis. High mortality rates are reported following therapy with busulfan, chlorambucil, and melphalan. Nitrosourea therapy is associated with delayed onset of pulmonary fibrosis, noted 17 years following treatment for pediatric intracranial tumors.[96] **Table 6** contain a comprehensive list of pulmonary toxins and their respective clinical effects.[99,100]

Clinical evaluation
Hypersensitivity pneumonitis typically manifests with bronchospasm and may entail other hypersensitivity symptoms, such as urticaria. Interstitial pneumonitis and pulmonary fibrosis are both associated with progressively worsening dyspnea and cough. Low-grade fever is common in patients with interstitial pneumonitis and may confuse the clinical picture in immunocompromised patients. The presence of hypoxia depends on the degree of pulmonary involvement. Pulmonary embolism (PE) and infection may present similarly and must be considered in the differential diagnosis of oncological patients with respiratory complaints.

Diagnostic evaluation
The following diagnostics are recommended for the assessment of chemotherapy-induced pulmonary toxicity:

- CXR
  - Interstitial pneumonitis: interstitial and alveolar infiltrates
  - Pulmonary fibrosis: initial lack of radiographic findings; bibasilar interstitial markings, ground-glass reticular pattern
- CT chest: may be more sensitive in early detection of disease; protocol for evaluation of PE when diagnosis is entertained
- Pulmonary function tests: typically demonstrate restrictive pattern with decreased lung volumes in pulmonary fibrosis

Table 6
Chemotherapeutic pulmonary toxins

Toxicity	Drug
BOOP	Bleomycin
	Cetuximab
	Chlorambucil
	Cyclophosphamide
	MTX
	Mitomycin C
Bronchospasm	Pentostatin[40]
	Vincristine[10]
Hemoptysis	Bevacizumab[5]
Hypersensitivity pneumonitis	Cetuximab
	Fludarabine[49]
	MTX
	Paclitaxel (Cremophor-EL)
	Vinblastine
Interstitial pneumonitis	Bleomycin
	Carmustine
	Cetuximab
	Chlorambucil
	Cyclophosphamide
	Dactinomycin[38]
	Docetaxel
	Erlotinib[6]
	Etoposide
	Gefitinib[97]
	Gemcitabine
	Gemtuzumab[98]
	Irinotecan[32]
	Lapatinib[74]
	Mitomycin C
	Mitoxantrone[69]
	MTX[11]
	Paclitaxel
	Panitumumab
	Procarbazine[42]
	Topotecan[52]
	Vinorelbine[12]
Noncardiogenic pulmonary edema	Cytarabine
	Dasatinib (volume retention)
	Docetaxel
	Erlotinib (volume retention)[6]
	Gemcitabine
	Gemtuzumab[98]
	Imatinib (volume retention)[30]
Pleural effusions	Dasatinib[39]
	Docetaxel
	Imatinib[30]
	MTX
	Palcitaxel
	Procarbazine[42]
Pulmonary arterial hypertension	Dasatinib[39]

(continued on next page)

Table 6 (continued)	
Toxicity	**Drug**
Pulmonary fibrosis	Azathioprine
	Bleomycin
	Busulfan
	Carmustine[31]
	Chlorambucil
	Cyclophosphamide
	Erlotinib
	Fludarabine
	Gefitinib
	Ifosfamide
	Lomustine
	Melphalan
	Mercaptopurine
	Mitomycin C
	MTX
	Oxaliplatin
	Panitumumab
	Procarbazine

- Bronchoscopy and biopsy: may be necessary for definitive diagnosis and exclusion of underlying infection or metastatic disease; emergent if patients present with hemoptysis

Management

The mainstay of management is the removal of the offending agent, institution of steroid therapy, and supportive care. Patients who present with cough, dyspnea, fever, and evidence of hypoxia following chemotherapy are at risk for the development of acute respiratory distress syndrome (ARDS). Empiric antibiotics with pulmonary coverage should be initiated in immunocompromised patients with cough, hypoxia, dyspnea, and fever. Although most cases of hypersensitivity and interstitial pneumonitis respond to steroid therapy, pulmonary fibrosis typically has a protracted course and poor response to conventional treatment. Although oxygen is considered a risk factor for worsening bleomycin-associated pulmonary toxicity, it should be administered during emergency management of patients with hypoxia. In most other circumstances, however, oxygen therapy is helpful.

Gastrointestinal Emergencies

Mucositis

Mucositis refers to inflammation of the oral mucosa. The extension of mucositis into the oral tissues, such as lips, teeth, and periodontal tissues, is referred to as stomatitis. Inflammation may extend the length of the gastrointestinal (GI) tract, manifesting as esophagitis, gastritis, enteritis, colitis, and proctitis. Mucositis is often seen following therapy with chemotherapeutic agents that affect the rapidly dividing gastrointestinal epithelium. The pathophysiology of mucositis entails injury to the mucosal barrier by reactive oxygen species (ROS).[101] Mucositis causes significant pain, impedes adequate nutrition and healing, impairs patients' quality of life. Ulcerations may serve as a nidus for infection in an immunocompromised patient.

Oral mucositis is frequently caused by MTX, dactinomycin, 5-FU, vincristine, and vinblastine. **Table 7** contains a comprehensive list of agents associated with oral mucositis.[101,102] If patients are taking MTX, the appearance of mucositis should

Table 7
Chemotherapeutic agents associated with oral mucositis

Class	Agents
Alkylating agents	Carboplatin Chlorambucil Cisplatin Cyclophosphamide Dacarbazine Lomustine Mechlorethamine Melphalan
Antimetabolites	Capecitabine Cytarabine Fludarabine 5-FU[51] Gemcitabine Mercaptopurine MTX Pentostatin Thioguanine
Antibiotics	Dactinomycin Daunorubicin Doxorubicin Epirubicin Idarubicin Mitomycin C
Antimitotic agents	Docetaxel Paclitaxel
Topoisomerase inhibitors	Etoposide
Tyrosine kinase inhibitors	Dasatinib Sorafenib Sunitinib

prompt an evaluation for MTX toxicity (see MTX section later). **Table 7** contains the a comprehensive list of agents that cause mucositis. Esophageal mucositis is caused by MTX, 5-FU, paclitaxel, and docetaxel. Mucositis of the small intestine is seen following therapy with MTX, bleomycin, and cyclophosphamide. Irinotecan is a unique chemotherapeutic agent that predisposes to colonic mucositis.

Nausea and vomiting
Chemotherapy-induced nausea and vomiting (CINV) is common and may lead to malnutrition, significant volume depletion, and may affect adherence to the chemotherapy regimen. Simulation of serotonergic receptors ($5\text{-}HT_3$) of the chemoreceptor trigger zone (CTZ) in area postrema in the fourth cerebral ventricle is the primary mechanism for nausea.[102,103] Other mechanisms included modulation of dopaminergic receptors in the CTZ and stimulation of the vomiting center in the reticular formation. In addition to vagal and cerebral cortical input, vomiting center is regulated by the interaction of substance P with a neurokinin-1 (NK-1) receptor. **Table 8** lists chemotherapeutic agents with high and moderate emetogenic potential.[104]

Diarrhea
Diarrhea is a frequent adverse effect of chemotherapy. Irinotecan and 5-FU induced diarrhea is associated with significant morbidity and mortality.[32,51,105,106] The

Table 8	
CINV high and moderate emetogenicity agents	
Emetogenicity	Drug
High (>90%)	Carmustine
	Cisplatin[15]
	Cyclophosphamide (>1500 mg/m^2)
	Dacarbazine[36]
	Dactinomycin
	Mechlorethamine
	Streptozotocin[44]
	Temozolomide[46]
Moderate (30%–90%)	Carboplatin
	Cyclophosphamide (<1500 mg/m^2)
	Cytarabine (>1 g/m^2)
	Daunorubicin
	Doxorubicin
	Epirubicin
	Idarubicin
	Ifosfamide
	Irinotecan
	Methotrexate
	Oxaliplatin

pathophysiology of chemotherapy-induced diarrhea is not well understood and is likely multifactorial. Bloody diarrhea may be an extension of mucositis seen with high doses of 5-FU, and has a high mortality rate.[102] Concomitant neutropenia may contribute to the risk for enteric sepsis. Cytotoxic damage to the intestinal epithelium may lead to increased permeability and translocation of gut bacteria.[105]

Constipation
Severe constipation may be precipitated by opioid therapy for management of cancer-related pain.

GI hemorrhage and perforation
Gastrointestinal hemorrhage is potential complications of bevacizumab, dasatinib, rituximab, erlotinib, imatinib, and sorafenib therapy.[5,6,17,30,39,68] GI perforation has been described with bevacizumab, rituximab, erlotinib, imatinib, and sorafenib therapy.[5,6,17,30,68]

Pancreatitis
L-asparaginase therapy is uniquely associated with hemorrhagic pancreatitis.[7]

Liver injury
Chemotherapy-induced hepatotoxicity is fortunately uncommon. However, it may alter metabolism of many drugs metabolized by the P450 hepatic microsomal system and evolve into hepatic failure. Mechanisms of injury are thought to be idiosyncratic and immunologic.[107] **Table 9** provides a comprehensive list of chemotherapeutic hepatotoxins.[107]

Clinical evaluation
Although several tools are available for grading oral mucositis by the National Cancer Institute Common Toxicity Criteria and the World Health Organization, the severity depends on the presence of pain and the ability to tolerate oral nutrition. Ulcerations are

Table 9
Chemotherapeutic hepatic toxins

Toxicity	Drug
Biliary stricture	Fluorodeoxyuridine (5-FU metabolite, intra-arterial)
Cholestasis	Cisplatin Gemcitabine Mercaptopurine
Granulomatous hepatitis	Procarbazine
Hepatic cirrhosis	MTX (chronic low dose)
Hepatic fibrosis	MTX (chronic low dose)
Hepatic necrosis	Dacarbazine[36] Mercaptopurine[37] Plicamycin Thioguanine[50]
Hepatocellular injury	L-asparaginase[7] Busulfan[20] Carboplatin Capecitabine Carmustine Chlorambucil Cisplatin Cytarabine Dactinomycin Docetaxel[108] Erlotinib[6] Etoposide 5-FU (IV) Fluorodeoxyuridine (5-FU metabolite, intra-arterial) Gefitinib[97] Gemcitabine[109] Imatinib[30] Irinotecan Lapatinib[74] Lomustine Melphalan Mercaptopurine MTX[11] Oxaliplatin Paclitaxel Plicamycin[144] Procarbazine[42] Sorafenib[68] Streptozotocin[44] Sunitinib[19] Tamoxifen Thioguanine Vinorelbine[12]
Hepatorenal syndrome	Erlotinib[6]
Sclerosing cholangitis	Fluorodeoxyuridine (5-FU metabolite, intra-arterial)
Venoocclusive disease	Dacarbazine[36] Dactinomycin[38] Gemtuzumab[98] Melphalan[35] Thioguanine[50]

typically present on the oral mucosa and may be painless or painful, and associated with or without erythema and edema. Severe edema may lead to airway compromise.

Esophagitis, gastritis, colitis, and proctitis typically present with pain in the affected region. Dysphagia and retrosternal pain are typical symptoms of esophagitis. Abdominal pain, nausea, vomiting, and diarrhea may be seen with gastritis, enteritis, and colitis.

The assessment of the frequency of emesis, ability to tolerate oral intake, and presence of blood are important in the evaluation of CINV. Although hematemesis is not an expected clinical finding of CINV, it may be suggestive of mucositis or an esophageal tear during forceful emesis. It is challenging to discern an infectious versus a drug-induced cause of diarrhea in immunocompromised patients. The severity of diarrhea depends on volume depletion, presence of blood, abdominal pain, fever, decrease in urine output, and change in mental status as a result of profound dehydration.

Constipation may be mild or severe. Patients who present to the emergency department for the management of opioid-induced constipation may have less than three bowel movements per week, sensation of incomplete evacuation, abdominal discomfort/pain, bloating, nausea, and emesis. Small-bowel obstruction should be considered in patients with risk factors, such as abdominal cancer, prior surgeries, and/or ill appearance.

GI bleed may be painless or painful. Significant blood loss may manifest with generalized weakness and signs of end-organ ischemia caused by a lack of oxygen delivery. Clinical examination may demonstrate abdominal pain and signs of peritonitis in gastrointestinal perforation.

Epigastric abdominal pain is a common clnical finding in pancreatitis. Pain may radiate to the back and may be associated with nausea and vomiting. Severe pancreatitis may lead to significant electrolyte abnormalities.

Clinical signs and symptoms of hepatic toxicity are typically a late finding unless routinely monitored with laboratory analyses. Nausea, vomiting, abdominal pain, ascites, jaundice, and peripheral edema may be signs of liver injury. Failure of coagulation factor synthesis may lead to bleeding, prolonged PT/INR, and thrombocytopenia with petechiae, ecchymosis, and/or purpura. Hepatic encephalopathy is a late finding and typically manifests with lethargy, confusion, and/or asterixis on physical examination.

Diagnostic evaluation

The following laboratory and diagnostic tests are suggested for the assessment of chemotherapy-induced GI conditions:

- Serum electrolytes
- CBC: evaluate for presence of infection or in the setting of acute blood loss
- LFTs: exclusion of biliary pathology
- PT/INR, PTT: evaluation of synthetic function
- Plain radiographs (including chest imaging): may be helpful in assessment of intraperitoneal air
- CT abdomen/pelvis: may be considered if suspicion for infectious enteritis/colitis or perforation not seen on plain radiograph
- Endoscopy or colonoscopy: establishment of diagnosis of esophageal/enteric/colonic mucositis

Management

Emergency department management of oral mucositis entails the assessment of the airway. In patients without evidence of airway compromise, outpatient management centers on good oral hygiene and avoidance of oral irritants. Topical viscous lidocaine and oral and IV opioids may be provided for pain relief in the emergency department.

Although there are no specific recommendations, caution is advisable in prescribing outpatient viscous lidocaine and benzocaine. Absorption may be enhanced through denuded skin, with the potential for systemic toxicity. Although outside the scope of emergency medicine management, mucosal coating agents and keratinocyte growth factor-1 agents have been used during inpatient and outpatient management of mucositis.[110–114]

Emergency department management of esophagitis and gastritis are symptomatic. Proton pump inhibitors or H2 blockers are recommended.[110,111,115] The management of enteritis and colitis is supportive. It is imperative to assess for presence of infectious enteritis/colitis in immunocompromised patient.

Supportive care is the mainstay of therapy for CINV. Patients are often volume depleted and require volume resuscitation with IV crystalloid. Antiemetics are critical in controlling nausea and vomiting. Ondansetron, a first-generation 5-HT$_3$ antagonist, is first-line therapy in the management of CINV.[116] Dexamethasone should be considered in patients with persistent emesis. Benzodiazepines, olanzapine, and metoclopramide have been used in the treatment of intractable emesis.[117] NK-1 antagonists, such as aprepitant, and fosaprepitant are used in both outpatient and inpatient settings and may be considered in patients with intractable emesis following the consultation with oncologist.

The treatment of chemotherapy-induced diarrhea is often supportive and entails volume and electrolyte repletion. Antibiotics may be warranted in patients with a concern for infectious diarrhea. Loperamide may be used with caution as a first-line therapy in patients with noninfectious chemotherapy-induced diarrhea. Reassessment within 24 to 48 hours is necessary for patients who are discharged to home with loperamide. Octreotide is advised as a second-line agent for severe and refractory diarrhea.[118]

Methylnaltrexone should be considered for the management of opioid-induced constipation in patients with advanced cancer receiving palliative care with a prior insufficient response to laxative therapy.[119] It is approved by the FDA for this indication. Only one dose should be administered in the emergency department. It is typically dosed every other day, without exceeding one dose in a 24-hour period. Subcutaneous administration of 8 mg is recommended for patients weighing 38 to 62 kg. Subcutaneous administration of 12 mg is recommended for those patients who weigh between 62 and 114 kg. Subcutaneous administration of 0.15 mg/kg is suggested for those patients who weigh less than 38 kg or greater than 114 kg. A pharmacist should be consulted to verify the correct dose for patients weighing more than 114 kg.

Supportive care, observation, reversal of coagulopathy with blood products, and gastroenterology consultation is the mainstay of management in GI hemorrhage.

Clinical signs of peritonitis should prompt an emergent surgical consultation. GI perforation warrants surgical management.

Withdrawal of the offending agent and supportive care are the mainstays of therapy in patients with chemotherapy-induced hepatotoxicity. In cases of severe hepatotoxicity, transplant consultation should be considered.

Renal Emergencies

Renal injury may be broadly classified into prerenal, intrinsic renal, and postrenal. Prerenal injury typically results from hypovolemia. Direct renal injury, precipitation of drugs or metabolites in the renal tubules, ischemia, glomerular disease, and damage to the renal vasculature may lead to intrinsic nephrotoxicity. Postrenal injury results from mechanical outflow obstruction. Chemotherapy may affect the tubules, renal parenchyma, and renal vasculature. Cisplatin is a well-recognized chemotherapeutic nephrotoxin. Drugs that affect the proximal tubule may result in Fanconi syndrome, which is characterized by renal wasting of phosphate, glucose, potassium, and bicarbonate.[120,121] Volume depletion and acidic urine predispose to the precipitation of MTX and metabolites into the renal tubules. HUS is a manifestation of thrombotic angiopathy, manifests with the constellation of microangiopathic hemolytic anemia, thrombocytopenia, fever, and renal injury, which is likely caused via fibrin deposition of afferent arterioles and glomeruli.[122–124] A list of nephrotoxins with the respective toxicity are outlined in **Table 10**.[120–122]

Clinical evaluation
Nephrotoxicity may manifest with decreased urine production as well as nausea and vomiting in cases of uremia. Electrolyte abnormalities may present with alteration of consciousness, effects on cardiac conduction, myopathy, or weakness.

Diagnostic evaluation
The following laboratory studies are suggested for the evaluation of chemotherapy-induced nephrotoxicity:

- Serum electrolytes
- Urinalysis: assessment of proteinuria, glucosuria
- Urine sodium, potassium, phosphorus, uric acid, and glucose: may be seen in Fanconi syndrome
- CBC, LFTs, PT/PTT, LDH, and peripheral smear: evaluation of HUS (thrombocytopenia, hemolysis with anemia and indirect hyperbilirubinemia, elevated serum LDH, and schistocytes)

Management
Management of intrinsic renal damage is supportive. The decision to initiate hemodialysis should be discussed with the consulting nephrologist. The hematological

Table 10 Chemotherapeutic nephrotoxins	
Toxicity	**Drug**
Acute renal insufficiency	Carboplatin[14]
	Erlotinib[6]
	Irinotecan[32]
	Nitrosoureas (carmustine, lomustine, streptozotocin)
	Oxaliplatin
	Pentostatin
Acute tubular necrosis	Cisplatin
	Ifosfamide
	Imatinib
Chronic kidney disease	Cisplatin
	Ifosfamide
	Nitrosoureas (carmustine, lomustine, streptozotocin)
Crystal nephropathy	MTX
HUS[123,124]	Bleomycin
	Cisplatin
	Gemcitabine
	Mitomycin C
Renal tubular acidosis	Streptozotocin[44]
Tubulopathy	Cisplatin[15]
	Ifosfamide (chloroacetaldehyde metabolite)

emergencies section reviews HUS management. Precipitation of MTX in the renal tubules may be treated with urinary alkalinization (see the MTX section). Amifostine is an antidote that is used for the prevention of cisplatin-induced nephrotoxicity.

Antidotal considerations: Amifostine

Amifostine is approved by the FDA for the prevention of cisplatin-induced nephrotoxicity.[82,83] Patients receiving cisplatin chemotherapy are pretreated with amifostine.[125] It is not part of the emergency department management of cisplatin-induced nephrotoxicity.

Genitourinary Emergencies

The most important complication of chemotherapy in the bladder is development of hemorrhagic cystitis. The acrolein metabolite of cyclophosphamide and ifosfamide is a causative agent.[121,122,126] Although several mechanisms have been proposed, acrolein promotes the generation of ROS, leading to oxidative cellular damage in uroepithelium.[126] Urinary retention may be seen during vincristine chemotherapy.[10]

Clinical evaluation

Hematuria and urinary discomfort are typically present with hemorrhagic cystitis. Painful and palpable bladder distention may be evident with urinary retention.

Diagnostic evaluation

The following diagnostics are suggested for the evaluation of hemorrhagic cystitis:

- Urinalysis with microscopic analysis: evaluation of hematuria
- CBC: monitor for anemia in patients with gross hematuria
- Urine culture

Management

Emergency department management for hemorrhagic cystitis is supportive. Foley insertion and bladder irrigation may be helpful in cases of obstructive hematuria and subsequent urinary retention. Mesna is an antidote used for the prevention of ifosfamide- and cyclophosphamide-induced hemorrhagic cystitis.

Antidotal considerations: Mesna (sodium 2-mercaptoethanesulfonate)

Mesna is approved by the FDA for the prevention of hemorrhagic cystitis in patients receiving ifosfamide or high-dose cyclophosphamide chemotherapy.[82,83] It is available in both oral and IV formulations. Mesna binds the acrolein metabolite, preventing it from entering the uroepithelium.[126] Mesna coadministration is recommended in patients receiving high-dose cyclophosphamide to prevent urothelial toxicity.[82,83] It is not part of the emergency department management of hemorrhagic cystitis.

Dermatologic Emergencies

Cutaneous reactions, such as alopecia, mucosal lesions, epidermal lesions, nail changes, and hypersensitivity reactions, are commonly seen following chemotherapy. This section focuses on drugs that cause erythema multiforme (EM), Stevens-Johnson syndrome (SJS), toxic epidermal necrolysis (TEN), and hypersensitivity reactions that are pertinent to emergency medicine.

The following chemotherapeutic agents are associated with EM/SJS/TEN:

- Chlorambucil[127]
- Dactinomycin[38]
- Erlotinib[6]
- Etoposide[47]

- Imatinib[30]
- Ibritumomab[27]
- Mechorethamine
- MTX[11]
- Plicamycin[144]
- Rituximab[17]
- Sorafenib[68]

Both immune and nonimmune mechanisms have been implicated in hypersensitivity reactions. Most reactions occur within several minutes to several hours of drug administration. The following chemotherapeutic agents may cause anaphylaxis:

- L-asparaginase[7]
- Carboplatin[14]
- Cisplatin[15]
- Cyclophosphamide[71]
- Docetaxel[108]
- Etoposide[47]
- 5-FU[51]
- Gemtuzumab[98]
- Ibritumomab[27]
- Irinotecan[32]
- Melphalan[35]
- Mechlorethamine
- Oxaliplatin[128]
- Paclitaxel[75]
- Teniposide
- Vincristine[10]

Paclitaxel and docetaxel are associated with non–immune-mediated anaphylactoid reactions.[129] Infusion reactions are characterized by hypotension, confusion, fever, chills, and wheezing.[94] They are commonly associated with bleomycin, alemtuzumab, ibritumomab, rituximab, panitumumab therapy.[17,27,130] Nonfatal infusion hypersensitivity reactions were reported with bevacizumab, cetuximab, gemtuzumab, tositumomab, trastuzumab, and teniposide.[5,48,54,73,76,98]

Clinical evaluation

EM typically presents as skin macules that develop into raised erythematous target lesions. EM minor lesions are limited to epidermis and are acral in distribution. EM major lesions involve one or more mucous membranes in addition to the epidermis, with epidermal detachment in less than 10% of the body surface area. SJS is a spectrum of EM with lesions extending into truncal and facial distribution, mucosal involvement, and epidermal detachment of 10% and 30% of the total body surface area. TEN is the most severe form, with diffuse lesions including both epidermis and mucosa, with epidermal detachment in more than 30% of the total body surface area. Clinical signs and symptoms of hypersensitivity range from urticaria to anaphylaxis. Hypoxia, pulmonary infiltrates, ARDS, myocardial infarction, dysrhythmia, and/or cardiogenic shock may be seen following severe infusion reactions.

Diagnostic evaluation

Laboratory studies and imaging are generally unhelpful in the diagnosis of hypersensitivity reaction, anaphylaxis, or EM/SJS/TEN. Dermatologic consultation for biopsy may be helpful, but is not typically a part of emergent management.

Management

The emergency department management of anaphylaxis involves discontinuation of the offending agent, treatment with histamine antagonists, and steroids. Epinephrine should be used in severe anaphylaxis with hemodynamic instability and/or airway compromise. SJS/TEN treatment necessitates immediate removal of the offending agent volume resuscitation, and aggressive wound care. Consultation with a burn center for potential transfer is warranted in cases of extensive epidermal detachment.

Extravasation Emergencies

Extravasation of chemotherapeutic agents may lead to skin irritation, devastating skin necrosis, and compartment syndrome.[131] Chemotherapeutic agents characterized as vesicants, such as anthracyclines, vinca alkaloids, and nitrogen mustard, cause an inflammatory response and have the potential to cause severe tissue damage.[129] Chemotherapeutic irritants, including platinoids, taxanes, anthracyclines, dactinomycin, mitomycin C, mitoxantrone, and topoisomerase inhibitors, cause skin irritation, swelling, and pain. The physical examination may demonstrate local skin erythema, edema, tenderness to palpation, blistering, ulceration, and tissue necrosis.[129]

The treatment involves immediate cessation of the infusion. The IV cannula should be left in place, with aspiration of the extravasated drug attempted rapidly through the cannula. Intermittent cooling may be effective in reducing pain and irritation from the irritant compounds. Direct ice compress application for 6 to 12 hours may be helpful following mechlorethamine extravasation.[132] Given the potential for severe toxicity and skin necrosis, extravasation of vesicant chemotherapeutic agents should be addressed rapidly.

Antidotes are available for the treatment of anthracyclines, vinca alkaloid, and nitrogen mustard extravasation. Intravenous dexrazoxane should be started within 6 hours of anthracycline extravasation. It is administered once daily over 1 to 2 hours for 3 consecutive days via large-bore IV opposite the affected extremity. A dose of 1000 mg/m^2 (max 2000 mg) IV should be administered within 6 hours of extravasation, followed by a repeat 1000 mg/m^2 IV (max 2000 mg) on the second day and a third dose of 500 mg/m^2 IV on the third day. Dose adjustments may be necessary is patients with renal impairment.[133] Hyaluronidase is locally injected at the site of vinca alkaloid extravasation, along with application of warm compresses, to promote diffusion of the agent. The recommended initial total dosing is 150 units subcutaneously with 25-ga or 27-ga needle divided in 5 different injections around the extravasation site. A local subcutaneous injection of one-sixth molar solution of sodium thiosulfate may be used for nitrogen mustard (mechlorethamine) extravasation. Please see the mechlorethamine package insert for sodium thiosulfate dilution instructions to achieve an appropriate concentration.

Patients who have sustained anthracycline, vinca alkaloid, and mechlorethamine extravasation injuries should be observed for a minimal period of 24 hours or longer depending on the type of extravasation and symptoms.

Patients with pain, erythema, or swelling at the site of an indwelling thoracic access port should be evaluated for infection or extravasation of chemotherapeutics caused by the formation of a fibrous sheath encapsulating the line. This condition is diagnosed by the inability to draw back on the line but relative ease in flushing the line. If this occurs, imaging of the chest with CT is warranted.

Methotrexate

MTX is widely used for treatment of rheumatologic disease, trophoblastic disease, malignancy, and as a part of an immunosuppressant regimen in organ transplantation. It is administered for therapeutic abortion. MTX is a structural analogue of folic acid. It prevents DNA and RNA synthesis by inhibiting dihydrofolate reductase (DHFR) and thymidylate synthetase, and inhibits de novo purine synthesis via the inhibition of 5-aminoimidazole-4-carboxamide ribonucleotide transformylase.[134] MTX toxicity depends on the dose, duration of administration, and renal clearance. Toxicity from MTX accumulation may be seen with impaired renal function or renal toxic medications. MTX forms crystals in the renal tubule acidic milieu.[135] Toxicity may be prolonged in patients with anasarca, pleural effusions, and ascites because of the prolonged redistribution from the third space compartment to the plasma during elimination.

Clinical evaluation
Clinical MTX toxicity may be challenging to recognize, especially in patients without a history of overt overdose. Nausea and vomiting may be seen within 2 to 4 hours of high-dose MTX (1000 mg/m^2 or more). Mucositis, stomatitis, and diarrhea may manifest within 1 to 2 weeks. Bone marrow toxicity and pancytopenia typically occur within the first 2 weeks. High-dose MTX may also lead to nephrotoxicity, further decreasing clearance and potentiating toxicity. Neurologic manifestations, such as acute and chronic leukoencephalopathy, paresis a transient acute neurologic syndrome, and seizures, may be noted following high-dose IV administration.[136]

Diagnostic evaluation
All patients undergoing therapeutic abortion with MTX should have an evaluation of renal function. The following laboratory and diagnostic studies may be helpful in evaluating patients with MTX toxicity:

- CBC with differential: assessment of bone marrow suppression
- Serum electrolytes
- LFTs: assessment of hepatotoxicity
- MTX concentration
- CT brain without contrast: workup of altered mental status
- LP: consider as a part of infectious workup in immunocompromised patients with altered mental status
- MRI brain: more sensitive in assessment of encephalopathy, nonemergent

Management
The treatment involves the cessation of MTX exposure and the administration of activated charcoal in cases of acute oral ingestion. IV hydration and urine alkalinization are important in preventing precipitation of MTX and its metabolites in the renal tubules. Sodium bicarbonate 150 mEq is added to 1 L of D5W and infused at 1.5 to 2.0 times the maintenance to alkalinize urine (pH 7–8). Serum potassium monitoring with sufficient repletion is important given intracellular potassium shifts seen with alkalinization. Hypokalemia leads to aciduria in exchange for potassium reabsorption in the tubules. Monitor serum pH closely to prevent a pH greater than 7.55.

Bone marrow suppression may be treated with GM-CSF. Leucovorin rescue should be initiated immediately on recognition of toxicity. Carboxypeptidase G_2 should be considered in patients with acute MTX overdose or significant toxicity caused by decreased renal clearance.

Antidotal considerations: Leucovorin (folinic acid)
Leucovorin is a reduced, active form of folic acid used to treat acute and chronic MTX toxicity. Unlike folic acid, it does not require DHFR for conversion for activation.[137] The administration of leucovorin bypasses DHFR inhibition and promotes

purine nucleotide and thymidylate synthesis. Leucovorin dosing should ideally match MTX serum concentration.[135] MTX concentrations greater than 1×10^{-8} mol/L (0.01 μmol/L) are associated with inhibition of DNA synthesis.[137] Because laboratory determinations of MTX concentrations may be delayed, an empiric dose of leucovorin 100 mg/m^2 IV over 15 to 30 minutes should be administered on recognition of MTX overdose or chronic toxicity.[138] It should be repeated every 3 to 6 hours. The administration rates should not exceed 160 mg/min because of leucovorin's calcium content.[139] Benzyl alcohol-free preparations are used for neonates. Treatment should be continued for at least 3 days. The duration of MTX toxicity depends on the dose and renal function. Longer leucovorin dosing may be required in patients with ascites, pleural effusions, and bone marrow toxicity because the half-life of MTX may not accurately reflect intracellular concentrations. A nomogram may be used as a guide for treatment.[140] Ideally, treatment should be continued until the serum MTX concentration is less than 1×10^{-8} mol/L in the absence of bone marrow suppression. Adverse effects are uncommon and limited to parenteral administration. Allergic or anaphylactoid reactions and rare seizures[141] have been reported. Hypercalcemia may be noted with high doses and prolonged administration. Leucovorin administration may enhance the toxicity of 5-FU. Leucovorin should never be administered IT.

Antidotal considerations: Carboxypeptidase G$_2$ (glucarpidase)

Carboxypeptidase G$_2$, a recombinant enzyme, inactivates folate and MTX by cleaving the C-terminal glutamate residues.[142] It cleaves MTX into 4-deoxy-4-amino-N^{10}-methylpteroid acid (DAMPA) and glutamate moieties. Carboxypeptidase G$_2$ received FDA approval in 2012 for the IV treatment of MTX toxicity in patients with a serum MTX concentration of greater than 1 μmol/L and the presence of impaired renal function. Aggressive therapy with leucovorin should be initiated before the consideration of carboxypeptidase G$_2$. The serum MTX concentration should be obtained before carboxypeptidase G$_2$ administration. The DAMPA metabolite interferes with MTX immunoassay and overestimates the serum MTX concentration for at least 48 hours. A single dose of 50 U/kg is administered over 5 minutes.[143] Leucovorin should not be administered 2 hours before or after carboxypeptidase G$_2$ therapy, given the risk of leucovorin inactivation. Adverse events are rare following IV administration. Paresthesias, flushing, nausea, and vomiting occur most commonly.

Unlike leucovorin, carboxypeptidase G$_2$ may be provided IT following IT MTX toxicity (off label); 2000 U is administered IT over 5 minutes (see also the IT section).[62]

SUMMARY

The recognition of the toxicity of chemotherapeutic agents is challenging. The use of combination therapy, the potential of a single agent to affect multiple body systems, and the resemblance of clinical symptoms to both cancer and non–cancer-related illness present a diagnostic dilemma. The emergency department management should focus on the evaluation of infectious cause of symptoms and other potential emergent conditions. IT emergencies should be immediately addressed because recognition and time to intervention are the most important factors in the prevention of significant neurologic morbidity and death. There are few specific antidotes that would change the course of illness in the emergency department setting: leucovorin for MTX overdose, carboxypeptidase G$_2$ for the management of IT MTX overdose, and dexrazoxane/hyaluronidase/sodium thiosulfate for the management of extravasation injuries. The Poison Control Center (1-800-POISONS) should be notified following overdose or unintentional erroneous route of administration. The management of most chemotherapy-induced adverse effects is supportive.

REFERENCES

1. World Health Organization. 2013. Available at: http://www.who.int/mediacentre/factsheets/fs297/en/index.html. Accessed April 15, 2013.
2. American Cancer Society. 2013. Available at: http://www.cancer.org/acs/groups/content/@epidemiologysurveilance/documents/document/acspc-036845.pdf. Accessed April 15, 2013.
3. Wang RY. Antineoplastic overview. In: Nelson LS, Lewin NA, Howland MA, et al, editors. Goldfrank's toxicologic emergencies. 9th edition. New York: McGraw-Hill; 2011. p. 770-7.
4. PQD® cancer information summaries: adult treatment. National Cancer Institute. Available at: www.cancer.gov/cancertopics/pdq/adulttreatment. Accessed May 13, 2013.
5. Bevacizumab solution for intravenous infusion [package insert]. San Francisco (CA): Genentech, Inc.; 2009.
6. Erlotinib tablets [package insert]. Melville (NY): Schwarz Pharma, OSI Pharmaceuticals Inc.; 2010.
7. Asparaginase [package insert]. Deerfield (IL): Lundbeck; 2013.
8. Ifosfamide for injection, USP [package insert]. Princeton (NJ): Baxter Healthcare Corporation for Bristol-Myers Squibb Company; 2007.
9. Ocean AJ, Vahdat LT. Chemotherapy-induced peripheral neuropathy: pathogenesis and emerging therapies. Support Care Cancer 2004;12:619-25.
10. Vincristine sulfate injection [package insert]. Lake Forest (IL): Hospira, Inc; 2013.
11. Methotrexate tablets, USP [package insert]. Fort Lee (NJ): Excella GmbH for DAVA Pharmaceuticals; 2010.
12. Vinorelbine tartrate injection [package insert]. Research Triangle Park (NC): Pierre Fabre Médicament Production for GlaxoSmithKline; 2002.
13. Jaggi AS, Singh N. Mechanisms in cancer-chemotherapeutic drug-induced peripheral neuropathy. Toxicology 2012;291:1-9.
14. Carboplatin for injection, USP [package insert]. Princeton (NJ): Bristo-Myers Squibb Company; 2010.
15. Cisplatin for injection, USP [package insert]. Princeton (NJ): Bristol-Myers Squibb Company; 2007.
16. Hildebrand J. Neurological complications of cancer chemotherapy. Curr Opin Oncol 2006;18:321-4.
17. Rituximab injection [package insert]. San Francisco (CA): Genentech Inc.; 2010.
18. Dasanu CA. Gemcitabine: vascular toxicity and prothrombotic potential. Expert Opin Drug Saf 2008;7:703-16.
19. Sunitinib malate capsules [package insert]. New York: Prizer, Inc.; 2012.
20. Busulfan for injection, USP [package insert]. Edison (NJ): ESP Pharma, Inc; 2007.
21. Vinblastine sulfate for injection, USP [package insert]. Bedford (OH): Ben Venue Labs, Inc for Bedford Laboratories; 2010.
22. Sioka C, Kyritsis AP. Central and peripheral nervous system toxicity of common chemotherapeutic agents. Cancer Chemother Pharmacol 2009;63:761-7.
23. Lyass O, Lossos A, Hubert A, et al. Cisplatin-induced non-convulsive encephalopathy. Anticancer Drugs 1998;9:100-4.

24. Patel PN. Methylene blue for management of ifosfamide induced encephalopathy. Ann Pharmacother 2006;40:299–303.
25. Ajithkumar T, Parkinson C, Shamshad F, et al. Ifosfamide encephalopathy. Clin Oncol (R Coll Radiol) 2007;19:108–14.
26. Alemtuzumab [package insert]. Cambridge (MA): Millenium and ILEX Partners, LP; 2001.
27. Ibritumomab tiuxetan [package insert]. San Diego (CA): IDEC Pharmaceuticals Corporation; 2001.
28. Idarubicin hydrochloride for injection, USP [package insert]. Glasgow (KY): Onco Therapies Limited for Amneal-Agila, LLC; 2012.
29. Capecitabine tablets [package insert]. Nutley (NJ): Roche Laboratories Inc; 2000.
30. Imatinib mesylate tablets [package insert]. East Hanover (NJ): Novartis Pharmaceuticals Corporation; 2013.
31. Carmustine for injection [package insert]. Princeton (NJ): Ben Venue Laboratories, Inc for Bristol-Myers Squibb Company; 2011.
32. Irinotecan injection [package insert]. New York: Pfizer, Inc.; 2011.
33. Lomustine capsules [package insert]. Princeton (NJ): Bristol-Myers Squibb Company; 2012.
34. Cytarabine for injection, USP [package insert]. Bedford (OH): Ben Venue Laboratories, Inc for Bedford Laboratories; 2008.
35. Melphalan hydrochloride for injection [package insert]. Research Triangle Park (NC): GlaxoSmithKline LLC; 2008.
36. Dacarbazine for injection, USP [package insert]. Irvine (CA): Teva Parenteral Medicines, Inc; 2007.
37. Mercaptopurine tablets [package insert]. Greenville (NC): Gate Pharmaceuticals for DSM Pharmaceuticals, Inc; 2011.
38. Dactinomycin injection [package insert]. Deerfield (IL): Baxter Oncology GmbH for Lundbeck; 2012.
39. Dasatinib tablets [package insert]. Princeton (NJ): Bristol-Myers Squibb Company; 2013.
40. Pentostatin for injection [package insert]. Lake Forest (IL): Hospira, Inc; 2009.
41. Daunorubicin hydrochloride for injection [package insert]. Bedford (OH): Ben Venue Laboratories, Inc for Bedford Laboratories; 1999.
42. Procarbazine hydrochloride capsule [package insert]. Gaithersburg (MD): AAI Pharma Inc for Sigma-tau Pharmaceuticals, Inc; 2008.
43. Doxorubicin hydrochloride injection, USP [package insert]. Irvine (CA): Teva Parenteral Medicines, Inc; 2008.
44. Streptozotocin sterile powder [package insert]. Irvine (CA): Teva Parenteral Medicines, Inc; 2007.
45. Epirubicin hydrochloride injection [package insert]. Irvine (CA): Teva Parenteral Medicines, Inc; 2013.
46. Temozolomide capsules [package insert]. Whitehouse Station (NJ): Merck Sharp & Dohme Corp for Merck & Co, Inc; 2005.
47. Etoposide phosphate for injection [package insert]. Princeton (NJ): Baxter Healthcare Corporation for Bristol-Myers Squibb Company; 2011.
48. Teniposide injection [package insert]. Princeton (NJ): Bristol-Myers Squibb Company; 1998.
49. Fludarabine phosphate for injection [package insert]. Montville (NJ): Ben Venue Laboratories for Berlex; 2003.

50. Thioguanine tablets [package insert]. Research Triangle Park (NC): DSM Pharmaceuticals for GlaxoSmithKline; 2009.
51. Fluorouracil injection, USP [package insert]. New York: Pfizer Inc; 2012.
52. Topotecan hydrochloride for injection [package insert]. Research Triangle Park (NC): GlaxoSmithKline LLC.; 2009.
53. Gemcitabine for injection [package insert]. Indianapolis (IN): Eli Lilly; 2013.
54. Tositumomab injection [package insert]. Wilmington (DE): GlaxoSmithKline, LLC.; 2013.
55. Dunford J. Fatal ascending tonic-clonic seizure syndrome. Ann Emerg Med 1998;32:624–62.
56. Al Ferayan A, Russell NA, Al Wohaibi M, et al. Cerebrospinal fluid lavage in the treatment of inadvertent intrathecal vincristine injection. Childs Nerv Syst 1999; 15:87–9.
57. Penn RD, Kroin JS. Treatment of intrathecal morphine overdose. J Neurosurg 1995;82:147–8.
58. Chidester S. Baclofen pump complications. Toxicol Lett 2011;16:1.
59. Coffey RJ, Burchiel K. Inflammatory mass lesions associated with intrathecal drug infusion catheters: report and observations on 41 patients. Neurosurgery 2002;50:78–86.
60. Coffey RJ, Edgar TS, Francisco GE, et al. Abrupt withdrawal from intrathecal baclofen: recognition and management of a potentially life-threatening syndrome. Arch Phys Med Rehabil 2002;83:735–41 [Erratum appears in Arch Phys Med Rehabil 2002;83:1479].
61. Rao RB. Special considerations: intrathecal medication errors. In: Nelson LS, Lewin N, Howland MA, et al, editors. Goldfrank's toxicologic emergencies. 9th edition. New York: McGraw Hill; 2011. p. 548–58.
62. Widemann BC, Balis FM, Shalabi A, et al. Treatment of accidental intrathecal methotrexate overdose with intrathecal carboxypeptidase G_2. J Natl Cancer Inst 2004;96:1557–9.
63. Shaikh AY, Shih JA. Chemotherapy-induced cardiotoxicity. Curr Heart Fail Rep 2012;9:117–27.
64. Outomoro D, Grana DR, Azzato F, et al. Adriamycin-induced myocardial toxicity: new solutions for an old problem? Int J Cardiol 2007;117:6–15.
65. Senkus E, Jassem J. Cardiovascular effects of systemic cancer treatment. Cancer Treat Rev 2011;37:300–11.
66. Jones RL, Swanton C, Ewer MS. Anthracycline cardiotoxicity. Expert Opin Drug Saf 2006;5:791–809.
67. van der Pal HJ, van Dalen EC, van Delden E, et al. High risk symptomatic cardiac events in childhood cancer survivors. J Clin Oncol 2012;30:1429–37.
68. Sorafenib tablets [package insert]. Wayne (NJ): Onyx Pharmaceuticals, Inc. for Bayer HealthCare Pharmaceuticals, Inc.; 2013.
69. Mitoxantrone for injection concentrate [package insert]. Seattle (WA): Lederle Parenterals, Inc. for Immunex Corporation; 2002.
70. Mitomycin C for injecton, USP [package insert]. Bedford (OH): Ben Venue Laboratories, Inc for Bedford Laboratories; 2000.
71. Cyclophosphamide for injection, UPS. Cyclophosphamide tablets, USP [package insert]. Princeton (NJ): Baxter Healthcare Corporation for Bristol-Myers Squibb Company; 2005.
72. Morandi P, Ruffini PA, Benvenuto GM, et al. Cardiac toxicity of high-dose chemotherapy. Bone Marrow Transplant 2005;35:323–34.
73. Trastuzumab [package insert]. San Francisco (CA): Genentech, Inc.; 2000.

74. Lapatinib tablets [package insert]. Research Triangle Park (NC): GlaxoSmithK-line LLC; 2007.
75. Paclitaxel injection [package insert]. Princeton (NJ): Bristol-Myers Squibb Company; 2011.
76. Cetuximab injection [package insert]. Indianapolis (IN): ImClone LLC.; 2013.
77. Tamoxifen citrate tablet [package insert]. Ft. Lauderdale (FL): Andrx Pharmaceuticals, Inc.; 2007.
78. De Pas T, Curigliano G, Franceschelli L, et al. Gemcitabine-induced systemic capillary leak syndrome. Ann Oncol 2001;12:1651–2.
79. Speyer JL, Green MD, Zeleniuch-Jacquotte A, et al. ICRF-187 permits longer treatment with doxorubicin in women with breast cancer. J Clin Oncol 1992; 10:117–27.
80. Swain SM, Whaley FS, Gerber MC, et al. Cardioprotection with dexrazoxane for doxorubicin-containing therapy in advanced breast cancer. J Clin Oncol 1997; 15:1318–32.
81. Marty M, Espie M, Llombart A, et al. Multicenter randomized phase III study of the cardioprotective effect of dexrazoxane (Cardioxane®) in advanced/meta-static breast cancer patients treated with anthracycline-based chemotherapy. Ann Oncol 2006;17:614–22.
82. Schuchter LM, Hensley ML, Meropol NJ, et al. 2002 update of recommendations for the use of chemotherapy and radiotherapy protectants: clinical practice guidelines of the American Society of Clinical Oncology. J Clin Oncol 2002; 20:2895–903.
83. Hensley ML, Hagerty KL, Kewalramani T, et al. American Society of Clinical Oncology 2008 Clinical practice guideline update: use of chemotherapy and radiation therapy protectants. J Clin Oncol 2008;27:127–45.
84. Walker RW, Rosenblum MK, Kempin SJ, et al. Carboplatin-associated thrombotic microangiopathic hemolytic anemia. Cancer 1989;64:1017–20.
85. Kwaan HC, Gordon LI. Thrombotic microangiopathy in the cancer patient. Acta Haematol 2001;106:52–6.
86. Blake-Haskins JA, Lechleider RJ, Kreitman RJ. Thrombotic microangiopathy with targeted cancer agents. Clin Cancer Res 2011;17:5858–66.
87. Kim SK, Demetri GD. Chemotherapy and neutropenia. Hematol Oncol Clin North Am 1996;10:377–95.
88. Dale DC. Advances in the treatment of neutropenia. Curr Opin Support Palliat Care 2009;3:207–12.
89. Fraunfelder FW. Corneal toxicity from topical ocular and systemic medications. Cornea 2006;25:1133–8.
90. al-Tweigeri T, Nabholtz JM, Mackey JR. Ocular toxicity and cancer chemotherapy. Cancer 1996;78:1359–73.
91. Rybak LP, Whitworth CA, Mukherjea D, et al. Mechanisms of cisplatin-induced ototoxocity and prevention. Hear Res 2007;226:157–67.
92. Yorgason JG, Fayad JN, Kalinec F. Understanding drug ototoxicity: molecular insights for prevention and clinical management. Expert Opin Drug Saf 2006; 5:383–99.
93. Brock PR, Knight KR, Freyer DR, et al. Platinum-induced ototoxicity in children: a consensus review on mechanisms, predisposition, and protection, including a new international society of pediatric oncology boston ototoxicity scale. J Clin Oncol 2012;30:2408–17.
94. Bleomycin for injection, USP [package insert]. Irvine (CA): Teva Parenteral Medicines, Inc.; 2007.

95. Fyfe AJ, McKay P. Toxicities associated with bleomycin. J R Coll Physicians Edinb 2010;40:213–5.
96. Abid SH, Malhotra V, Perry MC. Radiation-induced and chemotherapy-induced pulmonary injury. Curr Opin Oncol 2001;13:242–8.
97. Gefitinib tablets [package insert]. Wilmington (DE): AstraZeneca UK Limited for AstraZeneca Pharmaceuticals LP; 2010.
98. Gemtuzumab ozogamicin for injection [package insert]. Philadelphia: Wyeth Pharmaceuticals Inc.; 2005.
99. De Sanctis A, Taillade L, Vignot S, et al. Pulmonary toxicity related to systemic treatment of nonsmall cell lung cancer. Cancer 2011;117:3069–80.
100. Limper AH. Chemotherapy-induced lung disease. Clin Chest Med 2004;25: 53–64.
101. Wright J, Feld R, Knox J. Chemotherapy-induced oral mucositis: new approaches to prevention and management. Expert Opin Drug Saf 2005;4:193–200.
102. Mitchell EP. Gastrointestinal toxicity of chemotherapeutic agents. Semin Oncol 2006;33:106–20.
103. Inrhaoun H, Kullman T, Elghissassi I, et al. Treatment of chemotherapy-induced nausea and vomiting. J Gastrointest Cancer 2012;43:541–6.
104. Kris MG, Hesketh PJ, Somerfield MR, et al. American society of clinical oncology guideline for antiemetics in oncology: update 2006. J Clin Oncol 2006;24:2932–47.
105. Richardson G, Dobish R. Chemotherapy induced diarrhea. J Oncol Pharm Pract 2007;13:181–98.
106. Gibson RJ, Stringer AM. Chemotherapy-induced diarrhea. Curr Opin Support Palliat Care 2009;3:31–5.
107. King PD, Perry MC. Hepatotoxicity of chemotherapy. Oncologist 2001;6:162–76.
108. Docetaxel injection concentrate [package insert]. Bridgewater (NJ): Sanofi-Aventis U.S., LLC; 2013.
109. Robinson K, Lambiase L, Li J, et al. Fatal cholestatic liver failure associated with gemcitabine therapy. Dig Dis Sci 2003;48:1804–8.
110. Keefe DM, Gibson RJ, Hauer-Jensen M. Gastrointestinal mucositis. Semin Oncol Nurs 2004;20:38–47.
111. Keefe DM, Schubert MM, Elting LS, et al. Updated clinical practice guidelines for the prevention and treatment of mucositis. Cancer 2007;109:820–31.
112. Gibson RJ, Keefe DM, Lalla RV, et al. Systematic review of agents for the management of gastrointestinal mucositis in cancer patients. Support Care Cancer 2013;21:313–26.
113. National Cancer Institute. Oral mucositis. Available at: http://www.cancer.gov/cancertopics/pdq/supportivecare/oralcomplications/HealthProfessional/page5#Reference5.17. Accessed May 10, 2013.
114. U.S. Food and Drug Administration (FDA). Palifermin. Available at: http://www.fda.gov/Drugs/DrugSafety/PostmarketDrugSafetyInformationforPatientsandProviders/ucm110263.htm. Accessed May 10, 2013.
115. Sartori S, Trevisani L, Nielsen I, et al. Randomized trial of omeprazole or ranitidine versus placebo in the prevention of chemotherapy-induced gastroduodenal injury. J Clin Oncol 2000;18:463–7.
116. Grunberg S. Patient-centered management of chemotherapy-induced nausea and vomiting. Cancer Control 2012;19:10–5.
117. Basch E, Prestrud AA, Hesketh PJ. Antiemetics: American Society of Clinical Oncology clinical practice guideline update. J Clin Oncol 2011;29:4189–98.
118. Benson AB, Ajani JA, Catalano RB, et al. Recommended guidelines for the treatment of cancer-treatment induced diarrhea. J Clin Oncol 2004;22:2918–26.

119. Gatti A, Sabato AF. Management of opioid-induced constipation in cancer patients: focus on methylnaltrexone. Clin Drug Investig 2012;32:293–301.
120. Hanly L, Chen N, Rieder M, et al. Ifosfamide nephrotoxicity in children: a mechanistic base of pharmacological intervention. Expert Opin Drug Saf 2009;8:155–68.
121. Perazella MA, Moeckel GW. Nephrotoxicity from chemotherapeutic agents: clinical manifestations, pathobiology, and prevention/therapy. Semin Nephrol 2010;30:570–81.
122. Kintzel PE. Anticancer drug-induced kidney disorders. Drug Saf 2001;24:19–38.
123. Saif MW, McGee PJ. Hemolytic-uremic syndrome associated with gemcitabine: a case report and review of the literature. JOP 2005;6:369–74.
124. D'Elia JA, Aslani M, Schermer S, et al. Hemolytic-uremic syndrome and acute renal failure in metastatic adenocarcinoma treated with mitomycin: case report and literature review. Ren Fail 1987;10:107–13.
125. Santini V. Amifostine: chemotherapeutic and radiotherapeutic protective effects. Expert Opin Pharmacother 2001;2:479–89.
126. Korkmaz A, Topal T, Oter S. Pathophysiological aspects of cyclophosphamide and ifosfamide induced hemorrhagic cystitis; implication of reactive oxygen species and nitrogen species as well as PARP activation. Cell Biol Toxicol 2007;23:303–12.
127. Chlorambucil tablets [package insert]. Research Triangle Park (NC): Heumann Pharma GmbH for GlaxoSmithKline LLC; 2004.
128. Oxaliplatin for injection [package insert]. Bridgewater (NJ): Ben Venue Laboratories for Sanofi-Aventis U.S. LLC; 2009.
129. Huang V, Anadkat M. Dermatologic manifestations of cytotoxic therapy. Dermatol Ther 2011;24:401–10.
130. Panitumumab injection for intravenous infusion [package insert]. Thousand Oaks (CA): Amgen Inc.; 2013.
131. Wang RY. Special considerations: extravasation of xenobiotics. In: Nelson LS, Lewin NA, Howland MA, et al, editors. Goldfrank's toxicologic emergencies. 9th edition. New York: McGraw-Hill; 2011. p. 793–5.
132. Mechlorethamine hydrochloride powder for solution [package insert]. Deerfield (IL): Baxter Oncology GmbH for Lundbeck LLC; 2012.
133. Dexrazoxane for injection [package insert]. Bedford (OH): Ben Venue Laboratories for TopoTarget A/S; 2007.
134. Wang RY. Antineoplastics: methotrexate. In: Nelson LS, Lewin NA, Howland MA, et al, editors. Goldfrank's toxicologic emergencies. 9th edition. New York: McGraw-Hill; 2011. p. 778–82.
135. Widemann BC, Adamson PC. Understanding and managing methotrexate nephrotoxicity. Oncologist 2006;11:694–703.
136. Walker RW, Allen JC, Rosen G, et al. Transient cerebral dysfunction secondary to high-dose methotrexate. J Clin Oncol 1986;4:1845–50.
137. Chabner BA, Young RC. Threshold methotrexate concentration for in vivo inhibition of DNA synthesis in normal and tumorous target tissues. J Clin Invest 1973;52:1804–11.
138. Howland MA. Antidotes in depth. Leucovorin (folinic acid) and folic acid. In: Nelson LS, Lewin NA, Howland MA, et al, editors. Goldfrank's toxicologic emergencies. 9th edition. New York: McGraw-Hill; 2011. p. 783–6.
139. Leucovorin calcium injection, USP [package insert]. Bedford (OH): Ben Venue Labs Inc for Bedford Labs; 2008.

140. Bleyer WA. New vistas for leucovorin in cancer chemotherapy. Cancer 1989;63: 995–1007.
141. Meropol NJ, Creaven PJ, Petrelli N, et al. Seizures associated with leucovorin administration in cancer patients. J Natl Cancer Inst 1995;87:56–8.
142. Smith SW. Antidotes in depth: glucarpidase (Carboxypeptidase G_2). In: Nelson LS, Lewin NA, Howland MA, et al, editors. Goldfrank's toxicologic emergencies. 9th edition. New York: McGraw-Hill; 2011. p. 787–92.
143. US FDA. Voraxaze. FDA; 2012. Available at: http://www.accessdata.fda.gov/drugsatfda_docs/label/2012/125327lbl.pdf. Accessed June 12, 2013.
144. BC Cancer Agency. Plicamycin (Mithramycin). BCCA Cancer Drug Manual. Vancouver: BC Cancer Agency; 1994. p. 591–600. Available at: http://hemonc.org/docs/packageinsert/plicamycin.pdf. Accessed September 20, 2013.

Central Nervous System Toxicity

Anne-Michelle Ruha, MD[a],*, Michael Levine, MD[b,c]

KEYWORDS

- Agitated delirium • Altered mental status • CNS toxicity • CNS depression
- Drug-induced seizures

KEY POINTS

- Central nervous system (CNS) toxicity may manifest as a depressed level of consciousness, agitation, confusion, seizures, or psychosis; each existing along a spectrum, coexisting, or waxing and waning.
- History may be valuable in elucidating the cause of CNS toxicity but can often be misleading; the clinician must maintain skepticism when considering the history and place at least equal emphasis on physical findings when determining the cause of illness and managing patients.
- Identification of toxidromes, when present, or smaller constellations of physical and electrocardiographic findings may allow the identification of a toxicant or class of toxicants, aiding in management.
- Patients for whom there is any concern for nonconvulsive status epilepticus, such as those with a prolonged period of unconsciousness following a generalized seizure, sudden unexpected deterioration in level of consciousness, or motor activity of unclear significance, may benefit from electroencephalogram evaluation.

INTRODUCTION

Central nervous system (CNS) toxicity may result from exposure to a vast array of xenobiotics. The term *xenobiotic* describes any substance that is foreign to the human body. Sources of exposure may be medicinal, recreational, environmental, or occupational; the means of exposure may be intentional or unintentional. Whether toxic effects result from an exposure depends on the dose to which one is exposed. However, other factors may influence the development of toxicity, such as chronicity of exposure, the pharmacokinetics of the particular agent, genetic polymorphisms that may influence the pharmacokinetics, and concomitant exposure to other toxicants.

---

[a] Department of Medical Toxicology, Banner Good Samaritan Medical Center, Center for Toxicology and Pharmacology Education and Research, University of Arizona College of Medicine, 925 East McDowell Road, Phoenix, AZ 85006, USA; [b] Section of Medical Toxicology, Department of Emergency Medicine, University of Southern California, 1200 North State Street, Los Angeles, CA 90033, USA; [c] Department of Medical Toxicology, Banner Good Samaritan Medical Center, 925 East McDowell Road, Phoenix, AZ 85006, USA
* Corresponding author.
E-mail address: Michelle.ruha@bannerhealth.com

Emerg Med Clin N Am 32 (2014) 205–221
http://dx.doi.org/10.1016/j.emc.2013.09.004
0733-8627/14/$ – see front matter © 2014 Elsevier Inc. All rights reserved.

Clinical manifestations of CNS toxicity are diverse. Patients may present with CNS depression, agitation, confusion, psychosis, or seizures. *Altered mental status* is a vague term that is often used to describe disturbances in consciousness. Xenobiotic toxicity may manifest as altered thought content, resulting in psychosis or confusion; may vary the level of arousal, resulting in agitation, lethargy, stupor, or coma; or may affect both elements of consciousness.[1]

The goal of this article is to provide a rational approach to the assessment, diagnosis, and management of patients presenting with CNS toxicity resulting from xenobiotic exposure. CNS toxicity is categorized as CNS depression, indicating a decrease in the level of alertness, and agitated delirium, indicating a state of restlessness or excitation with confusion. Seizures are considered separately. The focus is on the more common causes of CNS toxicity that emergency health care providers are most likely to encounter in their practice because a comprehensive list and description of toxicants is beyond the scope of this article.

PATIENT HISTORY

In assessing patients with potential CNS toxicity, the history is a valuable component of the evaluation. Occasionally, history alone can provide a diagnosis and allow anticipation of the clinical course. However, the history may be limited, unavailable, or, in some cases, misleading because patients, friends, families, and caregivers may erroneously misattribute symptoms to an inconsequential agent or cause. It is not unusual for patients to present with an empty pill bottle, which may have been used to store a completely different medication than that listed on the label. Thus, although it is important to gather as much information as possible from patients, families, friends, bystanders, and prehospital personnel, it is equally important to maintain a degree of skepticism and to place more value on physical examination findings if they are inconsistent with the history provided.

Box 1 lists the historical elements to consider when assessing patients with possible CNS toxicity. The clinician should inquire about symptoms observed before the health care presentation, such as hallucinations, seizures, or confusion. The timing of the symptom onset may differentiate an acute overdose (with sudden development of symptoms) from chronic toxicity resulting from the gradual increase of a drug concentration to a toxic range. The use of new medications, whether over the counter or prescription, might point toward a drug interaction. Recent discontinuation of medications might suggest a withdrawal syndrome. Information regarding the availability of nonpharmaceutical toxicants, such as ethylene glycol or methanol, in addition to medications and illicit substances should be sought. Potential environmental

---

Box 1
Important historical information

- Symptoms before health care presentation
- Timing of onset of symptoms (sudden, gradual)
- Recent initiation or discontinuation of medications
- Availability of pharmaceutical and nonpharmaceutical toxicants
- Number and type of pills present in available containers
- Medical history of patient, relatives, and housemates
- Review of systems (ie, recent illnesses or complaints, suicidality)

or occupational exposures should be investigated. If medication containers are available, a pill identification and count should be performed to determine if more pills are missing than expected. Pill counts are primarily helpful only if a disproportionate number of pills are missing compared with the expected number. The past medical history of patients and the family members living in the same household may reveal additional medications available to patients.

The clinician should also inquire as to the patients' recent state of health and available review of systems because the history of a recent illness should prompt consideration of an evaluation for an infectious cause of CNS symptoms. A history of recent suicidal statements might support intentional self-poisoning.

CLINICAL PRESENTATION

CNS toxicity can present in diverse forms. Often vaguely described as *altered mental status*, CNS toxicity can manifest as a depressed level of consciousness, agitation, confusion, or psychosis. Each of these may exist along a spectrum, may coexist, and may wax and wane.[1] The degree of CNS depression may range from mild drowsiness to deep coma; agitation may display as mild restlessness or as a life-threatening syndrome referred to as *excited delirium*. Confusion may be present with or without CNS depression or agitation and with or without psychosis. CNS toxicity may also manifest as seizures. First, a determination of whether the patients' CNS findings are more consistent with CNS depression or agitated delirium will allow the clinician to begin to narrow the potential causes of toxicity (**Table 1**).

In addition to neurologic signs, the presence or absence of other physical and electrocardiographic findings can help to further narrow the cause of CNS toxicity. For example, vital signs, pupil size, and the presence or absence of diaphoresis may suggest a particular toxidrome. If a consistent toxidrome cannot be identified, other

Table 1
Drugs affecting consciousness

Drug Class	CNS Depression	Agitated Delirium	Seizures
GABA receptor agonists	++	+	(+ Baclofen)
Opioid receptor agonists	++	(+Meperidine)	(+ Tramadol, propoxyphene, meperidine)
Central alpha$_2$ agonists	++	—	—
Antipsychotics	++	(+ If concurrent M$_1$ receptor antagonism)	+
Anticonvulsants	++	+	+
[a]Nonopioid analgesics	+	—	(+ Salicylate, NSAIDs)
Muscarinic receptor antagonists	+	++	+
Serotonergic agents	+	++	+
Sympathomimetic agents	—	++	+

Abbreviations: +, may produce this effect but less common; ++, primary feature of toxicity; GABA, gamma-aminobutyric acid; M$_1$, muscarinic; NSAIDs, nonsteroidal antiinflammatory drugs.
[a] Nonopioid analgesics: acetaminophen, NSAIDs, and salicylate. These analgesics may produce CNS depression when taken in very large doses.

combinations of clinical findings may allow the clinician to identify a mini-toxidrome, leading to a more refined toxicologic differential diagnosis. For example, the presence of CNS depression, miosis, and tachycardia might suggest toxicity caused by a sedating medication with alpha$_1$-adrenergic antagonist effects (**Table 2**).

CNS Depression

CNS depression generally results from enhanced inhibitory neurotransmission in the brain. This process may result from direct interaction of a xenobiotic with neuronal receptors or ion channels or from indirect influence of a xenobiotic on neurotransmission. The clinical presentation may range from mild drowsiness, from which a patient may be easily aroused, to deep coma, in some instances mimicking brain death. Patients between these extremes may exhibit slurred speech, ataxia, incoordination, and confusion.

Gamma-aminobutyric acid agonists

Gamma-aminobutyric acid (GABA) is the primary inhibitory neurotransmitter in the CNS, with action at specific GABA receptors. Numerous xenobiotics target the GABA$_A$ receptor, enhancing the effect of GABA and clinically producing the classic sedative-hypnotic toxidrome, characterized by CNS depression and sometimes respiratory depression. GABA$_A$ receptor agonists include the benzodiazepines; the nonbenzodiazepine "Z" drugs (zolpidem, zopiclone, zaleplon); the barbiturates; meprobamate (the metabolite of carisoprodol); ethanol; and anesthetic agents, such as etomidate and propofol. The degree of CNS depression associated with exposure to the GABA$_A$ agonists depends on the particular agent and dose to which patients were exposed. For example, an isolated overdose of benzodiazepines typically results in only mild or moderate CNS depression, whereas an overdose of phenobarbital is more likely to produce profound CNS depression with respiratory compromise and loss of airway protective reflexes. GABA$_A$ receptor agonist toxicity is typically limited to CNS effects, although patients may develop mild bradycardia, hypotension, and hypothermia. Occasionally, patients exhibit agitated delirium in addition to, or alternating with, CNS depression. This result is a well-described effect of benzodiazepines, which sometimes produces paradoxic agitation, especially in children.[2]

Table 2 Mini-toxidromes		
Toxidromes	**Symptoms and Signs**	**Examples**
Alpha$_1$ antagonists	CNS depression, tachycardia, miosis	Chlorpromazine, quetiapine, clozapine, olanzapine, risperidone
Alpha$_2$ agonist	CNS depression, bradycardia, hypertension (early), hypotension (late), miosis	Clonidine, oxymetazoline, tetrahydrozoline, tizanidine
Clonus/myoclonus	CNS depression, myoclonic jerks, clonus, hyperreflexia	Carisoprodol, lithium, serotonergic agents, bismuth, organic lead, organic mercury
Sodium channel blockers	CNS toxicity, wide QRS	Cyclic antidepressants and structurally related agents, propoxyphene, quinidine/quinine, amantadine, antihistamines, bupropion, cocaine
Potassium channel blockers	CNS toxicity, long QT	Butyrophenones, methadone, phenothiazines, ziprasidone

Baclofen and gamma hydroxybutyrate (GHB) produce CNS depression via agonism at the GABA$_B$ receptor. Baclofen toxicity may result in a deep coma, which has been reported in some cases to mimic brain death.[3] In addition to CNS depression, patients with baclofen intoxication may also exhibit paradoxic seizures, hyperreflexia, clonus, cardiac dysrhythmias, bradycardia, and hypothermia.[4] GHB toxicity, although potentially severe enough to require life-supporting measures, tends to be short lived, with patients rousing from the coma within several hours of exposure. Emergence from the coma may be almost instantaneous, as compared with the gradual emergence typically seen with toxicity caused by other GABA agonists.

Opioid receptor agonists

Agonists at mu opioid receptors include natural alkaloids found in the poppy plant, such as morphine and codeine, as well as a large number of semisynthetic (eg, heroin, oxycodone, and buprenorphine) and synthetic chemicals (eg, methadone, fentanyl, and meperidine). Clinically, mu opioid receptor agonism by these agents, collectively described as opioids, produces the classic opioid toxidrome, consisting of CNS depression, respiratory depression, and miosis. These effects can be fully reversed by the administration of the mu opioid antagonist naloxone. Some opioids also act at additional receptors or ion channels, producing physical or electrocardiographic findings that can provide clues to which particular opioid patients were exposed. Methadone, for example, may block cardiac potassium channels, lengthening the QT interval and predisposing patients to torsades des pointes. Meperidine possesses anticholinergic activity, which may result in delirium. Tramadol, meperidine, and propoxyphene can all cause seizures. As with the GABA agonists, opioid agonist toxicity may result in mild bradycardia, hypotension, and hypothermia.

Central alpha$_2$-adrenergic agonists

Drugs that stimulate presynaptic alpha$_2$-adrenergic receptors in the brain inhibit the release of norepinephrine into neuronal synapses, ultimately increasing inhibitory neurotransmission. Examples of such agents include clonidine, tizanidine, guanfacine, and the parenterally administered dexmedetomidine. Toxicity mimics that produced by opioid receptor agonists, with CNS depression accompanied by miosis and, occasionally, respiratory depression. The effects that may distinguish central alpha$_2$ agonist toxicity from that caused by opioids include pronounced bradycardia and hypotension. However, in the event of a massive overdose of clonidine, such as might occur with a compounding error of a liquid formulation or an intrathecal pump malfunction, early hypertension may develop.[5,6] Unlike toxicity caused by opioids, central alpha$_2$ agonist effects are generally not reversed with the administration of naloxone, although a segment of the population may demonstrate improvement.

Antipsychotics

All antipsychotic medications may produce CNS depression in overdose. Antipsychotics are generally divided into a class of older typical agents, which have strong D$_2$ dopamine receptor antagonism, and newer atypical agents, which may antagonize D$_2$ receptors but have stronger binding properties at 5HT$_{2A}$ serotonin receptors. The typical antipsychotics include the butyrophenones (droperidol and haloperidol) and the phenothiazines, of which chlorpromazine, trifluoperazine, and fluphenazine are still in frequent use. Promethazine and prochlorperazine are phenothiazines that are often administered for their antiemetic effect. Atypical antipsychotic agents include clozapine, olanzapine, quetiapine, risperidone, ziprasidone, and others. With both classes of medications, CNS depression is dose dependent. These agents also possess activity at multiple other receptors and ion channels, which impart additional clinical effects.[7]

Cardiovascular effects are not uncommon following antipsychotic overdose. Some agents, including the phenothiazines, block sodium channels in the heart, leading to widening of the QRS interval on electrocardiogram (ECG) and predisposing to ventricular dysrhythmias. Many phenothiazines, as well as the butyrophenones, inhibit efflux of potassium through the delayed rectifier channel (K_{IR}), lengthening the QT interval on the ECG, and placing patients at risk for torsades des pointes. An additional property of some antipsychotics is alpha$_1$-adrenergic receptor antagonism, which leads to miosis, vasodilation, and reflex tachycardia. Hypotension may also occur.

Some antipsychotics, including chlorpromazine, clozapine, olanzapine, and quetiapine, antagonize muscarinic receptors. As a result, the anticholinergic effect of agitated delirium may predominate over CNS depression. However, in large overdoses, coma is still likely. In addition to muscarinic receptor antagonism, chlorpromazine and quetiapine also antagonize alpha$_1$-adrenergic receptors, which leads to miosis despite the presence of anticholinergic findings. Risperidone and ziprasidone also possess alpha$_1$-antagonist properties and produce miosis but lack antimuscarinic activity.

Lithium is commonly used in the management of bipolar disorder. CNS depression may occur in the setting of both acute and chronic intoxication with lithium. Typically, patients who acutely overdose on lithium develop gastrointestinal symptoms before the onset of neurotoxic effects. Neurotoxic signs may develop as CNS concentrations of lithium increase over time and include CNS depression, confusion, dysarthria, tremor, hyperreflexia, clonus, and seizures. Patients who develop lithium toxicity as a result of chronic use often develop CNS toxicity without prominent gastrointestinal symptoms.

All antipsychotics lower the seizure threshold. Although seizures may occur following exposure to these agents, they are not a common feature of most antipsychotic overdoses.

Anticonvulsants

Anticonvulsant medications act through various mechanisms to decrease excitatory neurotransmission and prevent seizures. Overdose of these agents often leads to CNS depression. Sedation is dose-dependent, but some agents, such as levetiracetam and gabapentin, have a wide therapeutic margin and are less likely to cause coma, even when taken in large overdose.[8,9] Significant CNS depression is a frequent event following acute or chronic exposure to many anticonvulsant medications. Phenytoin, carbamazepine, and valproic acid, for example, cause confusion, dysarthria, and coma at toxic concentrations. Patients with phenytoin or carbamazepine toxicity also frequently display cerebellar ataxia and nystagmus.

Although not a feature of phenytoin toxicity, many anticonvulsants produce seizures in overdose. Carbamazepine, lamotrigine, topiramate, and tiagabine are all associated with seizures, even in the absence of a baseline seizure disorder.

Carbamazepine possesses a structure analogous to that of cyclic antidepressants and, similar to those drugs, can produce both muscarinic receptor and sodium channel blocking effects. Tachycardia, anticholinergic delirium, and, in severe cases, widening of the QRS interval and cardiac dysrhythmias may all occur following carbamazepine overdose. Lamotrigine overdose may also produce sodium channel blockade with cardiac dysrhythmias.

Other anticonvulsants that produce unique clinical findings following overdose include topiramate, which causes a nonanion gap acidosis through the inhibition of carbonic anhydrase, and valproic acid, which is associated with hyperammonemia. CNS depression may result from valproic acid–associated hyperammonemia even when the serum concentration of valproic acid is therapeutic.

Nonopioid analgesics

Severe salicylate intoxication produces confusion, lethargy, and, ultimately, coma and seizures leading up to death. Patients with acute salicylate poisoning, who present early, will exhibit respiratory alkalosis, metabolic acidosis, tachycardia, diaphoresis, and tinnitus (or decreased hearing) before developing confusion and/or CNS depression. Patients with chronic salicylate toxicity are often older and present with the complaint of confusion or altered mental status.

Massive overdose of ibuprofen and acetaminophen may produce CNS depression. Coma may result following extremely large overdoses of ibuprofen and, when it occurs, is associated with metabolic acidosis.[10] Acetaminophen overdose may produce CNS toxicity in two circumstances. The first, and most common, is when acetaminophen-induced liver injury has progressed to hepatic failure and attendant hepatic encephalopathy. In such cases, patients present with elevated liver enzymes, coagulopathy, confusion, and CNS depression. Acetaminophen may be undetectable by the time encephalopathy develops. The second circumstance is when patients ingest a massive overdose of acetaminophen and present early following the ingestion. Acetaminophen levels are often very high (>500 mg/L), and metabolic acidosis is present. The mechanism for CNS depression in this setting is unknown.[11,12]

Marijuana is legal in many states as a treatment of pain and other conditions. Pediatric exposure to tetrahydrocannabinol in hashish, plant parts, or *Cannabis* edibles, such as candies and baked goods, may lead to CNS depression.[13,14]

Nonpharmaceutical agents

Numerous nonpharmaceutical agents can produce CNS toxicity. Ingestion of toxic alcohols, some pesticides, solvents, and essential oils may lead to varying degrees of CNS depression. Inhalation of gasses, including carbon monoxide, cyanide, and hydrogen sulfide, may produce CNS toxicity, ranging from agitation to CNS depression to coma. Exposure to several metals can result in CNS toxicity. The CNS effects of lead toxicity include seizure, encephalopathy, coma, or cerebral edema. Excessive exposure to mercury can produce insomnia, shyness, irritability, hallucinations, seizure, and movement disorders.

Agitated Delirium

Toxin-induced alterations in consciousness may manifest as agitation, which can range from mild anxiety or restlessness to severe agitation with combative behavior. Agitation may coexist or alternate with CNS depression. Patients with agitated delirium may be hallucinating, paranoid, and unable to remain still. Restless and agitated behavior places patients and health care staff at risk of harm and often requires control with chemical and physical restraints. The most severe manifestation of agitated delirium has been coined *excited delirium syndrome*.[15,16] In addition to extreme agitation and confusion, patients with excited delirium syndrome may exhibit diaphoresis, tachycardia, hypertension, hyperthermia, tachypnea, and pain tolerance. Patients are at risk for sudden cardiovascular failure, including cardiac arrest.

Muscarinic receptor antagonists

There are hundreds of xenobiotics that antagonize muscarinic receptors in the brain producing anticholinergic delirium. Examples of medications with strong antimuscarinic properties include the cyclic antidepressants and structurally related drugs (eg, cyclobenzaprine and carbamazepine), first-generation H_1 histamine receptor antagonists (eg, diphenhydramine, doxylamine), phenothiazines, several atypical antipsychotic agents, and the belladonna alkaloids (atropine and scopolamine). Patients who develop toxicity from these agents may exhibit delirium absent peripheral anticholinergic findings, termed *central* anticholinergic toxicity. More commonly, a constellation of peripheral antimuscarinic effects will be present, which may include tachycardia, flushing, mydriasis, decreased bowel motility, elevated body temperature, urinary retention, and impaired ability to sweat. The presence of peripheral findings on physical examination points toward an anticholinergic cause of delirium.

Atropine and scopolamine, which may be pharmaceutical or derived from plant species, such as *Datura* or *Brugmansia,* are pure muscarinic antagonists. Seeds or teas made from the leaves of these plants may be ingested for recreational purposes. Unlike these pure antimuscarinics, most muscarinic antagonists also act at additional receptors and ion channels. The resultant clinical findings can aid in the identification of the particular drug or drug class responsible for the presentation.

Cyclic antidepressants, including amitriptyline, nortriptyline, doxepin, clomipramine, and imipramine, all antagonize muscarinic receptors but also possess several other receptor and ion channel affinities. Perhaps the most important is the inhibition of sodium channels, which results in widening of the QRS interval on ECG and, when severe, ventricular dysrhythmias. Cyclic antidepressants may also prolong the QT interval via inhibition of potassium efflux in the heart and may antagonize alpha$_1$-adrenergic receptors, which may contribute to hypotension. Other effects include the inhibition of neuronal reuptake of norepinephrine and serotonin and, possibly, inhibition of GABA. Depending on the ingested dose, patients with cyclic antidepressant toxicity may exhibit mild CNS depression alone or severe CNS and cardiovascular effects, including wide-complex dysrhythmias and seizures. Amoxapine is especially recognized for producing seizures in overdose.

Serotonergic agents

CNS toxicity may result from excessive serotonergic activity in the brain. Medications that increase synaptic concentrations of serotonin, or otherwise lead to increased stimulation of $5HT_{2A}$ serotonin receptors, may predispose to serotonin syndrome. Serotonin toxicity may occur through the interaction of multiple serotonergic medications or following a large exposure to a single serotonergic agent. Symptoms of serotonin excess may include dizziness, anxiety and agitation, nausea, vomiting, diarrhea, and lethargy. As toxicity worsens, patients may develop serotonin syndrome, which involves altered levels of consciousness; autonomic hyperactivity, with associated tachycardia, hypertension, diaphoresis, and fever; and neuromuscular excitation, manifested by shivering, tremor, myoclonus, hyperreflexia, and clonus. In the most severe cases, patients exhibit coma, muscle rigidity, and life-threatening hyperthermia.[17] Hyperreflexia, rigidity, and clonus are often more pronounced in the lower extremities. This effect may help to distinguish the syndrome from neuroleptic malignant syndrome, from which it may be clinically indistinguishable, but is caused by decreased dopaminergic activity rather than excess serotonergic tone.

The selective serotonin reuptake inhibitors (SSRIs) and serotonin norepinephrine reuptake inhibitors (SNRIs) are the most abundant serotonergic agents in use today. SSRIs, including citalopram, escitalopram, sertraline, fluoxetine, and paroxetine, increase serotonin concentrations at neuronal synapses by inhibiting the serotonin reuptake transporter on presynaptic neuronal membranes. The SNRIs also inhibit reuptake and increase concentrations of synaptic norepinephrine. Most overdoses of SSRIs do not result in significant toxicity, but occasionally patients exhibit mild

CNS depression with tachycardia or gastrointestinal effects. Rarely, serotonin syndrome develops. Citalopram and escitalopram are unique among the SSRIs in that they are also associated with prolongation of the QT interval on ECG and seizures. The SNRIs are more likely to produce serious toxicity in overdose. Venlafaxine toxicity is associated with CNS depression, seizures, and cardiac effects, potentially prolonging both the QRS and the QT intervals on ECG and leading to cardiac dysrhythmias. Duloxetine toxicity is also likely to produce seizures.[17]

Other antidepressants that have serotonergic activity include the atypical antidepressants (trazodone and mirtazapine) and the monoamine oxidase inhibitors (MAOIs). Trazodone also possesses alpha$_1$-adrenergic receptor antagonist activity; patients may present with orthostatic hypotension. Mirtazapine toxicity is mainly limited to CNS depression and tachycardia.[18] The MAOIs have largely been replaced by newer antidepressants; but some drugs, such as phenelzine and tranylcypromine, are still prescribed. At therapeutic doses, MAOIs may interact with other serotonergic agents to produce serotonin syndrome. MAOI overdose may also cause severe CNS toxicity. Patients may have an extended asymptomatic period following MAOI overdose. However, for up to 24 hours they are at risk to develop agitation or CNS depression, which may progress to coma. Severe toxicity is also associated with myoclonus, hyperreflexia, rigidity, hyperthermia, and cardiovascular collapse. A particular ocular finding described with MAOI toxicity is a slow alternating movement of the eyes, the ping pong gaze.[19]

Non-antidepressant medications with serotonergic activity may interact with antidepressants to produce serotonin syndrome. Some of these include meperidine, dextromethorphan, linezolid, and tramadol. Drugs of abuse, such as amphetamines and their derivatives and cocaine, may contribute to serotonin excess.

Sympathomimetic agents

Xenobiotics that increase stimulation of alpha- and beta-adrenergic receptors are considered to be sympathomimetic. Although some drugs directly stimulate receptors (eg, norepinephrine and epinephrine), most xenobiotics increase the concentrations of norepinephrine available to agonize the receptor. Increased stimulation leads to the sympathomimetic toxidrome, which is characterized by CNS excitation, tachycardia, hypertension, diaphoresis, and mydriasis. Sympathomimetic agents often increase synaptic concentrations of dopamine and serotonin in addition to norepinephrine. Depending on the agent and dose to which patients were exposed, CNS symptoms may be limited to anxiety, restlessness, or psychosis. However, severe agitation, combative behavior, and seizures are common manifestations of sympathomimetic toxicity; lethal excited delirium syndrome has been associated with the recreational use of a variety of sympathomimetic agents. Rhabdomyolysis is a common secondary effect of sympathomimetic toxicity.

Amphetamine and its many derivatives, which possess a phenylethylamine backbone, are widely available as treatments for attention-deficit/hyperactivity disorder, narcolepsy, and as illicit drugs of abuse. In addition to the clinical effects resulting from stimulation of alpha- and beta-adrenergic receptors, signs of dopaminergic excess are commonly seen in the setting of toxicity. Patients may exhibit paranoia, repetitive behaviors, and choreoathetoid movements. Cardiac dysrhythmias may occur but are uncommon.

Cocaine toxicity may present very similarly to that caused by amphetamines. However, unlike amphetamines, cocaine inhibits cardiac sodium and potassium channels, which may result in wide-complex dysrhythmias and torsades des pointes. Seizures are also more common with cocaine toxicity.

Seizures

Many xenobiotics that produce CNS toxicity, whether in the form of CNS depression or CNS excitation, may lower the seizure threshold and are, to some degree, associated with seizures following overdose. Notable exceptions are the benzodiazepine and barbiturate classes of $GABA_A$ agonists, which increase inhibitory neurotransmission and are used to treat drug-induced seizures.

Xenobiotics can lead to seizures through a variety of interactions with neurons and neurotransmitter systems. As a result of these interactions, the balance between excitatory and inhibitory neurotransmission is altered. Xenobiotic-induced seizures are often generalized, occur within a few hours of overdose, and last only a few minutes. However, depending on the agent, dose, and, possibly, genetic factors, status epilepticus sometimes occurs. A significant concern is the potential for xenobiotic overdose to produce nonconvulsive status epilepticus. In such cases, patients do not demonstrate clinical evidence of seizure activity but do exhibit altered mental status. Epileptic activity is observed on electroencephalogram (EEG).[4,20]

Although many of the drugs previously discussed have the potential to produce seizures as part of their toxicity profile, there are particular xenobiotics and drug classes for which seizures are a primary feature of toxicity. Some of these are discussed later. There are many other agents that may produce seizures but that are less frequently encountered in the emergency department and are not included in this discussion. Some important ones for clinicians to be aware of include benzonatate, which is used to suppress cough, but may be fatal in exposed children, and camphor, which continues to be available in high concentrations as a cultural remedy.[21,22]

Bupropion

Bupropion is unique among the atypical antidepressants in that it inhibits the presynaptic reuptake of dopamine and norepinephrine but does not seem to inhibit serotonin reuptake. At therapeutic doses, bupropion is associated with seizures; patients with bupropion overdose are at a high risk for developing seizures. The seizure onset may be delayed up to 24 hours following ingestion of sustained-release preparations. Status epilepticus has been reported.[23] Other findings associated with bupropion toxicity include tachycardia, tremor, anxiety, and hallucinations.[24]

Isoniazid

Isoniazid is well known for producing seizures that are refractory to GABA agonists because isoniazid causes a functional pyridoxine deficiency. Because pyridoxine is an important cofactor in the metabolism of GABA, a GABA deficiency results, leading to the loss of GABA inhibitory neurotransmission and seizures.[25] In addition to seizures, patients with isoniazid overdose frequently develop coma and metabolic acidosis.[26] Seizures have also been reported following therapeutic use of isoniazid as have neuropsychiatric symptoms.[27]

Methylxanthines

Caffeine and theophylline antagonize adenosine receptors. Adenosine functions as an anticonvulsant in the brain; thus, adenosine antagonism leads to increased excitatory neurotransmission and seizures.[28] Overdose of the methylxanthines is associated with vomiting, tachycardia, acidosis, cardiac dysrhythmias, seizures, and death. Especially in the setting of theophylline toxicity, but also after large caffeine overdoses, seizures may be recurrent and status epilepticus may occur.[29,30]

Tramadol

Tramadol is classified as an opioid medication because of its agonist properties at the mu receptor, but it also inhibits serotonin and norepinephrine reuptake. Seizures are associated with both therapeutic use and toxicity caused by acute and chronic overdose.[24,31] Seizures may be recurrent. Other findings associated with toxicity include vomiting, CNS depression, and serotonin syndrome.

DIAGNOSTIC TESTING

In patients who present with an exposure history to a known toxicant, display CNS alterations consistent with the exposure, and who do not exhibit additional symptoms or findings, imaging and invasive diagnostic testing may not be warranted. For example, a child who is somnolent following a witnessed ingestion of a benzodiazepine or an adult who exhibits complete reversal of CNS depression following the administration of naloxone and admits to unintentional overdose of heroin do not warrant further diagnostic testing. However, most presentations are not this straightforward; in most situations when xenobiotic-induced CNS toxicity is a concern, further diagnostic testing is indicated.

Laboratory Analysis

Blood

When patients present with evidence of, or concern for, the development of CNS toxicity, routine laboratory testing can provide useful information. Although routine blood tests rarely provide direct evidence of CNS toxicity, information gained from both normal and abnormal laboratory values may help to identify a cause of CNS toxicity and guide management. Blood work should include a complete blood count, electrolytes, renal and liver function studies, and a creatinine phosphokinase. A prothrombin time may also be helpful if there is concern for anticoagulant exposure, acetaminophen toxicity, disseminated intravascular coagulation, or impaired hepatic function. Leukocytosis may suggest an infectious cause of symptoms or secondary infection, such as aspiration pneumonia, but is nonspecific and often encountered in patients who are agitated or who present after a seizure. Metabolic acidosis may suggest a recent seizure or indicate exposure to specific toxicants, such as toxic alcohols. Rhabdomyolysis may support a prolonged period of unconsciousness or, alternatively, agitation.

In patients for whom there is any concern for medication overdose or overuse, a serum acetaminophen concentration is recommended. Measurement of a salicylate concentration is also recommended because this is a potentially life-threatening cause of CNS toxicity. Specific drug concentrations can be very useful when available with a rapid turn-around time. For instance, lithium, phenytoin, carbamazepine, and valproic acid serum concentrations can be measured in many hospital laboratories and allow toxicity to be eliminated or further considered as a cause for CNS effects. If there is a concern for environmental lead exposure, a blood lead level should be obtained. For most xenobiotics, concentrations are not available rapidly enough to aid in acute management decisions. Depending on the situation, it may be worthwhile to send blood to specialty laboratories for measurement of specific drug concentrations in order to confirm or identify a cause of illness in retrospect.

Urine

Urine drug screen (UDS) immunoassays are widely available and have a relatively rapid turn-around time. They might be useful in the emergent setting by allowing the clinician to confirm or exclude the presence of certain drugs in the urine (more than a predetermined cutoff concentration). However, UDS testing does not confirm toxicity. A positive result may not represent the proximate cause of the presenting clinical condition; measured metabolites may demonstrate urinary persistence for days to weeks, depending on the substance and usage patterns, which limits the UDS utility in most cases. In addition, many false-positive and false-negative results can create significant confusion (particularly for opioids, benzodiazepines, other sedative-hypnotics, and amphetamines). False-positive results are especially common with the tricyclic antidepressant screen, which can be triggered by structurally related agents, such as diphenhydramine, cyclobenzaprine, carbamazepine, and quetiapine.[32,33]

Immunoassays detect a limited number of drugs and drug classes. If the identification of the specific agent responsible for a positive result on immunoassay or the identification of other xenobiotics present in urine is important for the diagnosis and care of patients, gas chromatography-mass spectrometry (GCMS) of urine can be performed. Very few hospital laboratories have this capability. Depending on the specific case, the confirmation or identification of intoxicants may be helpful, even in retrospect. In such cases, urine may be sent to a specialized laboratory for GCMS analysis.[33]

ECG

An ECG should be obtained in any patients with evidence of drug intoxication. The presence or absence of rate or rhythm disturbances can narrow the class of toxicant to which patients were exposed. Prolongation of the QRS and QT intervals provides evidence of exposure to medications with sodium channel or potassium channel blocking properties.

Radiology

If CNS depression is accompanied by respiratory depression or distress, a chest radiograph should be obtained to assess for aspiration or other pathologic conditions. A computed tomography (CT) scan of the head/brain is not routinely indicated in the assessment of CNS toxicity, unless diagnosis of toxicity is uncertain or there are findings on physical examination that are concerning for intracranial pathology, such as focal neurologic deficits or evidence of trauma. Routine head/brain CTs increase cost, prolong time spent in the emergency department, and subject patients to the risk of an adverse event occurrence during the transfer to radiology.[34]

EEG

Most drug-induced or drug withdrawal–induced seizures are self-limited or resolve easily with treatment and do not require an evaluation with EEG. However, occasionally it is unclear whether patients are experiencing seizures. Although clear-cut guidelines for when to obtain emergent EEG do not exist, it seems reasonable to obtain an EEG in such circumstances. Patients for whom there is any concern for nonconvulsive status epilepticus, such as those with a prolonged period of unconsciousness following a generalized seizure, sudden unexpected deterioration in level of consciousness, or motor activity of unclear significance, may benefit from an EEG evaluation.[35,36]

DIFFERENTIAL DIAGNOSIS

The differential diagnosis of CNS toxicity includes hypoglycemia, hypoxia, infection, trauma, endocrine disorders, electrolyte disturbances, and additional causes. Hypoglycemia should be ruled out immediately in every patient presenting with altered mental status. If hypoglycemia is present, toxicity from drugs, such as sulfonylureas, insulin, ethanol, and beta-adrenergic antagonists, must be considered. In patients who have experienced hypoperfusion or poor oxygenation, whether or not as a result of drug intoxication, hypoxic injury may be present and contribute to ongoing CNS depression. Evidence of infection must be investigated and treated, even if toxicity is also suspected. Any suspicion for trauma should also be appropriately investigated. Selected endocrinopathies, such as severe alterations in thyroid function (eg, myxedema coma and thyroid storm) may also require evaluation and treatment. Because several toxins and medical conditions may cause disturbances in fluids and electrolytes, these should be pursued.

MANAGEMENT

All patients who present with a history or findings concerning for drug toxicity should have an intravenous access obtained and be placed on a cardiac monitor. Any evidence of airway compromise mandates a definitive airway (ie, endotracheal intubation). Hypotension is initially treated with intravenous fluid resuscitation, followed by vasopressors if the blood pressure does not improve with 1 to 2 L of fluid. A good first choice of vasopressor in the setting of CNS toxicity is norepinephrine because many CNS intoxicants also antagonize $alpha_1$-adrenergic receptors. If hypotension is caused by central $alpha_2$ agonist toxicity, dopamine is a reasonable alternative. Hypoglycemia necessitates intravenous dextrose (0.5 - 1 g/kg). If QRS prolongation is noted on ECG, then boluses of intravenous sodium bicarbonate (1–2 mEq/kg) should be provided, along with consideration for a subsequent intravenous infusion. The remainder of care is largely supportive, with attention to other organ system toxicities that may directly result from the toxic exposure or develop as an indirect consequence of the exposure, such as aspiration pneumonitis and rhabdomyolysis. If the presentation is early after overdose, a dose of activated charcoal may be given, provided that the patients are able and willing to drink it and are not already exhibiting or anticipated to soon manifest CNS toxicity, which would place them at an increased risk for aspiration. Patients at risk for or suspected to have a deficiency of thiamine (vitamin B_1) should receive it in order to preclude Wernicke-Korsakoff syndrome.

CNS Depression

Patients presenting with a depressed level of consciousness are often also at risk for the development of respiratory depression and should have their airway protected if indicated. If CNS depression is the only physical examination finding, patients can often be observed clinically for improvement or deterioration. The time to resolution of symptoms will vary depending on the specific agent and dose ingested, and most symptomatic patients will require admission to a monitored unit. Whether asymptomatic patients can be medically cleared from the emergency department after a period of observation depends on the specific exposure. Some drugs, such as MAOIs, methadone, and bupropion, may have a delayed onset of toxicity.[37] Others, such as valproic acid, may exhibit slow and prolonged absorption, resulting in late peak levels and the onset of CNS toxicity.[38]

If an opioid toxidrome is identified, small doses of naloxone may be administered to awaken the patients and restore adequate respirations without producing withdrawal symptoms. Following ventilation to achieve a normal Pco_2, a reasonable starting dose in patients with anticipated opioid tolerance is 0.04 to 0.05 mg intravenously, which may be repeated and escalated as required. If withdrawal is not a concern based on the history, naloxone may be administered in 0.4- to 2.0-mg doses. A continuous infusion of naloxone can be initiated in patients with recurrence of respiratory depression, typically at two-thirds of the bolus dose required to reverse the opioid effects. Naloxone may also be useful diagnostically, if the cause of opioid toxicity is not certain.

Agitated Delirium

Patients presenting with mild restlessness or confusion may do well with reassurance, redirection, and minimal stimulation. When agitation is more severe and does not respond to these conservative measures, chemical sedation is necessary. Benzodiazepines are first-line agents, with midazolam, diazepam, and lorazepam all excellent choices, although each with different onsets and durations of action. If benzodiazepines alone are ineffective, the second-choice agent may depend on the cause of the delirium. Stimulant toxicity, when dopaminergic excess is a concern, may respond to haloperidol or ziprasidone, although seizures are a risk.[39,40] Phenobarbital may be preferable if a withdrawal syndrome is suspected. Cases of dexmedetomidine and ketamine as options for excited delirium syndrome are reported, although less substantiated.[41,42] If patients present with evidence of excited delirium syndrome, rapid control of agitation and hyperthermia are crucial. Sedation, paralysis, and endotracheal intubation may be required to control neuromuscular and autonomic hyperactivity, along with intravenous fluid administration and active cooling measures.

Patients who exhibit agitated delirium as part of the anticholinergic syndrome may be candidates for reversal with physostigmine. A 1 mg dose is given slowly over 2 to 3 minutes and may be repeated if mentation does not improve. Physostigmine should only be administered if there are no contraindications (such as a history of asthma or seizures) and there is no concern for intraventricular conduction delay. Physostigmine may be repeated as needed, with caution because cholinergic symptoms, such as vomiting or bronchospasm, may result.

Serotonin syndrome is best managed with the discontinuation of serotonergic agents and supportive care, including benzodiazepines for symptoms of neuromuscular excitation. Severe cases may require sedation, intubation, and paralysis for control of muscular hyperactivity and hyperthermia. Serotonin syndrome typically resolves within 24 hours. Although treatment with cyproheptadine may be considered, it has not been shown to improve outcomes and lacks a parenteral formulation.[17]

Seizures

The first-line therapy for drug-induced seizures is a benzodiazepine, such as midazolam, diazepam, or lorazepam. If seizures do not quickly resolve following 2 to 3 doses of benzodiazepines, the clinician should proceed to a barbiturate, such as phenobarbital. Phenytoin is not indicated for the treatment of drug-induced seizures except in cases of toxicity caused by 4-aminopyridine.[43] If seizures continue despite the administration of benzodiazepines and barbiturates, pyridoxine should be administered in addition to additional doses of GABA agonists. For patients who are known to have ingested isoniazid or another hydrazine (eg, *Gyromitra* mushrooms), pyridoxine is the first-line therapy for seizures.[25,26] If the dose of isoniazid ingested is known, the same dose of pyridoxine is administered (gram for gram). If the dose is unknown, 5 g may be given empirically. This dose can be repeated once.

SUMMARY

CNS toxicity caused by xenobiotic exposure is a common reason for presentation to the emergency department. There are countless potential sources of exposure, and the history is not always helpful in determining the diagnosis. Presentations of CNS toxicity vary widely, ranging along a spectrum from deep coma to an excited delirium syndrome. Identifying the characteristics of CNS toxicity as well as the corresponding effects on other organ systems will help to narrow the potential causes of illness and guide management. Care of patients with CNS toxicity caused by xenobiotic exposure is largely supportive, with a role for antidotes, including naloxone, physostigmine, and pyridoxine, in select cases. Benzodiazepines are the first-line therapy for agitated delirium and xenobiotic-induced seizures. Excited delirium syndrome may require sedation, intubation, and active cooling. Patients for whom there is concern for non-convulsive status epilepticus may benefit from an EEG evaluation.

REFERENCES

1. Han JH, Wilber ST. Altered mental status in older patients in the emergency department. Clin Geriatr Med 2013;29:101–36.
2. Golparvar M, Saghaei M, Sajedi P, et al. Paradoxical reaction following intravenous midazolam premedication in pediatric patients – a randomized placebo controlled trial of ketamine for rapid tranquilization. Paediatr Anaesth 2004;14: 924–30.
3. Sullivan R, Hodgman MJ, Kao L, et al. Baclofen overdose mimicking brain death. Clin Toxicol (Phila) 2012;50:141–4.
4. Weißhaar GF, Hoemberg M, Bender K, et al. Baclofen intoxication: a "fun drug" causing deep coma and nonconvulsive status epilepticus—a case report and review of the literature. Eur J Pediatr 2012;171:1541–7.
5. Perruchoud C, Bovy M, Durrer A, et al. Severe hypertension following accidental clonidine overdose during the refilling of an implanted intrathecal drug delivery system. Neuromodulation 2012;15:31–4.
6. Farooqi M, Seifert S, Kunkel S, et al. Toxicity from a clonidine suspension. J Med Toxicol 2009;5:130–3.
7. Levine M, Ruha AM. Overdose of atypical antipsychotics clinical presentation, mechanisms of toxicity and management. CNS Drugs 2012;26:601–11.
8. Larkin TM, Cohen-Oram AN, Catalano G, et al. Overdose with levetiracetam: a case report and review of the literature. J Clin Pharm Ther 2013;38:68–70.
9. Schauer SG, Varney SM. Gabapentin overdose in a military beneficiary. Mil Med 2013;178:e133–5.
10. Levine M, Khurana A, Ruha AM. Polyuria, acidosis, and coma following massive ibuprofen ingestion. J Med Toxicol 2010;6:315–7.
11. Roth B, Woo O, Blanc P. Early metabolic acidosis and coma after acetaminophen ingestion. Ann Emerg Med 1999;33:452–6.
12. Wiegand TJ, Margaretten M, Olson KR. Massive acetaminophen ingestion with early metabolic acidosis and coma: treatment with IV NAC and continuous venovenous hemodiafiltration. Clin Toxicol 2010;48:156–9.
13. Carstairs SD, Fujinaka MK, Keeney GE, et al. Prolonged coma in a child due to hashish ingestion with quantitation of THC metabolites in urine. J Emerg Med 2011;41:e69–71.
14. Wang GS, Roosevelt G, Heard K. Pediatric marijuana exposures in a medical marijuana state. JAMA Pediatr 2013;167:630–3.
15. Vilke GM, DeBard ML, Chan TC, et al. Excited delirium syndrome (ExDS): defining based on a review of the literature. J Emerg Med 2012;43:897–905.
16. Penders TM, Gestring RE, Vilensky DA. Excited delirium following use of synthetic cathinones (bath salts). Gen Hosp Psychiatry 2012;34:647–50.

17. Kant S, Liebelt E. Recognizing serotonin toxicity in the pediatric emergency department. Pediatr Emerg Care 2012;28:817–21.
18. LoVecchio F, Riley B, Pizon A, et al. Outcomes after isolated mirtazapine (Remeron) supratherapeutic ingestions. J Emerg Med 2008;34:77–8.
19. Erich JL, Shih RD, O'Connor RE. "Ping-pong" gaze in severe monoamine oxidase inhibitor toxicity. J Emerg Med 1995;13:653–5.
20. Ekicia A, Yakuta A, Kuralb N, et al. Nonconvulsive status epilepticus due to drug induced neurotoxicity in chronically ill children. Brain Dev 2012;34: 824–8.
21. Khine H, Weiss D, Graber N, et al. A cluster of children with seizures caused by camphor poisoning. Pediatrics 2009;123:1269–72.
22. McLawhorn MW, Goulding MR, Gill RK, et al. Analysis of benzonatate overdoses among adults and children from 1969-2010 by the United States Food and Drug Administration. Pharmacotherapy 2013;33:38–43.
23. Morazin F, Lumbroso A, Harry P, et al. Cardiogenic shock and status epilepticus after massive bupropion overdose. Clin Toxicol (Phila) 2007;45:794–7.
24. Wills BK, Barry JD. Neurotoxic emergencies. Neurol Clin 2011;29:539–63.
25. Alvarez FG, Guntupalli KK. Isoniazid overdose: four case reports and review of the literature. Intensive Care Med 1995;21:641–4.
26. Romero JA, Kuczler FJ Jr. Isoniazid overdose: recognition and management. Am Fam Physician 1998;57:749–52.
27. Kass JS, Shandera WX. Nervous system effects of antituberculosis therapy. CNS Drugs 2010;24:655–67.
28. Boison D. Methylxanthines, seizures and excitotoxicity. Handb Exp Pharmacol 2011;200:251–66.
29. Shannon M. Life-threatening events after theophylline overdose a 10-year prospective analysis. Arch Intern Med 1999;159:989–94.
30. Dietrich AM, Mortensen ME. Presentation and management of an acute caffeine overdose. Pediatr Emerg Care 1990;6:296–8.
31. Shadnia S, Brent J, Mousavi-Fatemi K, et al. Recurrent seizures in tramadol intoxication: implications for therapy based on 100 patients. Basic Clin Pharmacol Toxicol 2012;111:133–6.
32. Melanson SE. The utility of immunoassays for urine drug testing. Clin Lab Med 2012;32:429–47.
33. von Mach MA, Weber C, Meyer MR, et al. Comparison of urinary on-site immunoassay screening and gas chromatography-mass spectrometry results of 111 patients with suspected poisoning presenting at an emergency department. Ther Drug Monit 2007;29:27–39.
34. Patel MM, Tsutaoka BT, Banerji S, et al. ED utilization of computed tomography in a poisoned population. Am J Emerg Med 2002;20:212–7.
35. Fernández IS, Loddenkemper T, Datta A, et al. Electroencephalography in the pediatric emergency department: when is it most useful? J Child Neurol 2013. [Epub ahead of print].
36. Jordan KG, Schneider AL. Emergency ("stat") EEG in the era of nonconvulsive status epilepticus. Am J Electroneurodiagn Technol 2009;49:94–104.
37. LoVecchio F, Pizon A, Riley B, et al. Onset of symptoms after methadone overdose. Am J Emerg Med 2007;25:57–9.
38. Ingels M, Beauchamp J, Clark RF, et al. Delayed valproic acid toxicity: a retrospective case series. Ann Emerg Med 2002;39:616–21.
39. Ruha AM, Yarema MC. Pharmacologic treatment of acute pediatric methamphetamine toxicity. Pediatr Emerg Care 2006;22:782–5.

40. Spiller HA, Hays HL, Aleguas A Jr. Overdose of drugs for attention-deficit hyper-activity disorder: clinical presentation, mechanisms of toxicity, and management. CNS Drugs 2013;27:531–43.
41. Akingbola OA, Singh D. Dexmedetomidine to treat lisdexamfetamine overdose and serotonin toxidrome in a 6-year-old girl. Am J Crit Care 2012;21:456–9.
42. Ho JD, Smith SW, Nystrom PC, et al. Successful management of excited delirium syndrome with prehospital ketamine: two case examples. Prehosp Emerg Care 2013;17:274–9.
43. Stork CM, Hoffman RS. Characterization of 4-aminopyridine in overdose. J Toxicol Clin Toxicol 1994;32:583–7.

Marine Envenomations

Kamna S. Balhara, MD*, Andrew Stolbach, MD

KEYWORDS

- Jellyfish • Irukandji syndrome • *C fleckeri* • *Physalia physalis* • Spiny fish • Stingray
- Marine envenomation • Marine antivenom

KEY POINTS

- Marine fauna vary widely by geographic location. Antivenoms exist for stonefish, box jellyfish, and sea snake envenomation but vary in availability in North America.
- Bleeding and infection are the most significant complications of stingray exposure.
- Severe marine envenomations may cause hypertension, paralysis, or rhabdomyolysis.
- Box jellyfish, Irukandji jellyfish, sea snakes, blue-ringed octopi, and cone snail exposure can be fatal, but they do not typically naturally occur in North America. North American fatalities from *Physalia physalis* have been recorded, and spiny fish represent a large number of reported exposures in the United States.
- Acetic acid (4%–6%) application and hot-water immersion are advised for jellyfish exposures in North America.

INTRODUCTION

The marine environment poses many hazards for humans, including a myriad of organisms that have developed toxins for the purposes of defense or feeding. Organisms such as sea snakes, spiny fish, and certain species of jellyfish have the potential to cause significant human morbidity and, occasionally, mortality. The American Association of Poison Control Centers' 2010 and 2011 annual reports document approximately 1800 aquatic exposures in the United States alone each year, of which almost 500 annually were treated in health care facilities; however, this likely grossly underestimates the number of marine envenomations per year because it only takes into account those that were reported to poison control centers.[1,2]

Marine venoms comprise a wide array of toxins and are usually mixtures of high-molecular-weight proteins and low-molecular-weight compounds (histamine, bradykinin, indole derivatives). Although the pathophysiology of many venoms and the associated signs and symptoms remains unclear, in many cases envenomation leads to mast cell degranulation, disruption of cell metabolism, interference with neuronal

Department of Emergency Medicine, Johns Hopkins University, 1830 East Monument Street, Baltimore, MD 21287, USA
* Corresponding author. 1830 East Monument Street, Suite 6-100, Baltimore, MD 21287.
E-mail address: kbalhar1@jhmi.edu

Emerg Med Clin N Am 32 (2014) 223–243
http://dx.doi.org/10.1016/j.emc.2013.09.009
0733-8627/14/$ – see front matter © 2014 Elsevier Inc. All rights reserved.

emed.theclinics.com

transmissions, and myocardial depression. Subsequently, envenomations can cause significant pain, dermatitis, paralysis, cardiovascular collapse, and respiratory failure (**Box 1**). The appropriate treatment of many marine envenomations remains controversial, because much of our knowledge is based on animal models and human case reports.

The aim of this article is to highlight certain venomous vertebrate and invertebrate organisms that are either ubiquitous in causing morbidity or have the potential to cause mortality. The organisms to be considered are enumerated in **Boxes 2** and **3**. The epidemiology, clinical presentation, venom pathophysiology, and potential guidelines for the treatment of each of these organisms is reviewed. Although antivenoms are available for some of the deadlier marine creatures, none are approved by the Food and Drug Administration (FDA), and they vary in their availability in North America. Treatment guidelines and antivenoms are summarized in **Tables 1–3**.

VERTEBRATES
Stingrays (Class Chondrichthyes)

Epidemiology
Stingrays of the class Chondrichthyes are large, flat, cartilaginous fish with wings and a long, tapered, whiplike tail with bilateral retroserrated edges (**Fig. 1**). The tail is equipped with 1 to 6 sharp barbs and a ventrolateral groove containing venom glands that coat the spine with venom and mucus. They are found in tropical and subtropical waters worldwide; 11 species are found in the United States. One review described 17 fatalities from stingray exposure, two of which occurred in Australia.[3]

Venom
Stingray venom contains amino acids, serotonin, 5′-nucleotidase, and phosphodiesterase.[4] It is heat-labile and cardiotoxic in animal models. The heat lability of this venom has important implications for local analgesia at the site of injury.[5] Studies in Brazilian freshwater stingray venom in animal models have revealed toxins that may interact with membrane phospholipids, cause leukocyte rolling, and exert a potent vasoconstrictor effect.[6,7] The venom may also have proteolytic, gelatinolytic, and hyaluronidase activities, explaining severe wound necrosis and contributing to the local damage already caused by the sting.[8]

Presentation
These fish burrow under sand in shallow water, and most injuries occur from unintentional contact or unfouling fishing equipment. When the wings are stepped on, the tail

---

Box 1
Presentation pearls

Common Mechanisms of Morbidity and Mortality in Marine Envenomations

Stingray	Exsanguination
Spiny fish	Cardiotoxicity, neurotoxicity, hemolysis, edema
Sea snakes	Paralysis, respiratory failure, rhabdomyolysis
Box jellyfish (*Chironex fleckeri*)	Cardiotoxicity, catecholamine surge
Irukandji (*Carukia barnesi*)	Severe hypertension
Portuguese man-of-war (*Physalia physalis*)	Respiratory failure, hypotension
Cone snails	Paralysis, respiratory failure, cardiotoxicity
Octopus (*Hapalochlaena maculosa*)	Paralysis (without change in mental status), respiratory failure, hypotension

---

Box 2
Vertebrate marine organisms

Vertebrates

Stingray (class Chondrichthyes)

Spiny fish (families Scorpaenidae and Trachinidae)

   Stonefish (genus *Synanceia*)

   Lionfish (genus *Pterois*)

   Weeverfish (genus *Echiichthys* and genus *Trachinus*)

Sea Snakes (families Hydrophiidae and Laticaudinae)

---

whips forward reflexively, embedding spines in the victim's skin, tearing the stingray integument and, thus, releasing venom and often causing significant lacerations. The sting results in intense pain and edema, with symptoms peaking 30 to 90 minutes after the injury and lasting up to 48 hours. Local swelling, erythema, and cyanosis occur; the ruptured barb sheath leaves parts of the integument, barb, and venom-secreting glands in the wound, which may lead to necrosis and infection (**Fig. 2**).

Clinical manifestations include weakness, nausea, vomiting, diarrhea, headache, and cramps. In severe cases, patients present with vertigo, syncope, seizures,

---

Box 3
Invertebrate marine organisms

Invertebrates

Cnidaria

   Class Cubozoa

      Box jellyfish (*Chironex fleckeri*)

      Irukandji jellyfish (*Carukia barnesi*)

   Class Hydrozoa

      Portuguese man-of-war (*Physalia physalis*)

      Fire corals (*Millepora alcicornis*)

   Class Scyphozoa

      Thimble jellyfish (*Linuche unguiculata*)

Mollusca

   Class Gastropoda

      Cone snails (genus *Conus*)

   Class Cephalopoda

      Blue-ringed octopus (*Hapalochlaena maculosa*)

Echinodermata

   Sea urchins (*Diadema, Echinothrix, Asthenosoma*)

Porifera

   Sponges

Table 1
Marine vertebrate organism envenomations

Marine Organism	Treatment	Management Adjuncts
Stingray	Hemostasis Hot-water immersion Analgesia Wound exploration	Tetanus prophylaxis Antibiotic prophylaxis[a]
Stonefish	Hemostasis Hot-water immersion Analgesia Wound exploration Stonefish antivenom administration	Tetanus prophylaxis Antibiotic prophylaxis (controversial)
Lionfish	Hemostasis Hot-water immersion Analgesia Wound exploration	Tetanus prophylaxis Antibiotic prophylaxis (controversial)
Weeverfish	Hemostasis Hot-water immersion Analgesia Wound exploration	Tetanus prophylaxis Antibiotic prophylaxis (controversial)
Sea snakes	Patient stabilization Extremity pressure immobilization Rapid antivenom administration in envenomation	Laboratory analysis Creatinine kinase Electrolytes Creatinine Hematocrit/hemoglobin Urinalysis Fluid resuscitation (renal protection) Bedside epinephrine plus antihistamines in case of antivenom anaphylaxis

[a] Strongly consider.

fasciculations, hypotension, and dysrhythmia.[3,9] Mortality, however, is usually secondary to the effects of trauma, especially if patients are struck in the heart or if patients are in danger of exsanguinating from a significant chest or abdominal laceration.[9,10]

Treatment
Hemostasis should be addressed, and the wound should be immersed in hot water. In a systematic review of 119 cases, hot water (110°F–114°F or 43.3°C–45.6°C) was shown to be effective in relieving pain; a prospective study demonstrated total relief of pain in 73% of vertebrate fish stings.[11,12] Pain may be of such severity as to necessitate local anesthetic infiltration or regional nerve block.

Imaging should be performed to evaluate for embedded spines. Given that venom and tissue often remain in the wound, the tract should be explored for removal of foreign bodies, packed, and left to heal by secondary intention. The use of alginate-based wick dressing has been suggested to absorb the remaining venom and can be left in the wound for 8 to 10 days.[3] Surgical debridement may often be necessary.[13,14]

Tetanus prophylaxis should be administered if not current, and antibiotics (eg, sulfamethoxazole/trimethoprim) should be strongly considered because they may reduce the incidence of wound infection, especially in large lacerations.[10–12]

Table 2
Marine invertebrate organism envenomations[a]

Marine Organism	Treatment	Management Adjuncts
Chironex fleckeri (Box jellyfish)	Patient stabilization Decontamination (5% acetic acid) Immediate antivenom Respiratory and cardiac support	Bedside epinephrine plus antihistamines in case of antivenom anaphylaxis Cold pack application Analgesia Topical corticosteroids Topical antihistamines
Carukia barnesi (Irukandji)	Decontamination (5% acetic acid) Blood pressure control[b] Respiratory and cardiac support	Electrocardiogram Cardiac enzymes (troponin) Consider echocardiogram if troponins elevated Cold pack application Analgesia Topical corticosteroids Topical antihistamines
Physalia physalis (Portuguese man-of-war)	Patient stabilization Decontamination (5% acetic acid) Hot or cold pack application Analgesia Tentacle removal	Prolonged observation with systemic symptoms Topical corticosteroids Topical antihistamines
Millepora alcicornis (Fire corals)	Decontamination (5% acetic acid)	Topical corticosteroids Topical antihistamines
Linuche unguiculata (Thimble jellyfish)	Analgesia Topical corticosteroids Topical antihistamines Calamine lotion with menthol	Wash or discard clothes worn at time of eruption
Cone snails	Patient stabilization Extremity pressure immobilization Respiratory and cardiac support	—
Blue-ringed octopus	Patient stabilization Extremity pressure immobilization Respiratory and cardiac support	—
Sponges	Spicule removal	—
Sea urchins	Oral analgesia Hot-water immersion Visible spines/pedicellariae removal	Tetanus prophylaxis Surgical management for spines in joints or delayed granuloma

[a] Given the controversy regarding decontamination solution and temperature application, this table describes the American Heart Association's guidelines and the most recent literature for Indo-Pacific envenomation.
[b] Use easily titrable agents.

Family Scorpaenidae and Trachinidae

These two families of spiny fish, often found in tropical and temperate oceans, blend in with the rocky sea bottom. The Scorpaenidae family includes stonefish and lionfish, and the Trachinidae family's best-known species is the weeverfish. Fishermen, waders, and those with aquariums are most likely to present with envenomation from these fish. Only 5 deaths have been reported from spiny fish envenomation, all from stonefish; however, these are poorly documented.[3] Stonefish and lionfish have

Table 3
Marine antivenoms

Antivenom	Dosage	Potential Benefits
Chironex fleckeri Sheep-derived whole IgG	1 ampule (may dilute 1:10 by saline) intravenously 3 ampules may be given for coma, dysrhythmia, or respiratory depression Up to 6 ampules for patients receiving CPR with refractory dysrhythmia	May be effective against pain/scarring if given within 4–6 h Uncertain effect on cardiotoxicity
Sea snake Beaked sea snake and terrestrial tiger snake equine-derived IgG Fab fragment	1 ampule of either in 1:10 dilution with 0.9% saline	Reduction in mortality rate since introduction of antivenom Efficacy in all sea snake species
Stonefish Equine-derived IgG Fab fragment	1 vial for 1–2 punctures 2 vials for 3–4 punctures 3 vials for 5 or more punctures	Efficacy against pain Unknown efficacy against other spiny fish

Abbreviations: CPR, cardiopulmonary resuscitation; IgG, immunoglobulin G.

12 to 13 dorsal, 2 pelvic, and 3 anal spines, with paired glands at their base containing 5 to 10 mg of venom each. The related family of weeverfish tends to have 5 to 7 venom-containing spines on the front dorsal fin and a single spine on each gill cover. The toxins in spiny fish venom can remain stable for 1 to 2 days after the fish's death.[15,16]

Stonefish (genus Synanceia)

Epidemiology The stonefish include the Australian estuarine, Indian, and reef stonefish. These stationary bottom dwellers possess beady eyes and a gaping mouth and inhabit coastal waters with tropical temperatures (**Fig. 3**).

Venom The toxins produced by the stonefish include stonustoxin, verrucotoxin, and trachynilysin. These toxins have been shown to exert a variety of effects in animal

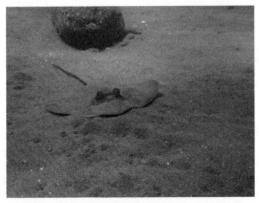

Fig. 1. Stingray. (*From* Fernandez I, Valladolid G, Varon J, et al. Encounters with venomous sea-life. J Emerg Med 2009;40:110; with permission.)

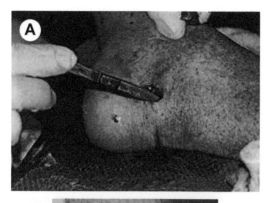

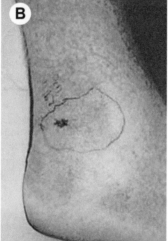

Fig. 2. Stingray injury to the ankle. Initial injury (*A*) and 10 days later with minor local infection (*B*). (*From* Isbister GK. Venomous fish stings in tropical northern Australia. Am J Emerg Med 2001;19:563; with permission.)

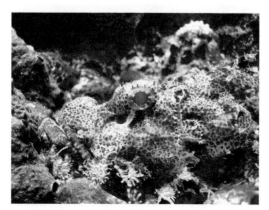

Fig. 3. Stonefish. (*From* Fernandez I, Valladolid G, Varon J, et al. Encounters with venomous sea-life. J Emerg Med 2009;40:109; with permission.)

models. They exhibit hyaluronidase activity, myotoxicity with muscle contracture, neurotoxicity, hemolysis, and vascular leakage and may cause decreased myocardial contractility.[17,18] Cardiotoxicity may result from action at muscarinic and adrenergic receptors.[19] Myotoxic, neurotoxic, and cardiotoxic effects have rarely been reported in humans.

Presentation Spines become embedded in the skin of unsuspecting victims who step on these fish in shallow water. Envenomation produces extreme pain, cyanosis, and edema, which is worst at 30 to 90 minutes and resolves within 6 to 12 hours (**Fig. 4**). The systemic effects, such as headache, abdominal pain, vomiting, delirium, seizures, paralysis, hypertension, congestive heart failure, respiratory distress, dysrhythmia, and hypotension, are rare. In fact, most systemic effects, such as syncope and nausea, may be a result of the severe pain rather than circulating venom. Stonefish spine wounds may take months to heal and may become necrotic if infected.[4]

Lionfish (genus Pterois)
Epidemiology These fish are most common in home aquariums and account for most poison center calls regarding fish envenomation in the United States. (**Fig. 5**). A 1985 review of poison control center cases found that of the 51 cases of scorpaenidae venom exposures recorded over five years, 45 were from lionfish and were sustained while handling them in an aquarium setting.[16]

Presentation Patients experience extreme pain, substantial swelling, and potential extension of pain to the entire limb. Some patients have systemic symptoms, such as diaphoresis, nausea, chest pain, abdominal pain, dyspnea, hypotension, and syncope. As discussed earlier, delayed wound healing and necrosis may occur.[16]

Weeverfish (family Trachinidae)
Epidemiology These saltwater dwellers include the lesser and greater weever (also known as adderpike, stingfish, or sea cat) and inhabit sandy or muddy, shallow, temperate waters around Europe.

Venom Dracotoxin, isolated from weeverfish venom, has been shown to cause hemolysis in rabbit models.[20] Other components of weeverfish venom include peptides, histamine, catecholamines, and mucopolysaccharide.[9]

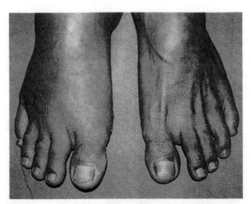

Fig. 4. Stonefish sting. The right foot demonstrates severe edema. (*From* Isbister GK. Venomous fish stings in tropical northern Australia. Am J Emerg Med 2001;19:562; with permission.)

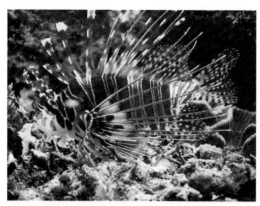

Fig. 5. Lionfish. (*From* Fernandez I, Valladolid G, Varon J, et al. Encounters with venomous sea-life. J Emerg Med 2009;40:109; with permission.)

Presentation The presentation of weeverfish envenomation mimics that described earlier, with excruciating pain similar to that inflicted by stonefish. In fact, the pain is so severe that there is an account dating from 1782 that describes a fisherman who cut off his finger to alleviate the pain from a weeverfish sting.[21] Pain usually subsides in 24 hours, although inflammation of the wound may last up to 14 days.[9,15]

Scorpaenidae and Trachinidae treatment Initial first aid is similar to that of stingray envenomation and involves bleeding control, immediate hot-water immersion, and potential local anesthesia or regional nerve block. The wound should be examined for foreign material, with imaging as suggested by the clinical presentation.

For stonefish, antivenom (equine-derived, immunoglobulin G [IgG] Fab fragment may be administered. In animal models, it has been shown to mitigate the toxin's hemolytic and vascular-leakage effects, and human clinical reports have reported its efficacy against pain.[17,22] Intramuscular administration is preferred over the intravenous route because of historical precedent; each ampule contains 2000 units and may neutralize 20 mg of venom.[22] The number of vials administered is determined by the number of puncture wounds: one vial should be provided for 1 to 2 punctures, 2 vials for 3 to 4 punctures, and 3 vials for 5 or more punctures. The antivenom is not FDA approved, although large regional aquariums may have a supply of this antivenom. The availability of antivenoms in North America can be found in the Antivenom Index maintained by the Association of Zoos and Aquariums (http://www.aza.org/antivenom-index/).

Epinephrine and antihistamines should be readily available in case of anaphylaxis, and the provider and patients should be aware of potential serum sickness within a week (5–24 days). The efficacy of stonefish antivenom against the toxins of other members of its family is uncertain. Tetanus prophylaxis should be provided.

Sea Snakes

Epidemiology

Sea snakes belong to the families Hydrophiidae and Laticaudinae. They are usually approximately one meter in length and are brightly colored with flat, paddlelike tails that allow them to move backward or forward at equally rapid speeds. All 52 species are venomous.[9] Unlike eels, they have scales but no fins or gills. They tend to inhabit the tropical and warm temperate waters of the Pacific and Indian Oceans, and none are found in the Atlantic Ocean or Caribbean Sea. Most envenomations occur in Southeast Asia, the Persian Gulf, and the Malay Archipelago. They are generally docile but can be aggressive during their mating season or if handled; most bites are incurred by fishermen handling nets. One-third to one-half of bites, however, may not result in envenomation.[9] The mortality rate from sea snake envenomations is approximately 3%, although it may have been as high as 10% before the introduction of antivenom.[3]

Venom
The simple venom apparatus of sea snakes consists of 2 or 4 hollow fangs with a pair of attached venom glands that open into ducts near the fang tips.[4] Sea snake venom has been shown to have neurotoxic, hemolytic, and myotoxic properties; the neurotoxin has been shown to target postsynaptic acetylcholine receptors, blocking the neuromuscular junction.[23]

Presentation
Patients may initially only note tiny puncture wounds in isolation or in a group of nearly 30. Local skin reaction is rare. Many bites are without venom. Systemic symptoms may present in an hour and can be delayed 6 to 8 hours; if systemic symptoms do not occur by then, envenomation has not occurred.[9] The main systemic manifestations are related to myalgia secondary to myotoxicity, although immobility may be caused by pain from muscle breakdown from myotoxins or caused by paralysis from neurotoxin. In some patients, the effect of one toxin may predominate over the other. Patients may have pain with movement, ascending paralysis, slurred speech, dysphagia, trismus, ptosis, and ophthalmoplegia, along with myoglobinuria that develops within three to four hours.[4,9] Renal function may be compromised and severe hyperkalemia may result. Ultimately, respiratory insufficiency, seizures, or coma may occur. Death results from ventilatory failure.

Sea snake treatment
The diagnosis of a sea snake bite is often delayed. The clinician should consider it in the presence of puncture wounds in waters where the snakes are found. Envenomation should be suspected if symptoms start to occur, such as myalgia or weakness. Patients should be closely monitored for paralysis and for compromised airway or respiratory effort. As with terrestrial snakebites, the limb should be immobilized and maintained in a dependent position; pressure immobilization may be considered as long as the arterial flow is not impeded.[9]

In the presence of envenomation, antivenom should be administered as soon as possible. The venom of beaked sea snakes and terrestrial tiger snakes has been used to derive equine IgG Fab fragment antivenom, and both have potency against the venom of almost all sea snakes. Ambiguity exists over which venom source is more effective and efficient, so it may be reasonable to use whichever antivenom is most readily available when envenomation is suspected. The manufacturer suggests starting with one ampule (1000 units) of sea snake antivenom, although no upper limit is established. A 1:10 dilution with 0.9% sodium chloride solution may be given intravenously over 30 minutes. One ampule (3000 units) of tiger snake antivenom should be given if beaked sea snake antivenom is not available. Neither antivenom is FDA approved; at writing, the Long Beach Aquarium maintains current sea snake antivenom; the Bronx, Houston, and Dallas zoos maintain current tiger snake antivenom. The provider should be prepared for potential anaphylaxis with epinephrine and antihistamines at bedside and should be aware of the potential for the development of serum sickness, within 1 to 2 weeks on average.

Laboratory studies are useful to identify rhabdomyolysis, hemolysis, and renal failure. Elevated liver function testing may accompany severe envenomation. Renal function should be supported with adequate fluid resuscitation.

INVERTEBRATES
The Jellyfish (Cnidaria, Formerly Coelenterates)

Cnidaria comprise four classes and contain 10 000 named species, more than 100 of which are dangerous to humans. All species have microscopic cnidae, which are organelles containing a hollow, sharply pointed, coiled thread tube that is about 200 to 400 μm long, surrounded by venom, and sharp enough to penetrate a surgical glove.[24] Thousands of these nematocysts are distributed along the tentacles and are discharged by contact with a victim's skin.[25] Intradermal injection of venom occurs when the flesh is penetrated.

The class Cubozoa includes box jellyfish, the class Hydrozoa includes the Portuguese man-of-war, the class Scyphozoa comprises the true jellyfish, and the class Anthozoa includes anemone and corals. The last class is the largest and least likely to cause systemic disturbance and is not covered here. Stings from jellyfish occur in the warmer months of the year and usually cause an acute dermatitis that resolves spontaneously. Cubozoan jellyfish, although often causing only minor effects, may cause the most severe envenomations leading to rapid mortality. In the Hydrozoa class, *Physalia* envenomation has been noted to result in deaths. The mechanisms suggested to explain the actions of jellyfish venom include pore formation, disturbances in sodium and calcium transport across membranes, and enzymatic activity with inflammatory mediators.[26]

Cubozoa

The class Cubozoa consists of 2 orders, Chirodropida and Carybdeida, whose species have a cube-shaped bell with tentacles at each corner.

Box jellyfish (Chironex fleckeri)
Epidemiology The box jellyfish (sea wasp) resides in the Indo-Pacific, primarily off the coast of Australia. Its bell measures 25 to 30 cm in diameter with 15 tentacles at each corner. It may be the world's most venomous animal, causing rapid death, potentially within 30 to 60 seconds.[27] A review of more than 100 years of data found 60 deaths.[28] At least one patient died with relatively minimal tentacle contact. Envenomation has resulted in rapid death; cardiac arrest and pulmonary edema may occur.[29]

Venom *C fleckeri* envenomation may initially cause transient hypertension, which may be a direct effect of the tentacle.[30] The venom itself causes rapid hypotension and cardiovascular collapse. The exact mechanism of action remains to be fully elaborated but has been suggested to be a pore-forming mechanism, with enhanced cation conductance leading to increased sodium and subsequently calcium entry into cells.[22,27,31] However, the toxin's effects in humans do mirror the cardiotoxicity seen in animal models.

Presentation Envenomation has caused arrhythmias and death. In fatal cases, death rapidly occurs from cardiac failure. Respiratory failure is also implicated in death, although the toxin does not affect the neuromuscular junction. Most cases cause no more than painful skin irritation.[22,28] Wheals and vesicles may be seen with a dark brown or purple whiplike flare pattern with stripes that are 8 to 10 mm wide, often referred to as a frosted ladder appearance. Blistering and superficial necrosis may be present in 12 to 18 hours. Sixty percent may have a delayed hypersensitivity reaction, with papular urticaria at sting sites.[22,28] Systemic symptoms include nausea, vomiting, spasms, headache, malaise, and fever. A rash may persist for days. In some, delayed hypersensitivity was noted and either resolved spontaneously or responded to oral antihistamines and topical corticosteroids.[28]

Irukandji jellyfish (Carukia barnesi)

Epidemiology The Irukandji jellyfish of the order Carybdeida is much smaller than the box jellyfish, with a 2.5-cm bell diameter. It is usually found in Australia and is known for causing the systemic Irukandji syndrome, which is named after an Aboriginal tribe that formerly inhabited the area near Cairns, Australia.[32] At least 2 deaths have been recorded from intracerebral hemorrhage secondary to severe hypertension from envenomation.[3]

Venom Hypertension may be a result of catecholamine release triggered by the venom.[33] However, extracts of the tentacle and nematocyst alone have also caused hypertension in animal models.[30,33]

Presentation Skin findings are typically absent, although some patients have mild local pain and redness. Severe systemic manifestations may occur within 30 minutes, consisting of severe pain in the head, trunk, and limbs, tachycardia, hypertension, sweating, piloerection, agitation, and spasms, especially in the back and abdomen.[34] The systolic blood pressure may exceed 200 mm Hg and may be followed by a second phase of hypotension with myocardial depression. Some case reports describe pulmonary edema,[25,32,35,36] which may be caused by stress cardiomyopathy from severe hypertension, disruption of cell function from membrane pore in myocardial cell membranes, or both.[32] In one retrospective study, marked troponin elevation was seen in patients whose pain did not resolve with one dose of opioid analgesia.[35] Full recovery may occur after one to two days.[32]

Hydrozoa

The Hydrozoa include the *Millepora* (fire corals) and *Physalia* (Portuguese man-of-war and bluebottle jellyfish) and are found worldwide.

Portuguese man-of-war (Physalia physalis)

Epidemiology The large number of *Physalia* species around the world may be responsible for thousands of envenomations. The members of this genus are often found in shallow water or washed onto the beach with the surf, and their nematocysts may remain active for months. The Portuguese man-of-war is found in the Atlantic Ocean and consists of a floating colony composed of several types of polypoid individuals attached to a free-floating stem, whereas the bluebottle jellyfish (*Physalia utriculus*) has single tentacles measuring 15 m and is found off the Australian coast.[37] The Portuguese man-of-war has very long tentacles (as long as 30 m), has a large float containing nitrogen and carbon monoxide, and has up to 750 000 nematocysts on each of its 40 tentacles. There have been at least two deaths reported from *Physalia physalis* envenomation along the US Atlantic coast.[38,39]

Venom In animal models, *Physalia physalis* toxins cause hemolysis, mast cell degranulation, vasodilation, and conduction disturbances.[25,40] Although the exact mechanisms for these are unknown, it has been suggested that histamine release occurs because of immediate exocytosis of granules from mast cells followed by a slow lysis of mast cells.[40]

Presentation Exposure may lead to immediate intense pain that radiates centrally and may fade in an hour, although it may last several hours with larger specimens. Characteristic linear erythematous skin irritation may be seen in a contact distribution, which, if severe, may lead to necrosis (**Fig. 6**). Delayed effects may also be present, beginning five minutes to several hours after the exposure. Systemic injury, in concert with an allergic reaction or even anaphylaxis, may be present. Patients may develop signs and symptoms ranging from malaise, nausea, myalgias, spasms, and headache to delirium, syncope, vertigo, and ataxia. Dysrhythmia, hypotension, and respiratory failure may occur.[36] In fatalities, death and respiratory failure may occur within minutes.[38,41–43]

Millepora alcicornis

Epidemiology The so-called fire coral is not a true coral. It is found in tropical shallow water and is often mistaken for seaweed.[24] Fire coral is smooth with a sharp lime carbonate exoskeleton, measuring 10 cm to two meters. Many tiny tentacles with nematocysts emerge from its gastropores and commonly cause stings in the southern United States and Caribbean.

Venom The venom of the fire coral is known to be a water-soluble protein, which induces convulsions, respiratory distress, and death in experimental mouse models, with a steep dose-response curve.[44] Recent studies have isolated proteinaceous toxins with cytotoxic and hemolytic effects in mouse models.[45]

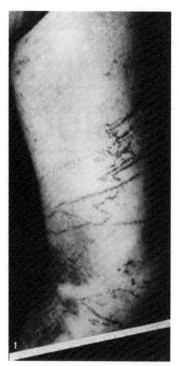

Fig. 6. Physalia physalis sting. Numerous erythematous linear tentacle marks on the right arm above the elbow, photograph taken at postmortem examination 5 days after envenomation. (*From* Stein M, Marraccini JV, Rothschild NE, et al. Fatal Portuguese man-ó-war (*Physalia physalis*) envenomation. Ann Emerg Med 1989;18:132; with permission.)

Envenomation Exposure results in immediate burning pain, which rarely radiates. Rubbing the area worsens pain by causing increased nematocyst discharge. Small papules may be present and become urticarial wheals over an hour; blistering does not usually occur. The skin irritation resolves over three to seven days if untreated, although hyperpigmentation may be present for up to eight weeks.[46]

Scyphozoa

The members of this class are what are considered true jellyfish. They include sea nettles (*Chrysaora* species), which rarely cause severe reactions with anaphylaxis or an immune-mediated response. This class also includes the extremely large hair jellyfish (*Cyanea*), which produce moderate pain and localized reaction and are especially prevalent in Australia.

Linuche unguiculata

Epidemiology This thimble jellyfish is responsible for sea bather's eruption (SBE), a vesicular and morbilliform pruritic dermatitis named in 1949. Although found everywhere, these jellyfish are often present in Florida and the Caribbean.

Venom Contact with the bather's skin causes discharge of nematocysts. SBE probably results from an immunologic response.[47]

Presentation SBE is likely caused by contact with the jellyfish's pinhead-sized larvae. The larvae become trapped under seams of swimwear where skin is covered. The dermatitis erupts within 1 day and can last up to 2 weeks with nocturnal pruritis.[47] Very rarely, headache, chills, malaise, conjunctivitis, and urethritis may occur. Recent studies have demonstrated that adult Linuche may also cause SBE.[48]

Cubozoa, hydrozoa, and scyphozoa treatment If patients are stable and serious box jellyfish envenomation or Irukandji syndrome are not suspected, efforts should be focused on decontamination and pain control. Decontamination is the first step for patients with isolated skin manifestations. Patients should be advised to refrain from rubbing the affected area to avoid nematocyst discharge. Hypotonic solutions, such as fresh water, should be avoided because they may trigger venom discharge. There are conflicting data regarding the best type of decontamination. Most research on treatment is based in the Indo-Pacific and not necessarily generalizable to species found near the continental United States and Hawaii. Household vinegar (5% acetic acid) is commonly suggested as a decontaminant, but studies in different populations of jellyfish in varying locales have demonstrated either pain relief or worsened nematocyst discharge. It is widely suggested that vinegar should be applied to inactivate nematocysts, especially when *Chironex* and other box jellyfish exposure is suspected.[32] Isopropyl alcohol should be avoided in *Chironex* envenomations.[25] For *Physalia*, it has been suggested that vinegar should be avoided because it may cause nematocyst discharge.[3] However, a recent review demonstrates pain relief with vinegar application in *Physalia* species.[49] Because *Physalia* is more common in the United States, some suggest that vinegar should potentially be avoided when the exposure source is unknown. Baking soda slurry may be used for *Chrysaora* or *Cyanea*. Once decontamination has been carried out, the provider may carefully remove the visible tentacles by scraping with a blunt object while wearing gloves for protection from undischarged nematocysts. Ice packs provide some relief and may be applied for analgesia; hot-water immersion has been shown to be effective in pain relief in *Carybdea alata* but not definitively established for the management of exposure to other species.[50–52]

Pressure immobilization should be avoided in Cnidaria exposure because it may further propagate venom delivery; however, it has been suggested that pressure immobilization may be of use once vinegar has been used to deactivate nemato-cysts.[24,53] The 2010 American Heart Association–American Red Cross International Consensus on First Aid for jellyfish stings in North America and Hawaii states that acetic acid (4%–6%) should be applied for 30 minutes, with baking soda slurry applied if acetic acid is unavailable. It is further advised that hot-water immersion should be undertaken; if not accessible, dry hot or cold packs should be applied. Pressure immobilization bandages are not recommended. The authors of the guidelines acknowledge the knowledge deficits on this issue.[54]

Analgesics and topical corticosteroids and/or antihistamines should be adminis-tered for further relief. For SBE, calamine lotion with menthol may be considered, fol-lowed by antihistamines and steroids if symptoms are severe.[24] In cases of more serious envenomation with systemic symptoms with box jellyfish, patients should be stabilized with attention to the airway, breathing, and circulation. Three ampules of box jellyfish antivenom should be administered as soon as possible for coma, dysrhythmia, or respiratory depression.[25] Three more ampules (to a total of 6) may be administered for refractory dysrhythmias.[22] The antivenom is a sheep-derived whole IgG antivenom raised against milked *C fleckeri* venom. Because death has occurred as early as five minutes after envenomation, the antivenom should be admin-istered as early as possible, although it is unclear if antivenom reduces mortality. Mortality has occurred despite antivenom administration, and patients have survived without antivenom administration. Case reports suggest that antivenom may reduce pain if given within four hours or limit scarring if given within 4 to 6 hours. There is no current report of box jellyfish antivenom being stocked in the United States. Mag-nesium, if given concurrently with antivenom, may improve hemodynamics.[27] The ef-ficacy of box jellyfish antivenom against its North Atlantic *Physalia* cousins is uncertain, and it has no effect on *Carukia barnesi* envenomation.[22]

The main goal of care for Irukandji syndrome is the control of pain and blood pres-sure. Because hypotension may occur later in the course of this envenomation, hyper-tension should be controlled with shorter-acting agents that are easily titratable. Some researchers recommend magnesium as an adjunct to reducing vascular resistance and suppressing catecholamine release.[55] However, a double-blind randomized-controlled trial demonstrated no difference in analgesia or blood pressure between affected groups who received magnesium and those who did not.[56] In patients with Irukandji syndrome, an electrocardiogram and cardiac enzymes (troponin) should also be obtained, especially in those patients with continued pain despite analgesia. These patients may be at a higher risk for cardiac complications.[35]

Mollusca

This phylum includes the classes Gastropoda (cone snails) and Cephalopoda (octopus, squid, and cuttlefish).

Cone snails (Gastropoda)

Epidemiology There are 400 species in the genus *Conus*, 18 of which have been known to cause human envenomation. They inhabit the Indo-Pacific and measure approximately 15 cm. They have a hollow proboscis containing a barb bathed in venom, which can extend from anywhere along the slit in the shell. When handled, the dartlike tooth may be fired. Multiple deaths from these univalve creatures have been reported worldwide; before 1980, 16 fatalities had been recorded, 12 of which were caused by *C geographus* (fish hunting cone).[3] Between 25% and 60% of exposures result in death.[57,58] *C geographus* is the most commonly implicated species, but the *Conus textile* species has also caused fatalities.[3]

Venom Each species has venom with 100 to 200 unique peptides, or conotoxins, that target voltage-gated and ligand-gated ion channels, as well as G protein–linked receptors.[59] These small 12 to 30 amino acid peptide ligands have affinity for nicotinic acetylcholine receptors, neuronal calcium channels, muscle sodium channels, vasopressin receptors, and N-methyl-D-aspartate receptors.[60] *C geographus* muconotoxin, for instance, targets the ion-conducting pore of voltage-gated Na channels by physical occlusion.[61] The venom paralyzes prey. One omega-conotoxin derivative, ziconotide, targets N-type calcium channels and has been approved by the FDA for intrathecal infusion for pain relief.[62]

Presentation Snail envenomation may produce discomfort that ranges from slight irritation to severe pain. Initial blanching at the envenomation site is followed by cyanosis, tissue ischemia, numbness, and swelling. Systemic manifestations including nausea, pruritus, muscle weakness, blurred vision, dysphagia, paralysis, respiratory failure, cardiovascular collapse may occur, leading to death within two hours.[37]

Octopi (Cephalopoda)
Hapalochlaena maculosa (blue-ringed octopus)
Epidemiology Found in the Indo-Pacific, the blue-ringed octopus develops blue rings when threatened but usually maintains a yellowish-brown color. Bites typically occur to the upper extremities during octopus handling.[37] Its beak creates small punctures in the skin, which are usually not painful. Most reported deaths have occurred in Australia; a 1983 review mentioned 14 cases of envenomations, with two deaths.[63]

Venom The salivary gland of the octopus produces tetrodotoxin (TTX), a sodium channel blocker. Evolved for immobilizing prey, TTX causes paralysis without cardiotoxicity or alteration in mental status because of TTX's lack of sensitivity for one of the major cardiac sodium channel isoforms, although reduced vasomotor tone may occur.[22,64]

Presentation Small puncture wounds result in minor discomfort. However, perioral and intraoral paresthesias, diplopia, dysphagia, ataxia, nausea, vomiting, flaccid paralysis, and respiratory failure may follow.[37] In some cases, death has occurred from cardiovascular collapse. In most cases, near-total reversal of paralysis may occur in 24 to 48 hours.[63,65]

Mollusca treatment
Patients should be assessed immediately for airway patency and sufficiency, breathing, and circulation. Severe cases necessitate mechanical ventilation. Pressure immobilization may limit the spread of venom.[3] The affected limb should be wrapped in a lymphatic-occlusive bandage and then splinted, which can be performed in a prehospital setting. Topical wound care and tetanus prophylaxis are advised. No specific antivenom exists for either cone snails or for octopi, and treatment is supportive. Assays for urine or serum TTX using high-performance liquid chromatography exist but are not readily available to most clinicians.

Echinodermata and Porifera

The phylum Echinodermata includes sea urchins, and the phylum Porifera is known for sponges. Envenomation, which occurs passively when the organism is handled or stepped on, usually results in only mild symptoms.

Sponges (Porifera)

Epidemiology The ubiquitous Porifera have an elastic, horny skeleton embedded with silicon dioxide or calcium carbonate spicules. They are stationary animals that live attached to the sea floor or coral beds and may be colonized by Cnidaria.

Venom The toxins produced by the sponges include halitoxin and okadaic acid, which may act as direct irritants.[4] Dried sponges may regain toxicity when wet.[66]

Presentation Contact with sponges, such as the fire sponge, poison-bun sponge, and red moss sponge, induces pruritic dermatitis. The pruritus may be accompanied by edema, local joint swelling, and vesicles. Symptoms usually resolve in one week. If extensive skin involvement is present, patients may experience fever, chills, muscle cramps, and, rarely, systemic erythema multiforme. Skin desquamation may occur at 10 days to two months and is usually caused by the fire sponge.[4,67] If the sponge is colonized with Cnidaria, patients may develop dermatitis and eventual skin necrosis, also known as *sponge diver's disease*.

Sea urchins (Diadema, Echinothrix, and Asthenosoma)

Epidemiology Sea urchins, found worldwide, are free-living, egg-shaped creatures with globular or flattened bodies with a hard shell surrounding their viscera. Their shell is covered with spines and triple-jawed pedicellariae. Pedicellariae are pincerlike grasping organs that are used to feed and defend. They contain more venom than spines and adhere tightly to wounds.

Venom Neurotoxins have been found in some venom types and are composed of steroid glycosides, serotonin, hemolysin, protease, and acetylcholinelike substances.

Presentation Unintentional contact with spines or contact from trying to touch the animal results in burning erythema. If the spine enters a joint, a severe synovitis can result; penetration over the metacarpal joint can cause fusiform finger swelling. Secondary infection and granuloma formation have been documented. There are less substantiated claims that, with multiple punctures (>15–20 spines), systemic effects may occur, including paralysis, bronchospasm, and hypotension.[4]

Echinodermata and Porifera treatment For exposure to urchins, oral analgesia and submersion in hot water are advised (105°F–115°F, 40°C–46°C).[3] Imaging should be considered for locating retained spines. Sea urchin spines can be challenging to remove and may disintegrate easily. Spines embedded in a joint may require surgical extraction. For visible spines, those that seem easily removable should be removed. Granulomas may need excision. Tetanus status should be brought up to date, and antimicrobials should be provided.

For sponges, spicules should be removed with tape or a blunt-edged object like a credit card. Most of these envenomations will run their course despite intervention, and antihistamines and steroids are rarely of use.[67,68]

SUMMARY

Most marine envenomations produce pain or few symptoms. However, clinical manifestations include paralysis, respiratory failure, hemodynamic collapse, anaphylaxis, and death. Organisms differ greatly by geographic location. Clinicians should be familiar with common marine organisms in their practice regions and with the availability and sourcing of marine antivenoms if they practice in an area inhabited by sea snakes, box jellyfish, or spiny fish. Vigilance should be maintained for systemic symptoms from envenomations. Further epidemiologic studies are needed to delineate exposures and presentations in North America. There is still significant opportunity for research, especially in the delineation of toxin mechanisms and in appropriate treatment, particularly in areas outside of Australia and Southeast Asia.

REFERENCES

1. Bronstein AC, Spyker DA, Cantilena LR, et al. 2010 annual report of the American Association of Poison Control Centers' National Poison Data System (NPDS): 28th annual report. Clin Toxicol (Phila) 2011;49:910–41.
2. Bronstein AC, Spyker DA, Cantilena LR, et al. 2011 annual report of the American Association of Poison Control Centers' National Poison Data System (NPDS): 29th annual report. Clin Toxicol (Phila) 2012;50:911–1164.
3. Fenner P. Marine envenomations: an update—a presentation on the current status of marine envenomations first aid and medical treatments. Emerg Med 2000;12:295–302.
4. Auerbach PS. Marine envenomations. N Engl J Med 1991;325:486–93.
5. Russell FE, Fairchild MD, Michaelson J. Some properties of the venom of the stingray. Med Arts Sci 1958;12:78–86.
6. Conceição K, Konno K, Melo RL, et al. Orpotrin: a novel vasoconstrictor peptide from the venom of the Brazilian stingray Potamotrygon gr. orbignyi. Peptides 2006;27:3039–46.
7. Conceição K, Santos JM, Bruni FM, et al. Characterization of a new bioactive peptide from Potamotrygon gr. orbignyi freshwater stingray venom. Peptides 2009;30:2191–9.
8. Haddad V Jr, Neto DG, de Paula Neto JB, et al. Freshwater stingrays: study of epidemiologic, clinic and therapeutic aspects based on 84 envenomings in humans and some enzymatic activities of the venom. Toxicon 2004;43:287–94.
9. McGoldrick J, Marx JA. Marine envenomations; part 1: vertebrates. J Emerg Med 1991;9:497–502.
10. Diaz JH. The evaluation, management, and prevention of stingray injuries in travelers. J Travel Med 2008;15:102–9.
11. Clark RF, Girard RH, Rao D, et al. Stingray envenomation: a retrospective review of clinical presentation and treatment in 119 cases. J Emerg Med 2007; 33:33–7.
12. Isbister GK. Venomous fish stings in tropical northern Australia. Am J Emerg Med 2001;19:561–5.
13. Barss P. Wound necrosis caused by the venom of stingrays. Pathological findings and surgical management. Med J Aust 1984;141:854–5.
14. Smarrito S, Smarrito F, Leclair O, et al. Surgical management of stingray injuries. About two clinical cases. Ann Chir Plast Esthet 2004;49:383–6 [in French].
15. Davies RS, Evans RJ. Weever fish stings: a report of two cases presenting to an accident and emergency department. J Accid Emerg Med 1996;13:139–41.
16. Kizer KW, McKinney HE, Auerbach PS. Scorpaenidae envenomation. A five-year poison center experience. JAMA 1985;253:807–10.
17. Kreger AS. Detection of a cytolytic toxin in the venom of the stonefish (Synanceia trachynis). Toxicon 1991;29:733–43.
18. Khoo HE. Bioactive proteins from stonefish venom. Clin Exp Pharmacol Physiol 2002;29:802–6.
19. Church JE, Hodgson WC. Dose-dependent cardiovascular and neuromuscular effects of stonefish (Synanceja trachynis) venom. Toxicon 2000;38:391–407.

20. Chhatwal I, Dreyer F. Isolation and characterization of dracotoxin from the venom of the greater weever fish Trachinus draco. Toxicon 1992;30:87–93.
21. Briars GL, Gordon GS. Envenomation by the lesser weever fish. Br J Gen Pract 1992;42:213.
22. Currie BJ. Marine antivenoms. J Toxicol Clin Toxicol 2003;41:301–8.
23. Walker MJ, Yeoh PN. The in vitro neuromuscular blocking properties of sea snake (Enhydrina schistosa) venom. Eur J Pharmacol 1974;28:199–208.
24. Auerbach PS. Envenomations from jellyfish and related species. J Emerg Nurs 1997;23:555–65.
25. Tibballs J. Australian venomous jellyfish, envenomation syndromes, toxins and therapy. Toxicon 2006;48:830–59.
26. Burnett JW, Weinrich D, Williamson JA, et al. Autonomic neurotoxicity of jellyfish and marine animal venoms. Clin Auton Res 1998;8:125–30.
27. Ramasamy S, Isbister GK, Seymour JE, et al. The in vivo cardiovascular effects of box jellyfish Chironex fleckeri venom in rats: efficacy of pre-treatment with antivenom, verapamil and magnesium sulphate. Toxicon 2004;43:685–90.
28. O'Reilly GM, Isbister GK, Lawrie PM, et al. Prospective study of jellyfish stings from tropical Australia, including the major box jellyfish Chironex fleckeri. Med J Aust 2001;175:652–5.
29. Lumley J, Williamson JA, Fenner PJ, et al. Fatal envenomation by Chironex fleckeri, the north Australian box jellyfish: the continuing search for lethal mechanisms. Med J Aust 1988;148:527–34.
30. Ramasamy S, Isbister GK, Seymour JE, et al. Pharmacologically distinct cardiovascular effects of box jellyfish (Chironex fleckeri) venom and a tentacle-only extract in rats. Toxicol Lett 2005;155:219–26.
31. Mustafa R, White E, Hongo K, et al. The mechanism underlying the cardiotoxic effect of the toxin from the jellyfish Chironex fleckeri. Toxicol Appl Pharmacol 1995;133:196–206.
32. Tibballs J, Li R, Tibballs HA, et al. Australian carybdeid jellyfish causing "Irukandji syndrome". Toxicon 2012;59:617–25.
33. Winkel KD, Tibballs J, Molenaar P, et al. Cardiovascular actions of the venom from the Irukandji (Carukia barnesi) jellyfish: effects in human, rat and guinea-pig tissues in vitro and in pigs in vitro. Clin Exp Pharmacol Physiol 2005;32:777–88.
34. Barnes JH. Cause and effect in Irukandji stingings. Med J Aust 1964;1:897–904.
35. Huynh TT, Seymour J, Pereira P, et al. Severity of Irukandji syndrome and nematocyst identification from skin scrapings. Med J Aust 2003;178:38–41.
36. Little M, Mulcahy RF. A year's experience of Irukandji envenomation in far north Queensland. Med J Aust 1998;169:638–41.
37. McGoldrick J, Marx JA. Marine envenomations; part 2: invertebrates. J Emerg Med 1992;9:71–7.
38. Stein MR, Marraccini JV, Rothschild NE, et al. Fatal Portuguese man-o'-war (Physalia physalis) envenomation. Ann Emerg Med 1989;18:312–5.
39. Burnett JW, Gable WD. A fatal jellyfish envenomation by the Portuguese man-o'war. Toxicon 1989;27:823–4.
40. Cormier SM. Exocytic and cytolytic release of histamine from mast cells treated with Portuguese man-of-war (Physalia physalis) venom. J Exp Zool 1984;231:1–10.
41. Kaufman MB. Portuguese man-of-war envenomation. Pediatr Emerg Care 1992; 8:27–8.
42. Loten C, Stokes B, Worsley D, et al. A randomised controlled trial of hot water (45 degrees C) immersion versus ice packs for pain relief in bluebottle stings. Med J Aust 2006;184:329–33.

43. Russo AJ, Calton GJ, Burnett JW. The relationship of the possible allergic response to jellyfish envenomation and serum antibody titers. Toxicon 1983; 21:475–80.
44. Wittle LW, Middlebrook RE, Lane CE. Isolation and partial purification of a toxin from Millepora alcicornis. Toxicon 1971;9:327–31.
45. Iguchi A, Iwanaga S, Nagai H. Isolation and characterization of a novel protein toxin from fire coral. Biochem Biophys Res Commun 2008;365:107–12.
46. Brown CK, Shepherd SM. Marine trauma, envenomations, and intoxications. Emerg Med Clin North Am 1992;10:385–408.
47. Wong DE, Meinking TL, Rosen LB. Seabather's eruption. Clinical, histologic, and immunologic features. J Am Acad Dermatol 1994;30:399–406.
48. Segura-Puertas L, Ramos ME, Aramburo C, et al. One Linuche mystery solved: all 3 stages of the coronate scyphomedusa Linuche unguiculata cause seabather's eruption. J Am Acad Dermatol 2001;44:624–8.
49. Ward NT, Darracq MA, Tomaszewski C, et al. Evidence-based treatment of jellyfish stings in North America and Hawaii. Ann Emerg Med 2012;60:399–414.
50. Exton DR, Fenner PJ, Williamson JA. Cold packs: effective topical analgesia in the treatment of painful stings by Physalia and other jellyfish. Med J Aust 1989; 151:625–6.
51. Atkinson PR, Boyle A, Hartin D, et al. Is hot water immersion an effective treatment for marine envenomation? Emerg Med J 2006;23:503–8.
52. Nomura JT, Sato RL, Ahern RM, et al. A randomized paired comparison trial of cutaneous treatments for acute jellyfish (Carybdea alata) stings. Am J Emerg Med 2002;20:624–6.
53. Pereira PL, Carrette T, Cullen P, et al. Pressure immobilisation bandages in first-aid treatment of jellyfish envenomation: current recommendations reconsidered. Med J Aust 2000;173:650–2.
54. Markenson D, Ferguson JD, Chameides L, et al. Part 13: first aid: 2010 American Heart Association and American Red Cross International Consensus on first aid science with treatment recommendations. Circulation 2010;122: 582–605.
55. Corkeron M, Pereira P, Makrocanis C. Early experience with magnesium administration in Irukandji syndrome. Anaesth Intensive Care 2004;32:666–9.
56. McCullagh N, Pereira P, Cullen P, et al. Randomised trial of magnesium in the treatment of Irukandji syndrome. Emerg Med Australas 2012;24:560–5.
57. Fegan D, Andresen D. Conus geographus envenomation. Lancet 1997;349: 1672.
58. Yoshiba S. An estimation of the most dangerous species of cone shell, Conys (Gastridium) geographus Linne, 1758, venom's lethal dose in humans. Nihon Eiseigaku Zasshi 1984;39:565–72.
59. Terlau H, Olivera BM. Conus venoms: a rich source of novel ion channel-targeted peptides. Physiol Rev 2004;84:41–68.
60. Olivera BM, Hillyard DR, Rivier J, et al. Conotoxins: targeted peptide ligands from snail venoms. In: Hall S, Strichartz G, editors. Marine Toxins. Washington, DC: American Chemical Society; 1990. p. 256–78.
61. Li RA, Tomaselli GF. Using the deadly mu-conotoxins as probes of voltage-gated sodium channels. Toxicon 2004;44:117–22.
62. Magbubah E, Bajic VB, Archer JA. Conotoxins that confer therapeutic possibilities. Mar Drugs 2012;10:1244–65.
63. Walker DG. Survival after severe envenomation by the blue-ringed octopus (*Hapalochlaena maculosa*). Med J Aust 1983;2:663–5.

64. Sheumack DD, Howden ME, Spence I, et al. Maculotoxin: a neurotoxin from the venom glands of the octopus *Hapalochlaena maculosa* identified as tetrodotoxin. Science 1978;199:188–9.
65. Sutherland SK, Lane WR. Toxins and mode of envenomation of the common ringed or blue-banded octopus. Med J Aust 1969;1:893–8.
66. Southcott RV, Coulter JR. The effects of the southern Australian marine stinging sponges, Neofibularia mordens and Lissodendoryx sp. Med J Aust 1971;2: 895–901.
67. Isbister GK, Hooper JN. Clinical effects of stings by sponges of the genus Tedania and a review of sponge stings worldwide. Toxicon 2005;46:782–5.
68. Burnett JW, Calton GJ, Morgan RJ. Dermatitis due to stinging sponges. Cutis 1987;39:476.

Ionizing Radiation Injuries and Illnesses

Doran M. Christensen, DO*, Carol J. Iddins, MD,
Stephen L. Sugarman, MS, CHP, CHCM

KEYWORDS

- Acute radiation syndrome • Hematopoietic syndrome • Cutaneous syndrome
- Cutaneous radiation syndrome • Acute local radiation injury • Radiological • Nuclear

KEY POINTS

- Ionizing radiation injuries and illnesses are usually delayed, with the exception of extremely high or fatal doses.
- Stabilize medical and surgical conditions before dealing with radiological issues.
- Remove victim from contaminated area and remove potentially contaminated clothing using radiation protection principles.
- Obtain medical history and physical examination to include pertinent negatives.
- Obtain incident history and summon physics expertise to assist with radiation dose estimations.

INTRODUCTION

The spectrum of information related to diagnosis and management of radiation injuries and illnesses is vast. It is assumed that most physicians in practice have little or no remembrance of materials taught in secondary school or college about physics and

Funding Sources: ORAU.
Conflict of Interest: None.
Declarations and disclaimers: This work was performed under Contract # DE-AC05-06OR23100 between Oak Ridge Associated Universities (ORAU) and the US Department of Energy (USDOE). REAC/TS is a program of the Oak Ridge Institute for Science & Education (ORISE), which is operated for the USDOE by ORAU. The opinions expressed herein are those of the authors and are not necessarily those of the US Government (USG), the USDOE, ORAU, or sponsoring institutions of ORAU. Neither the USG nor the USDOE, nor any of their employees, makes any warranty, expressed or implied, or assumes any legal liability or responsibility for the accuracy, completeness, or usefulness of the information contained herein or represents that its use would not infringe on privately owned rights.
Radiation Emergency Assistance Center/Training Site (REAC/TS), Oak Ridge Institute for Science and Education (ORISE), U.S. Department of Energy (DOE), Oak Ridge Associated Universities (ORAU), PO Box 117, MS-39, Oak Ridge, TN 37831, USA
* Corresponding author.
E-mail address: doran.christensen@orau.org

Emerg Med Clin N Am 32 (2014) 245–265
http://dx.doi.org/10.1016/j.emc.2013.10.002
emed.theclinics.com

units of measurement. A very brief overview will be provided. Ionizing radiation injuries and illnesses are very rare, as are contamination incidents involving radioactive materials (REAC/TS Radiation Accident Registry). Most health care providers have had little to no experience with such cases, with perhaps the exception of those working in radiation oncology or nuclear medicine, where diagnostic and therapeutic application normally occur.[1] Furthermore, many medical school curricula do not include information about Disaster Medicine including radiological and nuclear hazards[2]; this is despite the fact that radiation sources (radioisotopes) enjoy widespread use in industry (eg, oil, gas, electrical power, and engineering); food, blood, and medical supply treatment; the military; research, and medicine. The US Nuclear Regulatory Commission and the States maintain approximately 22,000 radioactive materials licenses.[3] Exposures to ionizing radiation and internal contamination with radioactive materials can cause significant tissue damage and conditions. Emergency practitioners unaware of ionizing radiation as the cause of a condition, may miss the diagnosis of radiation-induced injury or illness. A review of the pathophysiology and medical management of radiation injuries and illnesses is thus important to fill this gap.

APPLICABLE PHYSICS

Radiation is generally defined as energy that is propagated through space.[4] A basic understanding of physics is necessary to fully apprehend the injuries that may result from radiological incidents. Radioactive materials are substances that emit ionizing radiation in an effort to reach nuclear stability. Ionizing radiations have sufficient energy to create charged particles, that is, ions, by the removal of a negatively charged electron from an atom. Electrons circle in orbits around central atomic nuclei made up of positively charged protons and electrically neutral neutrons.[5–9] Removal of an electron from such an atom would create 2 ions: the negatively charged electron and the positively charged atomic remnant. If ionization occurs in a biologically important molecule like a strand of DNA, the genome may not be able to function properly.[10]

Types of Ionizing Radiation

There are only a few ionizing radiations of concern for practical medical purposes: alpha particles, beta particles, positrons, and neutrons, plus the pure electromagnetic energy radiations gamma rays and X rays. All of these radiations, with the exception of X rays, are emitted from the nuclei of unstable radioactive atoms. X rays can be machine produced or can occur when electrons drop to lower energy orbital shells due to "self-ionization" of radioactive atoms.[5–9]

Alpha (α)

An alpha particle consists of 2 protons and 2 neutrons and has a +2 charge associated with it. It is very effective at ionizing other atoms and deposits its energy rapidly across its linear path. For medical purposes, this is important because an alpha particle can travel no more than a few centimeters in air and, as a general rule, cannot penetrate the outer layer of dead human skin. Alpha particles are therefore an internal hazard only. Materials that emit alpha particles pose a radiological hazard only if taken into the body via inhalation, ingestion, or if they enter the body via a contaminated wound. A sheet of paper is an effective shield for alpha particles (**Fig. 1**).[5]

Beta (β)

A beta particle is identical to an electron; however, because of some nuclear transformations it is emitted from the nuclei of some radioactive materials. Negatively charged beta particles, typically thought of as negatively charged, can penetrate further than

SHIELDING

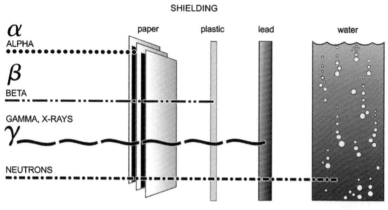

REAC/TS 2012

Fig. 1. Shielding requirements for various ionizing radiations.

alpha particles (several feet in air) and can penetrate human skin sometimes into subcutaneous tissues. Betas can therefore be an internal or an external hazard. A sheet of plastic, even plastic eyeglass lenses, can shield humans from most beta particles (see **Fig. 1**).[5]

Positron (β⁺)

Positrons are positively charged beta particles emitted from the nuclei of some radioactive materials. They are essentially the antiparticles of electrons. When a positron interacts with an electron (its antiparticle), their masses are converted to energy (annihilation) resulting in the release of 2 "coincident" 511 keV photons at 180° from each other. Shielding from these photons requires dense materials like lead, steel, or concrete (see **Fig. 1**).[5] Positron-emitters are commonly used in some medical procedures.

Neutron

Neutrons are emitted from some radioactive materials. Those materials, however, are rare. More commonly, neutrons are associated with a criticality, a term used for nuclear fission or "the splitting of the atom." Neutrons can occur across a wide range of energies and can travel very long distances in air. They are not very interactive, but depending on their energy, can cause much damage to tissues when they finally interact because of their mass. Hydrogen is an excellent material for neutron shielding because its nucleus is approximately the same mass as the neutron. Water and paraffin are excellent shields for neutrons because they contain a large number of hydrogen atoms (see **Fig. 1**).[5] Neutrons are the only kind of ionizing radiation that can make other matter radioactive by adding neutrons to other atomic nuclei called "neutron activation."

Gamma rays and X rays

Gamma rays and X rays are photons or pure electromagnetic energy that have no mass. For that reason, they are not very efficient at creating ionization in matter and are much more penetrating than alpha and beta particles. Generally, gamma rays are more energetic than X rays and are more penetrating. Shielding from gamma or X rays requires high atomic weight materials such as lead, steel, or concrete (see **Fig. 1**).[5]

Units of Measurement

Radioactive materials are quantified by their decay rate. This is referred to as activity and defined as the number of disintegrations occurring per unit time. One disintegration per second (dps) is a becquerel (Bq) in SI units (International System of Units of Measurement). This unit is so small that it is much more common to see units of millions of Bq (megabecquerels or MBq) or trillions of Bq (gigabecquerels or GBq) or even larger.

More commonly used in the United States is the conventional unit called the curie (Ci) which is equivalent to 3.7×10^{10} dps (or Bq). Common subdivisions of the curie include the millicurie (mCi, thousandth of a curie) and the microcurie (μCi, millionths of a Ci). Disintegrations per minute (dpm) are also commonly used. A simple conversion factor is 1 μCi = 2.22 million dpm = 37,000 dps = 37 kBq.[5] Specific activity is a concept that describes activity per unit mass. Common units include Ci/g and Bq/g.

Radiation Dose

When ionizing radiation deposits its energy in the human body, it is referred to as absorbed dose or simply dose. The unit of measure for dose used in the United States is the rad. The unit for radiation dose in the SI system is the gray (Gy). A gray is equivalent to 100 rad or 0.01 Gy is equivalent to 1 rad. Use of the SI units is recommended.[5]

Equivalent Dose

Some radiations are more effective at causing long-term effects than others. The method for equating the biologic effect and longer-term risk from exposure to the various kinds of ionizing radiation is called equivalent dose. Equivalent dose is calculated by multiplying the radiation dose in rads or Gy by a radiation weighting factor (W_R). The radiation weighting factor is different for each radiation based primarily on their abilities to interact with other materials, and it relates the amount of biologic damage, and thus resulting risk, caused by any type of radiation to that caused by the same absorbed dose of X rays or gamma rays. Equivalent dose is measured in the United States with a unit called the rem. The SI unit is the sievert (Sv). The relationship between rem and Sv is the same as the relationship between the radiation absorbed dose units rad and gray: 100 rem = 1 Sv and 0.01 Sv = 1 rem[5–9]

As an example, simply put alpha particle irradiation (by internalization) is 20 times more effective than gamma rays or X rays at causing long-term tissue damage **(Table 1)**.

RADIOBIOLOGY

Radiobiology is the study of effects of ionizing radiation on living creatures. The very basics assist in understanding ionizing radiation injuries and illnesses. Elements in this

Table 1
Radiation types and their weighting factors

Radiation Type	W_R (Weighting Factor)
Gamma- and X-rays	1
Alpha	20
Beta	1
Neutron	5–20

section are derived from a Hall and Giaccia text entitled "Radiobiology for the Radiologist,"[10] which is recommended reading for background in managing radiation-induced injuries and illnesses. A few of the major concepts follow.

Deterministic Effects of Ionizing Radiation

The short-term or relatively early effects of exposure to ionizing radiation are called deterministic effects because, essentially, the radiation dose "determines" the effect. There are also other factors that help determine radiation effects: total dose, dose rate, volume of tissue irradiated, type and quality of the radiation, presence of other disease conditions, concomitant physical trauma and/or thermal burns, and individual susceptibility.[10] Each of these factors contributes to worsening of the effects of radiation exposure. For deterministic effects, there is a "threshold" dose at which an effect is seen. As the dose is increased above that threshold, the effect worsens.

Stochastic Effects of Ionizing Radiation

Stochastic effects of radiation exposure are effects that occur by chance. An example of a stochastic effect is carcinogenesis. As the dose is increased, the likelihood that cancer will develop increases.[10] Counseling patients on the longer-term risk of radiation exposure is difficult and complex. In reality, several delayed effects need to be explained to exposed persons or families to help relieve anxiety. A few are mentioned in **Box 1**.

There are several information sources regarding the topics in **Box 1**. These include documents on the atomic bomb data and effects on survivors, hereditary effects in children of atomic bomb survivors, effects on children who were *in utero* at the time of the Japanese atomic detonations, cancer risk following low doses of ionizing radiation,[11–14] effects on personnel after the Chernobyl disaster such as thyroid cancer in children,[15] exposure of children to computed tomographic scans, and relationship to carcinogenesis.[16] Good sources of information about these matters are available in the Biologic Effects of Ionization Reports V–VII from the National Academy of Sciences and Sources and Effects of Ionizing Radiation from United Nations Scientific Committee on the Effects of Atomic Radiation (UNSCEAR), a 2-volume set most recently published in 2008. These sources should be accessed by anyone who might reasonably be expected to counsel patients and their families on the effects of ionizing radiation.

Exposure or Irradiation Versus Contamination

If one is in the presence of a source of ionizing radiation, one is being exposed or irradiated. There is *no transfer* of radioactive materials required for an exposure or

Box 1
Delayed effects of ionizing radiation
Radiation carcinogenesis
Genetic hazards
Late organ effects from therapeutic doses of radiation
Vascular changes, fibroatrophy
Cataracts
Infertility
Thyroid dysfunction

irradiation. As a reminder, an exposed or irradiated patient cannot contaminate others, equipment, or facilities. On the other hand, if something or someone has radioactive materials physically in them (internally contaminated) or on them (external contamination) they could cause contamination of others.[5,10] It is important to recognize that contamination with different materials results in differing risks. External contamination with an alpha-emitter will not pose a hazard unless that material is internalized, but contamination with a beta-emitter may be of concern because beta particles can penetrate beyond the outer, dead layer of skin, resulting in a potential risk for skin injury. Conversely, the level of concern is much higher for much smaller *amounts* of an internalized alpha emitter as compared to an internalized beta/gamma emitter because of the alpha's ability to create greater ionization/damage within cells as compared to that of a beta or gamma emitter.

Radiation Protection and ALARA

Protecting oneself, equipment, facilities, and the environment from exposure to ionizing radiation and/or contamination with radioactive materials is relatively easy when compared to chemical and biologic agents. This is because the energy from an ionizing radiation can easily be detected and identified with special instrumentation. Instrumentation that can give instantaneous levels of radiation or instantaneous identification of a radioactive material is readily available from several manufacturers.[5] There is also instrumentation available that will give accumulated dose to personnel or an area.

Health care providers should know that they can protect themselves from radioactive contamination relatively easily by using the same personal protective equipment (PPE) that is used as protection against biologic agents. The only difference between radioactive contamination and contamination with any other substance is that in the case of the former, some of the atoms emit radiation. A set of surgical scrubs, surgical mask, protective eyewear or face shield, head cover, shoe covers, and 2 pairs of nitrile gloves will generally meet protective needs. Be aware of protective clothing that does not "breathe" well, which may create a heat stress hazard during routine emergency activities. If the situation allows, PPE requirements can be lessened, thereby increasing responder comfort. On the rare occasion where respiratory protection will be required, an N95 mask or negative pressure HEPA-filtered respirator should suffice. Beware of interference of some of these PPE with ability to palpate, auscultate, and communicate with coworkers.[17]

The methods for minimizing the potential for exposure fall under the principles of ALARA, which is an acronym for "as low as reasonably achievable." These principles include the following: minimize *time* spent in the presence of a radiation source, maximize *distance* from a radiation source, maximize *shielding* between a source and persons, and minimize the *quantity* of radioactive materials in the area.[5]

Radiosensitivity and Radioresistance

Key to understanding the radiobiology of radiation injury is the concept of "radiosensitivity" and "radioresistance." These terms are the basis for an explanation of one of the oldest tenets of radiation medicine called the Law of Bergonié and Tribondeau (1906). This "law" simply states that cells that are actively dividing (are mitotically active or have a high mitotic index) and cells that are immature (or are not well-differentiated) are much more radiosensitive than other cells. The obverse is generally true: cells that are not actively dividing and those cells that are more differentiated are more radioresistant than others, with one major exception being mature lymphocytes (see the section "Hematopoietic Syndrome"). Radiosensitive cells of major clinical significance are hematopoietic stem cells, epidermal stem cells, endothelial cells, gastrointestinal stem cells, and cells of the neurovascular system (see the section "Acute Radiation Syndrome").

Median Lethal Dose 50/60 (LD$_{50/60}$)

The LD$_{50/60}$ is the acute dose of ionizing radiation that will cause the death of 50% of a human population within 60 days without medical treatment. This radiation dose is on the order of 3.5 to 4.5 Gy (350–450 rad).[10]

Chromatid Breakage and Mitotic Death

As has been mentioned previously, any atom or molecule can be ionized by radiation. If the molecule happens to be a biologically important molecule, for example, chromosomal DNA, the end results could be highly varied. The good news for damage to chromosomal DNA is that there are repair enzymes called endonucleases, that can repair a DNA single-strand break (SSB). If there is a break in only 1 strand of DNA and it is repaired properly, the chromosome may be able to function normally, although it is possible that its function could remain impaired.

If there is a break in both strands of chromosomes or sister chromatids, there is a double-strand break (DSB). The likelihood that repair would be accurate is much smaller than repair of an SSB. If DNA is transferred between sister chromatids and the sequences are not exactly the same, that is, the exchange is "asymmetrical", improper repair may result in the chromosomes not being able to function at all or may be impaired. Centromeres are important to mitosis because those sites are where microtubules attach to help pull sister chromatids apart at mitosis. If the asymmetrical exchange results in more than 1 centromere in a sister chromatid (a dicentric), the chromosomes will not be able to divide at mitosis and will die a "mitotic death" (**Fig. 2**).

Apoptosis

Another important method of cell killing is called apoptosis. Apoptosis is a term that is sometimes called "programed cell death." It is a normal physiologic process that allows an organism to rid itself of senescent cells, cells that are functioning abnormally, cancerous cells, or cells that are predestined to be eliminated. Apoptosis is a process

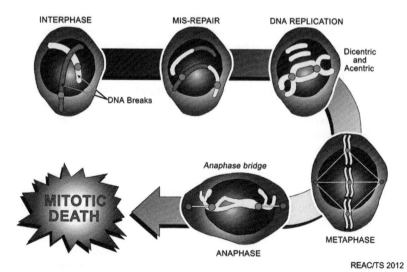

Fig. 2. Mitotic death.

of cellular death that is not accompanied by an inflammatory response, as opposed to necrosis. If a cell is damaged by a noxious agent such as ionizing radiation, it may initiate the apoptosis cascade and die. This is an abnormal physiological process that is sometimes called "cellular suicide." The genome is activated to produce the enzymatic sequence that will result in production of an executioner caspase enzyme that will result in cell death.[10]

Direct Ionization and Indirect Cellular Interactions

Direct ionization occurs when a radiation directly strikes a DNA sequence causing a break in the strand. The energy resulting from ionization, 33 eV, is more than enough to break a C=C bond with its bonding energy of 4.9 eV.[10] Direct ionization is more common with what are called "high linear energy transfer" (high LET) radiations like alpha particles. Indirect ionization occurs primarily when a "low linear energy transfer" (low LET) photon strikes a molecule of water generating a "free radical." A free radical is an atom or molecule that has an unpaired electron in its outer orbital. Free radicals are chemically very reactive, and they can cause DNA strand breaks. Their ionization is called indirect because it is not the original ionizing event that results in DNA damage, but rather the interaction of the free radical with the target molecule. Orbitals or sub-orbitals contain 2 electrons in each. Each electron has a spin on its own axis that is in the opposite direction of the other electron: one spins in a clockwise direction and the other in a counterclockwise direction. Lack of a paired electron in that orbital makes the atom more chemically reactive.[10]

INITIAL MANAGEMENT OF RADIATION CASUALTIES

There are some general rules for management of radiation casualties. Most importantly, the morbidity and mortality from ionizing radiation injuries increase dramatically in the face of physical trauma, thermal burns, and other significant medical conditions. Therefore, unstable medical and surgical conditions should be stabilized before radiological issues increase to any level of significance (**Box 2**).[17]

OVERALL MEDICAL MANAGEMENT OF RADIOLOGICAL EXPOSURES

The prime consideration for the radiation-injured or ill is to stabilize unstable medical or surgical conditions first. Then, and only then, do issues related to exposure or contamination rise to a level of priority. After emergent stabilization of any immediate life-threatening emergencies, the focus can turn to treatment of acute symptoms and the anticipation of later complications. Acute pain may be severe and may be managed with acetaminophen and opioids. It is generally advised to avoid nonsteroidal antiinflammatory agents, as the patient may be at risk of gastrointestinal bleeding due to mucosal damage if the estimated dose is >5-6 Gy. It is important to obtain a clear history of the timing of symptoms and a complete blood count as soon as possible to help approximate dose of radiation received by the patient (discussed in detail in the later discussion). Type and screen/crossmatch is also indicated for the possible administration of blood products. HLA typing should be done as soon as possible if the dose is expected to be >2 Gy in preparation for bone marrow or stem cell transplantation for pancytopenia. Those who survive the acute phase following a large exposure will be at risk for severe infectious (i.e. sepsis), gastrointestinal, and metabolic complications.

Acute Radiation Syndrome

There is a spectrum of predictable processes that occur in the organ systems of the body after a radiological exposure (irradiation) and/or contamination. These are often

---

Box 2
Sequence for managing contaminated injured/ill patients

In the field, ensure that the scene is safe for entry of responders

Attend to unstable medical and surgical conditions if the area is safe to conduct such activities

Remove a casualty from any source of further potentially dangerous radiation exposure or contamination with radioactive materials: remove the victim from the radiation area, remove contaminated clothing, and leave clothing at the scene if possible

Obtain a standard medical history as for all injuries and illnesses

Obtain a history of the radiation incident and call for health physics support to assist with incident recreation and dose estimation

Obtain vital signs, including temperature and weight

Complete physical examination, including documentation of pertinent negatives

Survey radiological contamination of open wounds, the face, and intact skin

Obtain nasal swab of each naris and count with radiation detector as soon as possible (if alpha emitter is suspected let swabs dry and resurvey)

Diagnostic imaging as indicated

Laboratory: routine trauma and medical laboratory analyses

Laboratories: initial CBC with WBCs and differential, then serially every 8 hours until decrease is stable, then daily; initial serum amylase (if head and neck region are involved) then daily for 3 days; initial CRP then daily for 3 days

Urinalysis

Begin collection of excreta for radioassay

Treat other significant medical conditions as appropriate

Call REAC/TS for assistance (865-576-1005)

Abbreviations: CBC, complete blood count; CRP, C reactive protein; WBC, white blood cell.

---

grouped into subsyndromes based on the affected organ system and have some fairly predictable dose thresholds at which the "classic" subsyndrome presents. It must be understood that all tissues/organs involved in the injury may have some degree of pathophysiologic process of damage occurring during this time.[17–20]

Fig. 3 shows recommended sequence of treatment priorities for a radiation incident patient. The top red box indicates that medical/surgical stabilization is the absolute top priority. After stabilization, radiological issues can rise to a level of priority. The lower left-hand 2 columns shows the sequence of activities required for the patient who might be internally contaminated. The lower right-hand column shows the sequence of activities for someone who might have been exposed or irradiated. In some cases, all 3 columns will need to be followed because a patient could well be contaminated and irradiated.

Hematopoietic Syndrome

The bone marrow produces billions of cells per day making this tissue one of the most prolific in the human body; it is highly metabolically active. Also, most of the cells in the bone marrow are relatively immature. These 2 features make the bone marrow one of the most radiosensitive organs in the human body, damage to which can result in a multitude of symptoms and signs, some of which can be lethal.

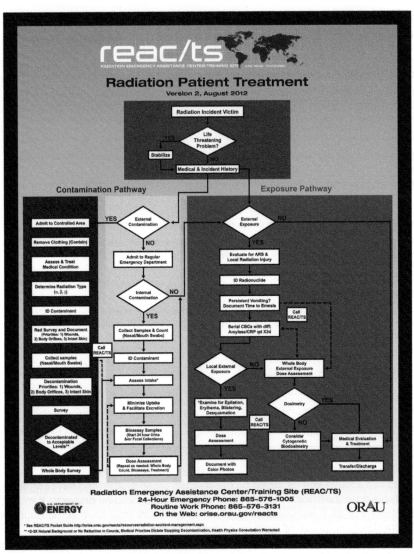

Fig. 3. REAC/TS Radiation Patient Treatment algorithm chart. (*Courtesy of* Oak Ridge Institute for Science and Education, Oak Ridge, TN.)

The lowest radiation dose that can produce changes in the bone marrow is about 0.20 Gy; however, clinical findings are not apparent until an absorbed dose of 0.75 to 1.00 Gy has been reached. The effects of ionizing radiation on the hematopoietic systems are deterministic, that is, as the dose increases, the hematopoietic acute radiation syndrome (H-ARS) becomes worse. The "classic" presentation will begin at doses greater than 2 Gy, but patients may be symptomatic at doses greater than 1 Gy.

Each type of blood cell has its own relative radiosensitivity. Of greatest concern initially following a radiation exposure is the damage that results to lymphocytes. The radiosensitivity of lymphocytes is the exception to the Law of Bergonié and Tribondeau mentioned earlier. Lymphocytes are terminally differentiated, and they are not mitotically active, yet they are exquisitely radiosensitive. The radiosensitivity of lymphocytes is also dose dependent, which is the basis for dose-response curves that have been developed to allow health care practitioners to use reductions in the absolute lymphocyte count (ALC) (lymphocyte depletion kinetics) to estimate how much of a whole-body exposure a casualty experienced. As the dose of ionizing radiation exposure increases, the faster the lymphocyte count drops and the lower its nadir (**Fig. 4**).

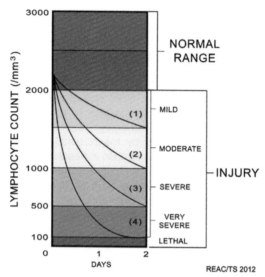

Fig. 4. Lymphocyte depletion kinetics. These lymphocyte depletion curves are called the "Andrews' curves" and are named after an early radiation medicine pioneer, Gould Andrews MD. (*Adapted from* Andrews GA, Auxier Jr, Lushbaugh CC. The importance of dosimetry to the medical management of persons accidentally exposed to high levels of radiation. In: Personnel Dosimetry for Radiation Accidents. Vienna: International Atomic Energy Agency; 1965.)

Absolute neutrophil count

The dose estimate from evaluating lymphocyte depletion kinetics can be used to predict another very important parameter, the drop in the "absolute neutrophil count (ANC)". As the immunocompetence of the casualty is degraded with the loss of lymphocytes, the loss of neutrophils can even further reduce the victim's immunologic competence. Infections will therefore become one of the greatest causes of morbidity and mortality in ionizing radiation incident victims.[18] The reduction of neutrophils usually occurs during a so-called critical period approximately 1 to 2 weeks after the exposure.

Enucleated cells

Mature red blood cells (RBC) and platelets are radioresistant. In keeping with the Law of Bergonié and Tribondeau, they are not mitotically active because they have no nuclei. They are also terminally differentiated. Their mitotically active and immature precursor cells, megakaryocytes and erythroblasts, are, however, sensitive to ionizing radiation. The time of appearance of significantly low levels of RBCs and platelets is also largely dependent on that cell's life cycle. For example, the developmental life cycle of RBCs is on the order of 4 months; therefore, an anemia caused by ionizing radiation does not usually appear for weeks at survivable doses, whereas a thrombo-cytopenia appears much earlier.

Medical management of the H-ARS

Management of the H-ARS depends on 2 major considerations: bridging cytopenic gaps and management of infections. Therefore, a hematologist and an infectious disease specialist should be consulted on these cases.

Bridging cytopenic gaps

Bridging the cytopenic gaps can be tackled currently in 3 ways: provision of cytokines or colony stimulating factors; administration of bone marrow cells from a closely matched relative; or stem cell transplants.

Cytokines or colony-stimulating factors

Granulocyte colony-stimulating factor (G-CSF) and granulocyte monocyte colony-stimulating factor stimulate immature granulocytes to proliferate, differentiate, and mature in the bone marrow. The Radiation Injury Treatment Network (RITN) is supported by the US Navy and managed by the National Marrow Donor Program. They recommend consideration of administration in healthy patients without other injuries at doses from 3 to 10 Gy (perhaps 2 Gy for children or the elderly). If multiple trauma or burns are present, lower doses may be more ideal thresholds for treatment, which ranges from 2 to 6 Gy. The World Health Organization (WHO) consultancy recommends consideration of initiating cytokine therapy for exposures of greater than or equal to 2 Gy within 24 hours of exposure, if possible: granulocyte CSF (filgrastim), 5 mcg/kg/d; granulocyte-macrophage (monocyte) CSF (sargramostim), 250 mcg/m^2/d; pegylated G-CSF (pegfilgrastim), in a 6 mg single subcutaneous dose. They extend this recommendation to include a decrease of ALC less than 500 that will persist for more than or equal to 7 days.[21]

The administration of CSFs must be timely, that is, preferably within several days of exposure. Administration will, of course, depend on having reasonable documentation that the acute whole body dose is 2 Gy or greater. The RITN website (www.ritn.net/) provides a more extensive discussion of managing cytopenias.

Bone marrow or stem cell transplants

Bone marrow transplants might be an acceptable treatment modality if there is an available allogeneic histocompatible donor. Patients with significant marrow injury estimated to be on the order of 2 to 9 Gy who become neutropenic within 5 to 7 days may need stem cell transplants (RITN). To be successful, these patients' other injuries such as physical trauma and/or thermal burns must be quite limited. The RITN website can be consulted for valuable information concerning the centers available for such transplants and other more detailed management guidelines. The WHO consultancy recommends consideration of stem/progenitor cell replacement (allogeneic hematopoietic stem cells from marrow, peripheral blood, or cord blood) if there is a lack of bone marrow recovery after 2 to 3 weeks of cytokine treatment and when that patient does not have other organ injuries.[21]

Prophylactic antimicrobials

Before the critical period of neutropenia, patients may need prophylactic antimicrobials to avoid reemergence of dormant viruses and other commensal organisms, for example, herpes simplex viruses, cytomegalovirus, Candida spp. These patients will need antimicrobials, antivirals, antifungals, and occasionally, antiparasitic agents if certain parasites are endemic.

Treatment of other infections

There are no guidelines *specifically* directed to management of infections related to the immunologic incompetence of *irradiated* patients. Therefore, most experts recommend the use of guidelines that have been developed by the Infectious Diseases Society of America for neutropenias from other causes.[22]

Cutaneous Radiation Syndrome or Local Radiation Injury

There are many terms to describe radiation injury to one of the body's largest organ systems, the skin. The terms cutaneous radiation syndrome (CRS), local radiation injury (LRI), radiodermatitis are all used in describing skin injury from radiation exposure. These injuries may be concurrent with total body irradiation or partial body irradiation (CRS), may be extensive enough in an area with other organs to cause a partial body irradiation, may be isolated to an area without major damage to other organ systems (eg, an extremity) (LRI), or may result from radiotherapy-induced erythema and edema. Radiodermatitis usually only describes skin effects of radiotherapy. These injuries may result in extensive disability, morbidity, and mortality. About 16 of the 28 acute deaths in Chernobyl were attributed to CRS.[23]

The inability to repopulate cell lines secondary to damage to epidermal stem cells in the basal layer of the epidermis occurs. The endothelial cells are also damaged and result in damage to the microvasculature as well as the extravasation of cytokines, neutrophils, macrophages, and other mediators into the surrounding tissues. The proinflammatory response seems to occur in successive waves. These injuries are best described as evolving. There is continued inflammation, tissue destruction, and often necrosis. The effects seen with time are excessive fibrosis into the affected tissues and even into the vasculature, poor wound healing, reinjury with the slightest of insult, and atrophy.

The threshold dose for deterministic effects in the skin is greater than 3 Gy (300 rad) for epilation or temporary loss of hair. The erythema dose for skin is about 6 Gy (600 rad). As the dose increases, skin effects worsen: dry desquamation at about 10–15 Gy (1000–1500 rad): moist desquamation at about 15–20 Gy (1500–2000 rad) ulcer formation and radionecrosis greater than 25 Gy (2500 rad).[17]

The clinical course of CRS is rather variable in that there may be a prodrome of erythema, pruritus, or burning/tingling sensation that can appear within the first 48 hours. There may be a latent phase in which the symptoms lessen or abate. Then, classically, the manifest illness phase occurs. Part of the variability with these injuries is that the patient may progress to manifest illness, skipping other phases. As a rule, the higher the dose, the faster this progression and worse the prognosis of the injury.

Medical management of CRS

Traditional treatment techniques for thermal burns are used in managing these patients. However, there are some differences for these injuries. The burn treatment modalities of dressing constructs such as Biobrane (UDL Laboratories Inc., Sugar Land, TX) and Integra (Integra LifeSciences Corporation, Plainsboro, NJ), surgical debridement, and grafting absolutely have a role in these injuries. The differences lie in the difficulty of demarcating the extent of the radiation injury. As the injury is evolving and ongoing, the naked eye cannot distinguish this line of demarcation. Various imaging techniques for evaluating extent of injury to the tissues and microvasculature should be considered before surgical treatment of these injuries. Another technique for demarcating the extent of injury is to do dose mapping. This technique along with another treatment modality was used by Lataillade and colleagues.[24] They combined dose mapping of extent of injury with injection of mesenchymal stem cells into the area of injury with good results. There are other countries doing small case studies of mesenchymal-derived or adipose-derived stem cell injections into injuries.

Other treatment modalities may be helpful in these injuries. The World Health consultancy (WHO) gave a strong recommendation for use of Class II and Class III steroids used topically, topical antibiotics, and topical antihistamines.[25] Other techniques include hyperbaric oxygen therapy, use of pentoxifylline/vitamin E, aloe vera, and other topicals used in radiation oncology.

Gastrointestinal Subsyndrome

The small intestine is uniquely designed and has increased its surface area for absorption of material many-fold by a design of elevations of intestinal villi and deep crypts. The most sensitive cells in the gastrointestinal system are the stem cells in the crypts of Leiberkühn between small intestinal villi.[10] These stem cells are the precursors of both enterocytes and goblet cells. These cells proliferate and mature in 3 to 5 days and then they will slough off with the passing fecal material. The higher the radiation dose, the greater the destruction and damage to the villi such that the tissues may become totally disorganized, thus disrupting the absorptive ability of the small intestine afforded by the crypts and villi. Damage to the epithelial lining is a primary defect in gastrointestinal subsyndrome (G-ARS) that allows translocation of bacteria with resultant infections.

The G-ARS like the CRS has the "classic" clinical presentation of prodrome, latent period, and manifest illness phase and like CRS is highly variable. The prodrome is characterized by nausea, emesis, occasionally diarrhea, and abdominal cramping. As the dose increases, the presentation of the prodrome may be more severe. Similar to the CRS, the higher the dose, the shorter the latent period. At higher doses there may be no latent period at all. As the dose increases, the effects become worse with severe nausea, emesis, hematemesis, hematochezia, fluid/electrolyte shifts, hypovolemia, obstruction, renal failure, and eventually cardiovascular collapse.[26]

Management of G-ARS

Emesis in the prodrome or the manifest illness phase of G-ARS is treated with 5-HT$_3$ receptor antagonists such as ondansetron 2 to 4 mg intravenously (IV) every 8 hours as needed for nausea or emesis.[25] Decontamination of the gut may be accomplished with the use of antibiotics, essentially to reduce the number of pathogenic bacteria that may become displaced to other parts of the body to cause infection. Nutritional support is absolutely essential if the patient is to survive, which may require total parenteral elemental nutrition (TPN) including the amino acid L-glutamine.[20] Despite being classified as "weak" recommendation by the recent WHO consultancy, antiemetics, antibiotics, and aggressive alimentary supplementation with TPN are reasonable efforts to initiate.[21,25]

Neurovascular Syndrome

The neurovascular syndrome (N-ARS) certainly occurs with total body irradiation greater than 20 Gy (>2000 rad).[17] Other authors say N-ARS can start at greater than 10 Gy (1000 rad).[25] Still others say N-ARS requires a higher than even 20 Gy (2000 rad). Significant cognitive, balance, and other neurologic signs and symptoms can be expected. The syndrome is universally fatal, so supportive, palliative care is indicated. A key point is that ionizing radiation does not cause neurologic signs and symptoms such as convulsions, coma, or extreme neurologic signs and symptoms at *survivable* doses. If neurologic findings are present and the dose of ionizing radiation is known to be less than 10 Gy (1000 rad), other causes should be sought.

Internal Contamination with Radioactive Materials

Internal contamination with radioactive materials is essentially a medical toxicology issue or the treatment of poisonings. This issue is very complicated and will require the assistance of REAC/TS, medical toxicologists, or health physicists, and physicians with experience with these injuries. Additionally, NCRP Report No. 161, Management of Persons Contaminated with Radionuclides: Handbook – Recommendations of the National Council on Radiation Protection and Measurements[27] should be available in emergency departments, radiation safety office, and/or occupational medicine clinic. Additionally, each of these facilities should have a copy of the REAC/TS Pocket Guide: Medical Aspects of Radiation Incidents,[17] which provides guidance on internal contamination, radiation protection, contamination control, and other valuable topics; this may be obtained by downloading in PDF or e-Pub form from the REAC/TS web page (https://orise.orau.gov/reacts/radiation-accident-management.aspx) or by attending a REAC/TS training course. The REAC/TS 24/7 emergency contact phone number is 865-576-1005.

Management of internal contamination with radioactive materials

A foreign material can enter the body in 4 ways, including inhalation, ingestion, absorption through a puncture or injection wound, or percutaneous absorption across normal skin. Because of the scope of this work, only management of more common radionuclides will be covered. General principles of management of internal contamination include the following: reduce absorption and internal deposition; enhance elimination or excretion; and begin treatment as soon as a credible and significant dose has been determined (**Box 3**).

Specific treatment methods

Intakes can be minimized by controlling contamination, removal of victims from contaminated environments, and removal of contaminated clothing.[27] Absorption may be reduced or inhibited by using some standard toxicologic therapies some of which have fallen or are falling from favor: gastric placement of activated charcoal, gastric

---

Box 3
Specific treatment methods for internal contamination

Minimize intake

Reduce and/or inhibit absorption

Block uptake

Isotopic dilution

Promote excretion

Alter chemistry of the substance

Displace isotope from receptors

Chelate

Bronchoalveolar lavage

Surgical removal

From International Atomic Energy Agency. Dosimetric and medical aspects of the radiological accident in Goiania in 1987. Vienna (Austria): International Atomic Energy Agency; 1998. IAEA-TECDOC-1009. Available at: http://www-pub.iaea.org/MTCD/publications/PDF/te_1009_prn.pdf. Accessed May 29, 2013. Copyright © 1998 IAEA.

lavage, the use of emetics, and the use of purgatives and laxatives. The use of oral stable iodine to saturate the metabolic processes of radioiodine incorporation into the thyroid hormone is an example of a blocking agent. Forced diuresis with IV fluids for ^3H (or tritium, the radioactive isotope of hydrogen) demonstrates the dilution technique.

Reduction or inhibition of absorption of some radionuclides can be accomplished using ion exchange resins orally (eg, Prussian blue or ferric [III] hexacyanoferrate [II] for internalization of radiocesium, radio thallium, or nonradioactive thallium). The chemistry of some substances can be changed, for example, barium sulfate or aluminum-containing antacids orally for ingested radiostrontium to result in strontium sulfate, which will be eliminated in the feces.

Chelation in the United States is generally accomplished with diethylene triamine pentaacetic acid (DTPA) of which there are 2 salts: Ca-DTPA and Zn-DTPA. Ca-DTPA is about 10 times as effective at chelation as the zinc salt; therefore, the first dose of DTPA is given 1 g IV and later doses are given 1 g IV as the zinc salt. DTPA is approved by Food and Drug Administration only for internal contaminations with plutonium, americium, and curium. Although DTPA may be effective for other heavy radioactive metals, its use in those cases would be off-label. Other chelators are available such as deferoxamine and penicillamine. There is no specific antidote for uranium. Depending on the amount of internalized uranium, alkalinization of the urine to 8 to 8.5 may be helpful. At larger internal burdens, uranium is dialyzable. Bronchoalveolar lavage used in experienced hands could be used for larger pulmonary intakes of various radionuclides. Amputations may be the last result for injuries that are not amenable to other therapies because of massive radiation tissue damage and/or complications.

Potassium iodide

After the Fukushima Japan 2011 nuclear power plant accident, many people sought out potassium iodide for "post-exposure" prophylaxis, even as far as on the US west coast. Radioactive I-131 can be suspended in the air or contaminated food and water supplies, so exposure occurs through inhalation and ingestion.

The EPA estimates that the risk of inhalational exposure is no more than a 10-mile radius surrounding a nuclear power plant, but ingestion can occur over a broader area (50 miles).[28] I-131 has a relatively short radioactive half-life of about 9 days, where nearly all of its radiation is dissipated within 3 months. Potassium iodide is used to block the uptake of I-131 into the thyroid tissue, decreasing the malignancy. But it is most effective when administered before I-131 exposure, and the benefits are significantly decreased after the exposure. The best evidence for the use of potassium iodide is in infants, children, and pregnant women. The risk of thyroid cancer is minimal in patients exposed to radioactive iodine after the age of 20 years and virtually no risk after 40 years of age.[29] Despite these facts, the sale and demand for potassium was very high after this nuclear incident and in most cases was not warranted. **Box 4** provides potassium iodide indications.

RADIOLOGICAL AND NUCLEAR INCIDENTS OF MEDICAL AND PUBLIC HEALTH CONCERN

There are several scenarios about which emergency planners, health care providers, and public health officials need to be aware. Some have the potential for massive destruction and multiple casualties, whereas some have the potential only for causing minor, although sometimes major injuries/illnesses in only a few persons.[30–35] Some scenarios present the challenges associated with managing mass casualties, many of whom will not be physically injured. Issues related to managing masses of persons

---

Box 4
Indications for potassium iodide administration

Predicted thyroid exposure

5 cGy in children, pregnant women, and breastfeeding women

10 cGy in adults between 18 and 40 years of age

500 cGy in those older than 40 years of age, solely to prevent radiation-induced hypothyroidism

From Center for Drug Evaluation and Research (CDER), U. S. Food and Drug Administration. Potassium Iodide as a Thyroid Blocking Agent in Radiation Emergencies. Rockville (MD): U.S. Department of Health and Human Services; 2001. Available at: http://www.fda.gov/downloads/Drugs/GuidanceComplianceRegulatoryInformation/Guidances/UCM080542.pdf. Accessed September 30, 2013.

---

who have anxiety, fear, and/or confusion may well interfere with the ability to practice medicine or recover from such an incident.[36,37]

Radiological Exposure Device

A radiological exposure device is conventionally thought of as surreptitious placement of a radiation source in an area that will expose unwary victims. Depending on the source activity and the time of exposure, several untoward consequences can occur. CRS and acute LRI might be expected. More significant exposures could result in H-ARS or even G-ARS depending on the circumstances. The numbers of affected persons would depend on how well the source was hidden and how wary public health and safety officials were about recognizing radiation injuries and illnesses. Several cases in the past couple of decades involving persons unwittingly handling dangerous radioactive sources have resulted in deaths of several people: 1996 Gilan, Iran, 1 seriously injured[38]; 1994 Tammiku, Estonia, 1 death, several seriously injured[39]; 2000 Samut Prakarn, Thailand, 3 deaths (7 seriously ill, hundreds significantly exposed),[40] among others.

Radiological Dispersal Device

A radiological dispersal device (RDD) is any device designed to spread radioactive materials. The 1987 Goiania, Brazil, cesium-137 accident in which 4 people died and 20 more became seriously ill can give an idea how a non-explosive RDD might cause havoc.[41,42] Many think of RDDs as explosive devices commonly called "dirty bombs" such as improvised explosive devices (IED) to which radioactive materials have been added. IEDs are relatively easy to make; all components can be purchased at farm supply stores. They are detonated daily around the world and cause untold injuries and deaths. RDDs do not need to explode; however, any device that could be used to spread radioactive materials is technically an RDD. The consequences from deployment of an RDD would depend on the amount and activity of the radioactive material and how widely the material is disseminated.

Nuclear Power Plant Incident

Nuclear reactors use a controlled fission process to generate electrical energy. The reactor core, where the fission process occurs, is the heat source that provides the elevated temperatures necessary for steam generation and electricity production. **Fig. 5** shows a pressurized water reactor, which can generate huge amounts of heat. If cooling of the reactor is interrupted, degradation of the components can occur

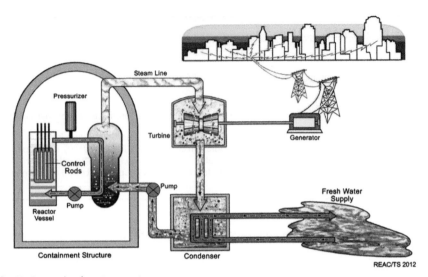

Fig. 5. Pressurized water reactor.

potentially, resulting in the release to the environment of radioactive materials such as radioiodines, ^{137}Cs, among others.

Improvised Nuclear Device/Nuclear Weapon

Nuclear reactors use heat generated to make electricity, but nuclear weapons use the criticality reaction to produce a detonation. Regardless of whether state-sponsored or as a result of a terrorist attack, a nuclear detonation would have catastrophic effects. If detonated in a populated urban area, even a small IND of less than 20 kT could be expected to cause tens of thousands of prompt deaths and many more within weeks. Wounds in survivors of the blast will likely be serious, including physical trauma, thermal burns, and eye injuries. Significant physical trauma including total blunt bodily trauma, ruptured tympanic membranes, and ruptured pleurae (pneumothoraces and pneumomediastinum) may be seen. Thermal burns can result from ignition of clothing or physical structures. Eye injuries can result from infrared exposure of the retina with temporary or permanent blindness. Many eye injuries could also result with foreign bodies from flying debris.

SUMMARY

Medical management of radiation exposure requires careful consideration of the route and type of exposure. Concomitant medical and surgical conditions require strict attention, as these increase morbidity and mortality. H-ARS, G-ARS, and CRS may be amenable to various therapies, although consultation is advised. N-ARS treatment is palliative.

REFERENCES

1. Benjamin GC, McGeary M, McCutchen SR, editors. Assessing medical preparedness to respond to a terrorist nuclear event: workshop report. Washington, DC: National Academies Press; 2009.

2. Association of American Medical Colleges. Training future physicians about weapons of mass destruction: report of the expert panel of bioterrorism education of medical students. Washington, DC: Association of American Medical Colleges; 2003.
3. Office of Public Affairs, U.S. Nuclear Regulatory Commission. The regulation and use of radioisotopes in today's world. NUREG/BR-0217 Revision 1. Washington, DC: U.S. Nuclear Regulatory Commission; 2000.
4. Borders RJ. The dictionary of health physics & nuclear sciences terms. Hebron (CT): RSA Publications; 1991.
5. Gollnick DA. Basic radiation protection technology. 6th edition. Altadena (CA): Pacific Radiation Corporation; 2011.
6. Turner JE. Atoms, radiation, and radiation protection. 2nd edition. Weinheim (Germany): Wiley-VCH Verlag GmbH & Co. KGaA; 2004.
7. Cember H, Johnson TE. Introduction to health physics. 4th edition. New York: McGraw-Hill; 2008.
8. Shapiro J. Radiation protection: a guide for scientists and physicians. 3rd edition. Cambridge (MA): Harvard University Press; 1990.
9. Stabin MG. Radiation protection and dosimetry: an introduction to health physics. New York: Springer; 2008.
10. Hall EJ, Giaccia AJ. Radiobiology for the radiologist. 7th edition. Philadelphia: Lippincott Williams & Wilkins; 2012.
11. International Commission on Radiological Protection. 1990 recommendations of the International commission on radiological protection. Oxford (United Kingdom): Pergamon Press; 1991. ICRP Publication 60.
12. National Council on Radiation Protection and Measurements. Risk estimates for radiation protection. Bethesda (MD): National Council on Radiation Protection and Measurements; 1993. NCRP Report No. 115.
13. Cardis E, Vrijheid M, Blettner M, et al. The 15-country collaborative study of cancer risk among radiation workers in the nuclear industry: estimates of radiation-related cancer risks. Radiat Res 2007;167:396–416.
14. Cardis E, Vrijheid M, Blettner M, et al. Risk of cancer after low doses of ionising radiation: retrospective cohort study in 15 countries. BMJ 2005;331:77.
15. Stsjazhko VA, Tsyb AF, Tronko ND, et al. Childhood thyroid cancer since accident at Chernobyl. BMJ 1995;310:801.
16. Mathews JD, Forsythe AV, Brady Z, et al. Cancer risk in 680 000 people exposed to computed tomography scans in childhood or adolescence: data linkage study of 11 million Australians. BMJ 2013;346:f2360.
17. Radiation Emergency Assistance Center Training Site, Sugarman SL, Goans RE, et al. REAC/TS pocket guide: the medical aspects of radiation incidents. Available at: http://orise.orau.gov/files/reacts/medical-aspects-of-radiation-incidents.pdf.
18. Fliedner TM, Friesecke I, Beyrer K, editors. Medical management of radiation accidents: manual on the acute radiation syndrome. London: British Institute of Radiology; 2001.
19. Flynn DF, Goans RE. Triage and treatment of radiation and combined-injury mass casualties. In: Mickelson AB, editor. Textbooks of military medicine: medical consequences of radiological and nuclear weapons. Fort Detrick (MD): Borden Institute; 2012. p. 17–72.
20. Ricks RC, Berger ME, O'Hara FM, editors. The medical basis for radiation-accident preparedness: the clinical care of victims. New York: Parthenon Publishing Group; 2002.

21. Dainiak N, Gent RN, Carr Z, et al. First global consensus for evidence-based management of the hematopoietic syndrome resulting from exposure to ionizing radiation. Disaster Med Public Health Prep 2011;5:202–12.
22. Freifeld AG, Bow EJ, Sepkowitz KA, et al. Clinical practice guideline for the use of antimicrobial agents in neutropenic patients with cancer: 2010 update by the infectious diseases society of america. Clin Infect Dis 2011;52:e56–93.
23. Gottlober P, Steinert M, Weiss M, et al. The outcome of local radiation injuries: 14 years of follow-up after the Chernobyl accident. Radiat Res 2001;155:409–16.
24. Lataillade JJ, Doucet C, Bey E, et al. New approach to radiation burn treatment by dosimetry-guided surgery combined with autologous mesenchymal stem cell therapy. Regen Med 2007;2:785–94.
25. Dainiak N, Gent RN, Carr Z, et al. Literature review and global consensus on management of acute radiation syndrome affecting nonhematopoietic organ systems. Disaster Med Public Health Prep 2011;5:183–201.
26. Mettler FA, Upton AC. Medical effects of ionizing radiation. 3rd edition. Philadelphia: Saunders Elsevier; 2008.
27. National Council on Radiation Protection and Measurements. Management of persons contaminated with radionuclides: Handbook. Bethesda (MD): National Council on Radiation Protection and Measurements; 2009. NCRP Report No. 161.
28. Adalja AA. Use of potassium iodide (KI) in a nuclear emergency. Biosecur Bioterror 2011;9:405–7.
29. Nauman J, Wolff J. Iodide prophylaxis in Poland after the Chernobyl reactor accident: benefits and risks. Am J Med 1993;94:524–32.
30. American College of Radiology. Disaster preparedness for radiology professionals: response to radiological terrorism: a primer for radiologists, radiation oncologists and medical physicists. Reston (VA): American College of Radiology; 2006.
31. Buddemeier BR, Dillon M. Key response planning factors for the aftermath of nuclear terrorism. Washington, DC: Lawrence Livermore National Laboratory; 2009. Available at: https://narac.llnl.gov/uploads/IND_ResponsePlanning_LLNL-TR-410067web.pdf. Accessed June 11, 2013.
32. International Atomic Energy Agency. Preparedness and response for a nuclear or radiological emergency: safety requirements. Vienna (Austria): International Atomic Energy Agency; 2002. STI/PUB/1133.
33. Mickelson AB, editor. Textbooks of military science: medical consequences of radiological and nuclear weapons. Fort Detrick (MD): Borden Institute; 2012.
34. National Council on Radiation Protection and Measurements. Management of terrorist events involving radioactive material. Bethesda (MD): National Council on Radiation Protection and Measurements; 2001. NCRP Report No. 138.
35. National Council on Radiation Protection and Measurements. Key elements of preparing emergency responders for nuclear and radiological terrorism. Bethesda (MD): National Council on Radiation Protection and Measurements; 2005. NCRP Commentary No. 19.
36. Radiation Studies Branch, National Center for Environmental Health, Center for Disease Control and Prevention. Population monitoring in radiation emergencies: a guide for state and local public health planners. Atlanta (GA): Centers for Disease Control and Prevention; 2007. Available at: http://emergency.cdc.gov/radiation/pdf/population-monitoring-guide.pdf. Accessed June 11, 2013.
37. Ansari A. Radiation threats and your safety: a guide to preparation and response for professionals and community. Boca Raton (FL): CRC Press; 2010.

38. International Atomic Energy Agency. The radiological accident in Gilan. Vienna (Austria): International Atomic Energy Agency; 2002. IAEA STI/PUB/1123.
39. International Atomic Energy Agency. The radiological accident in Tammiku. Vienna (Austria): International Atomic Energy Agency; 1998. STI/PUB/1053.
40. International Atomic Energy Agency. The radiological accident in Samut Prakarn. Vienna (Austria): International Atomic Energy Agency; 2002. STI/PUB/1124.
41. International Atomic Energy Agency. The radiological accident in Goiânia. Vienna (Austria): International Atomic Energy Agency; 1988. STI/PUB/815. Available at: http://www-pub.iaea.org/MTCD/publications/PDF/Pub815web.pdf. Accessed May 29, 2013.
42. International Atomic Energy Agency. Dosimetric and medical aspects of the radiological accident in Goiania in 1987. Vienna (Austria): International Atomic Energy Agency; 1998. IAEA-TECDOC-1009. Available at: http://www-pub.iaea.org/MTCD/publications/PDF/te_1009_prn.pdf. Accessed May 29, 2013.

Index

Note: Page numbers of article titles are in **boldface** type.

A

Acetaminophen, 114–115
Acetaminophen toxicity, management of, 115–116
Acid, absorbable, ingestion of, 157
Acid-base disorder(s), mixed, and isolated anion gap acidosis, distinguishing between, 151
   primary, identification of, 150
   toxicologic, **149–165**
Acid-base physiology, 149–150
Acute radiation syndrome, 252–253
Airways, direct injury to, 135–136
    thermal, 136
Alcohol (Ethanol), hepatotoxicity due to, 119–120
   management of, 120
Alcoholic ketoacidosis, ketones and, 161–162
Alcohols, toxic, 162–163
Amphetamines, 86–87
Anabolic steroids, hepatotoxicty due to, 121
Analgesics, nonopioid, as cause of central nervous system depression, 211
Anaphylaxis, chemotherapy-induced, 193
   management of, 194
Anion gap, metabolic acidosis association with, 151
Anion gap acidosis, isolated, and mixed acid-base disorder, distinguishing between, 151
Anion gap metabolic acidosis, 158
Anti-Xa inhibitors, 61–62
Anticonvulsants, as cause of central nervous system depression, 210–211
Antimicrobials, prophylactic, for irradiated patients, 256
Antipsychotics, as cause of central nervous system depression, 209–210
Apixaban, 61–62
Apoptosis, 251–252
Arterial blood gas, interpretation of, 150–152
Asbestos, as pulmonary toxicant, 137
Asphyxiants, simple, 131
Atropine, in toxicologic bradycardia, 91

B

Beryllium, as pulmonary toxicant, 138
Beta-adrenergic antagonists, 84–85
Blood analysis, in central nervous system toxicity, 215
Bone marrow or stem cell transplants, 256
Bone marrow suppression, chemotherapeutic agents associated with, 180
Bradycardia, agents causing, 83

Emerg Med Clin N Am 32 (2014) 267–275
http://dx.doi.org/10.1016/S0733-8627(13)00124-7
0733-8627/14/$ – see front matter © 2014 Elsevier Inc. All rights reserved.

emed.theclinics.com

Bradycardia (*continued*)
  toxicologic, 82–85
    management of, 91–97
Bupivacaine toxicity, intravenous lipid emulsion in, 95–96
Bupropion, as cause of seizures, 214

C

Calcium, in toxicologic bradycardia, 92
Calcium channel blockers, 83–85
Cannabinoids, clinical effects of, 5–7
  history and epidemiology of, 3–5
  pharmacology of, 5
  synthetic, description of, 3
    street/brand names for, 4
  testing and imaging for, 7
  treatment following use of, 7
Carbon dioxide, as cause of lung injury, 132
  carbonic acid, and bicarbonate, relationship of, 149–150
Carbon dioxide toxicity, 141
Carbonic anhydrase inhibition, 157
Carboxypeptidase G_2 (glucarpidase), 196
Cardiovascular emergencies, chemotherapy-associated, 176–179
    clinical evaluation in, 177
    management of, 177
Cardiovascular events, adverse, 80
  after drug overdose, 80
Cardiovascular failure, toxin-induced, **79–102**
    diagnostic testing in, 89–90
    gastrointestinal decontamination in, 90
    management approach to, 89–97
Cardiovascular toxins, chemotherapeutic, 178–179
Cathinones, synthetic (bath salts), clinical effects of, 10–11
    common, 7–8
    history and epidemiology of, 8–9
    pharmacology of, 9–10
    street names for, 8
    testing and imaging for, 11
  treatment following use of, 11
Caustic agents, ingested, as cause of airway injury, 135–136
Central alpha$_2$-adrenergic agonists, as cause of central nervous system depression, 209
Central nervous system depression, in central nervous system toxicity, management of, 217–218
Central nervous system toxicity, **205–221**
  central nervous system depression in, 208–211
    management of, 217–218
  clinical manifestations of, 206
  clinical presentation of, 207–215
  diagnostic testing in, 215–217
  differential diagnosis of, 216–217
  exposures causing, 205

history taking in, 206–207
management of, 217–218
Chemotherapeutic agents, classification of, 168–171
Chemotherapeutic emergencies, neurologic, 171–174
Chemotherapeutic neurotoxins, 173
Chemotherapeutic regimens, adult, 170–171
Chemotherapy-associated toxicity, approach to, **167–203**
Child abuse, by poisoning, 32–33
Child(ren), pathophysiologic considerations in, 33–34
    poisoned, antidotal therapy for, 41–43
        assessment of, 40
        cause, epidemiology, and prevention of, 30–33
        detoxification issues in, 40–41
        emergency management overview of, 34–44
        enhanced elimination for, 43–44
        evaluation, decontamination, and supportive care of, 38
        in emergency department, 30
        laboratory and ECG evaluation of, 38–40
        physical examination of, 38
        supportive care for, 44
    poisonings in, cases of, 45–47
    substances often involved in exposures, 31
    well-appearing, with poison exposure, 44–45
Cholestasis, 106–108
Cirrhosis, 108–110
Clopidogrel (Plavix), 56–57
Coagulopathy, toxin-induced, **53–78**
        anticoagulation, measures of, 54–55
        coagulation cascade and, 54
        platelet inhibitors in, 56–58
        reversal strategies in, 62–68
        targeted therapies in, 55–56
Cocaine, 86
Cone snails (Gastropoda), 237–238
Consciousness, drugs affecting, 207
Contraction alkalosis/chloride depletion alkalosis, 155
Cubozoa, 233–234
    envenomation by, treatment of, 236–237
Cutaneous radiation syndrome, 257
    medical management of, 257–258
Cytokines or colony-stimulating factors, 256

D

Dabigatran, 60–61
Delirium, agitated, in central nervous system toxicity, 211–213
        management of, 218
Dermatologic emergencies, following chemotherapy, 192–194
Dexrazoxane, in cardiovascular emergencies, 177–178
Diarrhea, toxins causing, 156–157
Digoxin toxicity, and cardioactive steroid toxicity, 87–89

Dilutional acidosis, 157
Drug overdose, cardiovascular events after, 80
Drugs and chemicals, fatal in small doses, 45–46
Drugs of abuse, emerging, **1–28**
    management principles in, 17–19

E

Echinodermata, 238–239
    envenomation by, treatment of, 239
Electrocardiogram, in central nervous system toxicity, 216
Electroencephalography, in central nervous system toxicity, 216
Enucleated cells, 255–256
Epidermal necrolysis, toxic, chemotherapeutic agents associated, 192–193
Ergot alkaloids, 87
Erythema multiforme, chemotherapeutic agents associated, 192–193
    clinical evaluation in, 193
Extravasation emergencies, chemotherapy-induced, 194

F

Factor VIIa, 67–68
Fire smoke, as pulmonary toxicant, 139
Fresh frozen plasma, in reversal of anticoagulation, 65–66

G

Gamma-aminobutyric acid agonists, as cause of central nervous system depression, 208–209
Gases, as respiratory irritant, 132–135
Gastrointestinal emergencies, chemotherapy-associated, 185–190
    clinical evaluation in, 187–189
    management of, 189–190
Gastrointestinal subsyndrome, 258
    management of, 258
Genitourinary emergencies, as complication of chemotherapy, 191
Glucagon, 94

H

Hapalochlaene maculosa (blue-ringed octopus), 238
Hawaiian baby woodrose (*Argyreia nervosa*), 17
Hematopoietic emergencies, chemotherapy-associated, 179–181
    management of, 181
Hematopoietic syndrome, 253–255
Hemodialysis, as antidote to drug poisoning, 68
Henderson-Hasselbalch equation, 149–150
Heparin, 58–59
Hepatic injury, toxin-induced, **103–125**
    clinical presentation of, 111
    epidemiology of, 103–105

imaging in, 113
incidence of, 104
laboratory evaluation in, 112–113
management of, 111–112
morbidity and mortality associated with, 104–105
pathology of, 113
physiology of, 105–111
scope of problem of, 103
specialized care transfer in, 113–114
toxins responsible for, 114–121
Hepatic necrosis, acute, 106
Hepatic toxins, chemotherapeutic, 188
Hepatitis, chronic, 108
Hepatotoxicity, forms of, 106–111
Hydrocarbon aspiration, causing airway injury, 136
Hydrozoa, 234–236
envenomation by, treatment of, 236–237
Hyperventilation, due to impaired oxygenation, 152
Hypoventilation, due to respiratory acidosis, 152–154

I

Insulin euglycemia therapy, high-dose, 94–95
Intrathecal (IT) emergencies, chemotherapy-associated, 174–176
management of, 176
Ionizing radiation, alpha (α), 246–247
beta (β), 246–247
chromatid breakage and mitotic death, 251
delayed effects of, 248
deterministic effects of, 249
direct ionization and indirect cellular interactions, 252
equivalent dose, 248
exposure to, or irradiation, versus contamination, 249–250
gamma rays and X rays, 247
injuries and illnesses due to, **245–265**
median lethal dose 50/60, 251
neutron, 247
positron ($\beta+$), 247
radiation dose, 248
stochastic effects of, 249
types of, 246–247
units of measurement of, 248
Irukandji jellyfish (Carukia barnes), 233–234
Isoniazid, as cause of seizures, 214

J

Jellyfish (Cnidaria, formerly Coelenterates), 233

K

Ketones, alcoholic ketoacidosis and, 161–162
Kratom, 15

L

Lactate, elevated, metabolic acidosis with, 159–161
Leucovorin (folinic acid), 195–196
Licorice abuse, acidosis in, 155
Linuche unguiculata, 236
Lionfish (genus Pterois), 230
Lipid emulsion, intravenous, in bupivacaine toxicity, 95–96
Liver, function of, 106
    injury of, agents causing, 109–110
        enzymes associated with, 106–107
    pathophysiology of, 106
    structure of, 105–106
Liver failure, acute, 110–111
Lungs, anatomy of, and physiology, and response to injury, 128–131
    cellular airway components and, 129–131
    gas exchange by, 128
    injury to, agents causing, 131–135
    ventilatory capacity of, 128
    ventilatory mechanics of, 128–129
Lymphocyte depletion kinetics, 255

M

Marine antivenoms, 228
Marine envenomations, **223–243**
    hazards posed by, 223–224
Marine organisms, invertebrate, 225
    vertebrate, 225
        envenomations by, 226
Metabolic acidosis, anion gap, 158
    association with anion gap, 151
    causes of, 155
    non-anion gap, 155–156
        from tolene and ethylene glycol, 157
    with elevated lactate, 159–161
Metabolic alkalosis, due to increased bicarbonate intake, 154–155
    underlying mechanisms of, 154
    vomiting in, 154
Metal fume fever, 139
MetHb inducers, 140–141
Methemoglobinemia, 140–141
Methotrexate, toxicity associated, 194–195
    clinical evaluation in, 195
    management of, 195
Methylene blue, in toxin-induced encephalopathy, 174
Methylxanthines, as cause of seizures, 214
Millepora alcicornis, 235–236
Mollusca, 237–238
    envenomation by, treatment of, 238
Mucositis, chemotherapy-associated, 185–186
    management of, 189–190

Muscarinic receptor antagonists, as cause of agitated delirium, 211–212
Mushrooms, 16–17
    hepatotoxicity due to, 118
        management of, 119

N

Nephrotoxins, chemotherapeutic, 191
Neurovascular syndrome, radiation therapy and, 258
Neutrophil count, absolute, 255
Nonpharmaceutical agents, as cause of central nervous system depression, 211
Nuclear device/nuclear weapon, improvised, 262
Nuclear power plant, pressurized water reactor, 261–262
Nuclear power plant incident, 261–262

O

Octopi (Cephalopoda), 238
Ocular toxins, chemotherapeutic, 182
Ophthalmologic emergencies, chemotherapy-associated, 181
Opioid receptor agonists, as cause of central nervous system depression, 209
Opioids, and hypoventilation, 153
Otolaryngologic emergencies, as complication of chemotherapy, 182–183
Oxygen, inhibition of use of, by tissues, 142
Oxygen transport, toxins inhibiting, 140–141
Oxygenation, impaired, hyperventilation due to, 152
Oxyhemoglobin dissociation curve, 140

P

Paraquat, as pulmonary toxicant, 136–137
Pediatric toxicology, **29–52**
Pediatric toxidromes, major, 39
Phenethylamines (2C drugs), clinical effects of, 13
    pharmacology of, 12–13
    testing of, 13
    treatment following use of, 13
    use of, 12
Phosgene, as respiratory irritant, 132–135
Phytonadione, 64–65
Piperazines, 14
Platelets, bleeding events associated with, 65
Porifera, 238–239
    envenomation by, treatment of, 239
Portuguese man-of-war (Physalia physalis), 234–235
Potassium iodide, for radiation exposure, 260–261
Prasugrel, 57
Prescription drug abuse epidemic, 2–3
Protamine sulfate, 63–64
Prothrombin complex concentrate, 66–67
Pulmonary carcinogens, 139–140

Pulmonary emergencies, chemotherapy-induced, 183–185
    management of, 185
Pulmonary toxicants, 131, 136–140
Pulmonary toxins, chemotherapeutic, 184–185

R

Radiation, casualties due to, initial management of, 252–253
    definition of, 246
    ionizing. See *Ionizing radiation*.
    protection from, and ALARA, 250
    types of, and weighting factors, 248
Radiation injury, biology of, radiosensitivity and radioresistance, 250–251
    local, 257
Radiation Patient Treatment algorithm chart, 253–254
Radioactive materials, internal contamination with, 259
        treatment methods for, 259–260
Radiobiology, 248–252
Radiological and nuclear incidents, of medical and public health concern, 260–262
Radiological dispersal device, 261
Radiological exposure device, 261
Radiological exposures, overall medical management of, 252–260
Radiology, in central nervous system toxicity, 216
Renal emergencies, chemotherapy-associated, 190–192
        management of, 191–192
Renal tubular acidosis, toxins causing, 156
Respiratory acidosis, 152–154
Respiratory alkalosis, 152
Respiratory disorder, chronic or acute determination of, 150
Respiratory distress, toxin-induced, **127–147**
Respiratory irritants, 132–135
Respiratory system, complaints or signs, assessment of, 142–143
Respiratory tract, systemic delivery of toxins by, 142
Rivaroxaban, 61

S

Salicylates, as cause of anion gap metabolic acidosis, 162
    as cause of respiratory alkalosis, 152
Salvia, 15–16
Scorpaenidae family, envenomations by, 227–233
        treatment of, 231
Scyphozoa, 236–237
    envenomation by, treatment of, 236–237
Sea snakes, 231–233
    envenomations by, presentation of, 232
        treatment of, 232–233
Sea urchins (Diadema, Echinothix, and Asthenosoma), 239
Sedatives/hypnotics, and hypoventilation, 153–154
Seizures, drugs causing, 214–215
    in central nervous system toxicity, 214–215
        management of, 218

Serotonergic agents, as cause of agitated delirium, 212–213
Shock, caused by drug overdose, 81
Silica, as pulmonary toxicant, 137–138
Smog, as pulmonary toxicant, 139
Spiny fish, envenomations by, 227–228
Sponges (Porifera), 239
Statins, 120–121
    hepatotoxicity due to, 121
        management of, 121
Steatosis, 108
Steroid toxicity, cardioactive, digoxin toxicity and, 92–94
Stevens-Johnson syndrome, chemotherapeutic agents associated, 192–193
Stewart strong ion theory, 151–152
Stingrays (Class Chondrichthyes), 224–226
    wound caused by, 228
        treatment of, 226–229
Stonefish (genus Synanceia), 228–230
Sympathomimetic agents, as cause of agitated delirium, 213

T

Tachycardia, toxicologic, 81–82
Thrombin (FactorII) inhibitors, direct, 59–61
Ticagrelor, 57–58
Tobacco smoking, as pulmonary carcinogen, 139–140
Tolene, and ethylene glycol, non-anion gap metabolic acidosis from, 157
Trachinidae, envenomations by, 227–233
        treatment of, 231
Tramadol, as cause of seizures, 215

U

Urine chloride, metabolic alkalosis caused by, 154
Urine drug screen immunoassays, in central nervous system toxicity, 215–216

V

Valproic acid, 116–117
    hepatotoxicity due to, management of, 117–118
Vasoconstriction, toxicologic, 85–87
        management of, 91
Venoocclusive disease, hepatic, 108
Vitamin K antagonists, 59

W

Weeverfish (family Trachinidae), 230–231

EmergencyMed **Advance**

All the latest emergency medicine news and research you need, all in one place

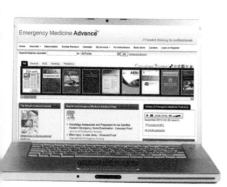

EmergencyMedAdvance.com is a new essential online resource offering valued high-quality content and news for the global community of Emergency Medicine professionals to save time and stay current—from physicians and nurses to EMTs.

Stay current
- Emergency Medicine news

Save time
- Access relevant articles in press from 16 participating journals

And more...
- Journals' profiles
- Personalized search results
- Emergency Medicine bookstore

- Upcoming meetings and events

- Search across 500+ health sciences journals
- Learn how to submit a manuscript

- Sign up for free e-Alerts
- Emergency Medicine jobs

Bookmark us today at
EmergencyMedAdvance.com

Printed and bound by CPI Group (UK) Ltd, Croydon, CR0 4YY

03/10/2024

01040409-0009